Other Volumes in This Series

Complications of Surgery of the Upper Gastrointestinal Tract

Complications in Surgery Series
Edited by John A. R. Smith

Complications of Surgery of the Upper Gastrointestinal Tract

R. M. Kirk
MS, FRCS

Consultant Surgeon, Royal Free Hospital, London

C. J. Stoddard
MD, FRCS

Consultant Surgeon, Royal Hallamshire Hospital, Sheffield
Formerly Senior Lecturer in Surgery, University of Liverpool
and Honorary Consultant Surgeon, Royal Liverpool and
Broadgreen Hospitals, Liverpool

 Baillière Tindall   London Philadelphia Toronto
Mexico City Rio de Janeiro Sydney Tokyo Hong Kong

Baillière Tindall   1 St Anne's Road
W. B. Saunders   Eastbourne, East Sussex BN21 3UN, England

West Washington Square
Philadelphia, PA 19105, USA

1 Goldthorne Avenue
Toronto, Ontario M8Z 5T9, Canada

Apartado 26370—Cedro 512
Mexico 4, DF Mexico

Rua Evaristo da Veiga 55, 20° andar
Rio de Janeiro—RJ, Brazil

ABP Australia Ltd, 44–50 Waterloo Road
North Ryde, NSW 2113, Australia

Ichibancho Central Building, 22-1 Ichibancho
Chiyoda-ku, Tokyo 102, Japan

10/fl, Inter-Continental Plaza, 94 Granville Road
Tsim Sha Tsui East, Kowloon, Hong Kong

First published 1986

Printed in Great Britain at the Alden Press, Oxford

British Library Cataloguing in Publication Data

Kirk, R.M.
    Complications of surgery of the upper
    gastrointestinal tract.—(Complications in
    surgery)
    1. Intestines—Surgery 2. Stomach—Surgery
    I. Title II. Stoddard, C.J. (Christopher James)
    III. Series
    617'.553 RD540.5

ISBN 0-7020-1138-X

Contents

Series Foreword

All doctors who are involved in the care of surgical patients are all too aware of the hazards of the operation and the morbidity and mortality that can result from an ill considered or ill managed procedure, and of the complications, whether related directly to the operation, the disease process, the patient or even to the hospital environment. It is also true to say that many hospitals are now mindful of these difficulties and have introduced a pattern of regular medical audit through which the extent and the significance of the problem can be identified and which, when necessary, can point to the remedy.

The majority of complications are of course preventable by careful preoperative preparation, by skilled operative technique and by proper postoperative care, but when they do occur, it is the early recognition, the immediate and correct investigation, and the awareness of the operative treatment that will decide the eventual outcome and the likelihood of early recovery.

Obviously every surgeon would like to believe that in his own practice complications will be, at the least, occasional events and hopefully this is the case in most hospitals. The corollary of this is, however, that the personal experience of many surgeons in these serious potential or actual problems is not great and the opportunities for the trainee surgeon to learn about them, and about their clinical significance and management, are less than adequate.

This deficiency of experience in the average surgeon, whether general surgeon or specialist, has now been appreciated and John Smith in this series of texts has set out to provide what has been termed a 'reference point' from which the surgeon will be able to increase his awareness of the problems and increase his knowledge in areas where he is unlikely to gain experience from clinical practice. The prime aim of the series has been to ensure that knowledge of the existence of complications increases, that prevention can become more widely accepted and that the recognition and management of established complications can be undertaken with skill and competence.

Each of the volumes in the series considers a specific area of surgical practice and, in each, authorities in the field have presented their experience and their views in such a way that it will not only instruct but will also stimulate the reader to study the subject further.

It is undoubtedly an area of surgical practice that is of major importance and which has been somewhat neglected in the past. This is the first time that there has been an attempt to present a comprehensive account covering all aspects of practice and it will undoubtedly be a significant contribution to patient care in its broadest interpretation.

Sir James Fraser Bt, PPRCS (Ed)
Nicolson Street
Edinburgh

Editor's Foreword

Most textbooks of surgery acknowledge that postoperative complications exist and some describe methods of prevention or options for their further management. However, it is clear to me from conversations with junior staff, candidates for higher degrees and trainees in all branches of surgery that there is no reference to which they can turn where the complex problem of complications is adequately considered, i.e. covering details of aetiology, predisposition and methods of prevention, together with advice on which complications are likely to be encountered and how they may be recognized, investigated and managed.

This series is directed at all surgical trainees and also at the consultant working outside specialist referral centres. The latter may not often encounter the complications which are under consideration, but when they are encountered the surgeon needs advice on what to do, what not to do and, finally, when specialist referral is indicated.

The authors in this series are all consultants with a specialist practice in teaching hospitals. Each has been asked to provide the necessary information and to be dogmatic where that is possible, but to advise on the options where the situation is less clear. Points of persisting controversy have been identified.

The multi-authored text has been avoided, specifically to preclude confusion through differences of opinion within an individual volume. Each volume is self-sufficient, except that *Complications of Surgery in General* deals with all general surgical complications to avoid detailed repetition in the other, more specialist, volumes. Inevitably there is some overlap between volumes but I feel this to be preferable to omitting topics that may be important. Detailed references have not been included as a deliberate policy of the series, but suggestions for further reading are provided.

Finally, not all the complications described have been created by the authors; the selection of topic reflects, rather, their ability to deal with such problems as are referred to them!

The concept of a single volume on *Complications in Surgery* arose from discussions involving, on separate occasions, Mrs Ann Saadi (lately of Baillière Tindall), Mr R. M. Kirk (Royal Free Hospital, London) and myself. The volume has grown into a series but acknowledgements are due to Mrs Saadi and Mr Kirk for the idea and to Mrs Saadi for the enthusiasm which ensured the launch. I am most grateful to Dr Geoffrey Smaldon of Baillière Tindall who has now assumed responsibility for the entire series and has encouraged or cajoled as necessary. The artistic talent of Mr Pat Elliott is clear for all to see and is greatly appreciated. Finally, I am happy to acknowledge the support and encouragement of my wife and family.

John A. R. Smith
Northern General Hospital
Sheffield

Preface

There are three types of surgeon: the first easily gets into trouble and does not know how to get out of it, the second gets into trouble but knows how to deal with it, and the third avoids trouble. All of us aspire to join the last category and a few of the masters of our profession approach it. We do not claim membership of the third group. If we did, we should not see any difficulties or complications in surgery. It is only by recalling our own mishaps that we hope to advise others on how to avoid them.

In spite of the availability of improved techniques and diagnostic aids, success in surgery depends essentially on clinical skills. A visit to one of the many outstanding surgeons working in a poor country drives home the truth of this. Such a surgeon appreciates his own limitations and those of his patients, and accepts the constraints placed on him by the circumstances in which he works. He is forced to compromise on the selection of the procedure. In contrast, there is no compromise in the perfection with which he accomplishes the chosen technique. He has appreciated that the time to deal with complications is before and during the operation, not afterwards.

Most textbooks of surgery describe operations carried out in idealized circumstances. We have concentrated on the selection of patients, procedures, instruments and techniques, and the preparation of the patient to reduce the risks of operation. We describe how to anticipate and avoid disasters and how to recognize and cope with catastrophes during the operation. We discuss the early recognition and management of postoperative complications.

All of us agonize over our decisions and our performance of operations when disaster strikes. We hope that this book will help our colleagues to spend fewer sleepless nights remorsefully considering what went wrong. We hope that our colleagues will also be comforted by the fact that in writing it, we are acknowledging the fact that we too have spent sleepless nights—and continue to do so, on occasion. When we no longer question our own actions after one of our patients develops a complication or fails to improve, then we should retire from the demanding career of surgery.

We wish to thank our respective secretaries, Mrs Geeta Wynne and Mrs Susan Ellis, for their outstanding skill and accuracy in typing the manuscript. We are also grateful to Mr Pat Elliot for the clear artwork throughout. Dr Geoffrey Smaldon, Senior Medical Editor at Baillière Tindall, has given great support in helping to achieve the objectives of the series of which this volume forms a part, while Mr Peter Gill, Senior House Editor at Baillière Tindall, has edited the manuscript with skill and speed. The Radio-diagnostic and Medical Physics Departments of the Royal Free Hospital, London, and the Royal Liverpool Hospital have generously provided the X-ray films and scans.

R. M. Kirk
C. J. Stoddard

1 Introduction

Complications in the upper gastrointestinal tract are frequently serious and may be fatal. They may be predisposed to before any procedure is carried out, may develop or may be caused during the procedure, and occur or become manifest afterwards. There is no time when vigilance can be relaxed. To some extent the succinct American aphorism 'Choose well, cut well, get well' sums up the three phases.

Choose well   Unfortunately we cannot select those patients upon whom we wish to operate. They select themselves because they suffer from a surgical condition or conditions. The risk can be cut to the minimum by carefully assessing the condition that requires surgery, the general condition of the patient, and the preliminary selection of an appropriate procedure—accepting that this may be modified at the time of the operation. The timing of the operation is also determined by the need to prepare the patient for operation, but urgent surgery is occasionally demanded without the luxury of preparation. In most cases, however, a previously ill patient can be improved by careful preoperative treatment. Aim to attain the best respiratory, cardiovascular, renal, metabolic and psychological states whenever possible. Anticipate the possibility of bleeding and postoperative sepsis, as well as general complications such as deep venous thrombosis, and the cardiovascular and respiratory effects of the operation and anaesthetic.

The condition of the patient before operation has an important influence on the vitality of the tissues and their subsequent healing. Age, sex, obesity, and the presence of malignancy, jaundice, anaemia, diabetes, uraemia and sepsis only partially explain the outcome of an operation. Some people are truly made of 'good stuff', with an almost incredible ability to heal and survive, while others succumb to comparatively trivial setbacks.

Cut well   Well-trained surgeons who are familiar with the tissues and the technique of the operation are likely to achieve better results than those who have been poorly trained and who are unfamiliar with the state of the tissues in the pathological state requiring surgery and with the technique of the operation. Many qualities of a successful surgeon cannot be assessed objectively. He cannot make once for all decisions but must continually reassess them, being willing to compromise, remembering that technical success is not the end of the matter. Compromise may seem to be the antithesis of what is required from a surgeon, who likes to think of himself as resolute. However, blind determination to complete a selected operation in the face of circumstances that presage disaster is not resolution but inflexibility. For a patient in bad condition, a less demanding procedure may be less effective but safer. Another surgical aphorism is 'A living problem is better than a dead certainty'.

Couch et al. (1981) identified four causes for surgical error:

1 Misplaced optimism ('I think we can get away with it').
2 Unwarranted urgency ('The only chance the patient has').
3 Urge for perfection (too much surgery, not minimal effective surgery).
4 'Vogue' therapy (stylish new technique, not simple, well-established method).

Of course these are retrospective judgements. For example, the minimal treatment is often not the most effective, and if it fails the surgeon may be accused of being faint-hearted.

There is one aspect of 'cut well' on which there is no room for compromise, namely the standard of technical performance. This includes gentle handling of the tissues, surgical tidiness, perfect haemostasis, recognition and avoidance of impending trouble, and careful checking for any mistake so that it can be corrected. Surgeons must resist the pressure to 'get on with it', when an unexpected difficulty arises. Operating lists are planned on the assumption that everything goes smoothly. The information that the next patient is 'premedicated' must not deter the surgeon from proceeding methodically with the present patient. Equally, he must resist pressures from within himself, regarding future commitments.

Surgeons in training are particularly vulnerable because they do not wish to appear incapable of accomplishing a major procedure under difficulty. It is important that when the master delegates responsibility to his apprentice, he should make it clear that the trainee must carry out surgery within the patient's capability to withstand it and within his own capability to carry it out. The apprentice must feel that the demands upon him to attend on time for subsequent duties are not absolute. Finally, he should feel reassured that calls for help, guidance or moral support, are not signs of incompetence but rather signs of surgical maturity.

Get well   It is unfortunately not a reliable outcome that the patient will get well following careful selection, preparation and operation. As the operation draws to its conclusion the patient must be carefully monitored so that impending complications are detected, prevented or treated. Whenever possible defunction the part that has been operated upon. This can usually be achieved in the upper gastrointestinal tract by stopping oral feeding and often by instituting nasogastric aspiration with replacement of fluids, electrolytes and metabolic needs by the parenteral route.

All patients subjected to an operation are prone to develop

general complications, particularly of cardiovascular, respiratory and renal function. These are dealt with in *Complications of Surgery in General*.

Audit

It is said that Billroth, the famous German surgeon, was the first member of our profession to admit mistakes, having carefully followed his patients for up to 5 years. Many surgeons are reluctant to declare their failures, but each surgeon should at the least carefully monitor his results. It is fortunate that in the literature reports can be found from centres with a particular interest in the field, against which the results of individual surgeons may be compared. It is surely part of our professional responsibility to ensure that we are not falling below acceptable standards of surgery. Most surgeons who carry out self-assessment find that the very intention to assess their results somehow improves their performance. Possibly, the knowledge that this result will weigh in the balance draws from us all a greater determination to avoid complications.

Misjudgements cost lives, cause severe and often permanent disability, and at best may require prolonged and expensive treatment to recover the damage. It is essential that we learn from our own mistakes but it is better if we can learn from the mistakes of others, and this ideally requires the wide exposure of the outcome of every operation, with careful analysis of all complications. Morbidity and mortality conferences need to be conducted with great discretion to encourage each surgeon to be explicit to his colleagues about his mishaps, without fear that he will be pilloried. On the other hand, there are isolated instances when a surgeon who is having more than an extended 'bad patch' must be monitored and restrained by his colleagues.

Nutrition

There is some, though not incontrovertible, evidence that postoperative complications are reduced in patients who are in a good nutritional state at the time of operation. Whenever possible correct the patient's nutritional state before operation and maintain it afterwards, especially if in spite of every precaution, a major complication develops.

Patients with upper gastrointestinal disease may be nutritionally deficient because of failure to take in food if they have anorexia, dysphagia or vomiting. If there is ulceration or general mucosal disease, blood and protein may be lost into the gut. Inflammation and particularly sepsis produce marked catabolism. Neoplasia appears to be associated with weight loss and nutritional deficit out of proportion to the size of the tumour. Metabolism may be different in the cachexia of malignant disease from cachexia in other diseases.

Because enteral feeding must be interrupted following surgery on the upper gastrointestinal tract it is advantageous for the patient to start in a good nutritional state, since any complication may further delay the start of normal feeding.

Assessment Weight loss is a most important indicator and must be related to age, sex, height, occupation, previous obesity, triceps skin fold thickness and muscle power.

Liver function tests including serum proteins should show albumin higher than 30 g/l (3 g per 100 ml). Urinary nitrogen excretion is normally 10–15 g per day: it may fall to 6 g per day when intake is reduced, but rises to 18–25 g per day in the presence of increased catabolism following injury, inflammation and sepsis.

Assessment of nutritional state
1 Weight
2 Triceps skin fold
3 Mid-arm muscle circumference
4 Muscle power
5 Serum albumin
6 Urinary nitrogen excretion

Correction Whenever possible prefer preoperative nutritional correction by the oral route using normal diet, if necessary augmented by some of the many supplements that are available. It may be necessary to dilate strictures, pass tubes through them or create stomas such as a jejunostomy to allow enteral feeding (Fig. 1.1). Do not attempt to give large volumes of high osmotic fluids immediately into the jejunostomy or intractable diarrhoea will result. Start by cautiously instilling small volumes of diluted nutrients, such as half-strength milk, and gradually increase the volume and strength.

Parenteral nutrition is expensive, less efficient, but sometimes necessary either alone or to augment inadequate enteral feeding. It is given through a central feeding catheter, such as a Hickman catheter (Fig. 1.2). This has a long subcutaneous track and a felted annular cuff along the track to cause fibrosis and help exclude infection. It is usually inserted through the internal jugular or subclavian vein into the superior vena cava, although the external jugular, axillary and cephalic veins have been used.

Each day 0.15 g of protein nitrogen (0.9 g of protein) and 30–35 kcal are required per kg body weight, together with minerals and vitamins. Of the twenty aminoacids, eight are essential. Of course the amount given and the time taken to restore a normal nutritional state depends on the initial state of the patient and continuing catabolism, tolerance to intravenous feeding, and the amount that can be given enterally. Usually total parenteral nutrition requires 9–13 g of protein, 200–350 g of carbohydrate and up to 3 g of fat per kg each day.

Figure 1.1
Creation of a
jejunostomy.

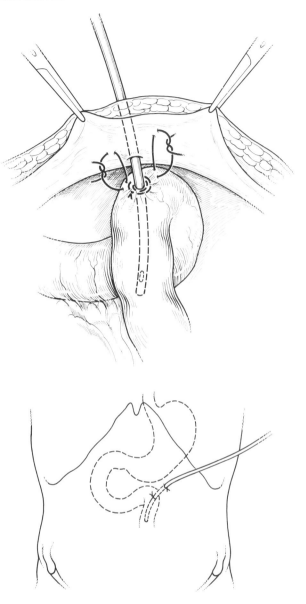

The patient's improvement is reflected in the weight gained, increase in triceps skin fold thickness, and muscle power, which can be conveniently assessed using a grip-testing apparatus. Monitor the plasma protein, electrolytes, osmolality, urea, glucose and urinary nitrogen regularly. Check the liver function tests, serum calcium, phosphate and magnesium at intervals.

It is essential to continue nutritional support after the operation. Following most operations on the upper gastrointesti-

Internal jugular vein

Figure 1.2
Hickman catheter.
The long
subcutaneous track
and felted cuff help to
exclude infection.

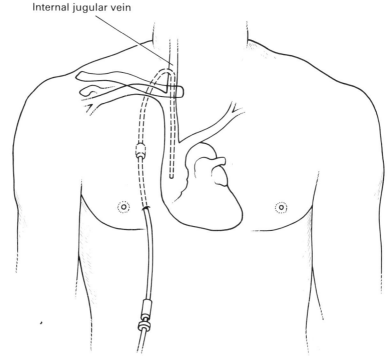

Internal jugular vein

nal tract enteral nutrition must cease until gut function returns. In this case parenteral feeding can be maintained until the bowel recovers. If preoperative jejunostomy feeding was initiated, it can be restarted soon after the operation. Alternatively, a jejunostomy can be created at the time of the operation.

If, in spite of all precautions, a further operation becomes necessary because sepsis, leak, obstruction or adynamic ileus develops, the nutritional demands may rise spectacularly. Increased catabolism allied to diminished intake and utilization have a disastrous effect on the patient and muscle mass can almost visibly dissolve away. Recovery often hinges on the surgeon's ability to maintain the nutritional state of the patient by parenteral feeding, usually through a central venous line, if possible augmented by small bowel feeding through a jejunostomy.

General principles of reoperative surgery
Do not be overwhelmed by despair. The realization that the first procedure has failed tends to make surgeons pessimistic about the outcome of a second operation. It is sometimes valuable to discuss the problem with a trusted colleague and if you are inexperienced, do not hesitate to ask him to take over the care of the patient. In the past it was considered an admission that one lacked self-confidence, but it is now more widely accepted that

this shows great maturity to admit that someone else might achieve better results than oneself in certain circumstances.

It is rare for a really emergency procedure to be necessary without preliminary resuscitation, theatre preparation, the cross matching of blood and the arrangement of preliminary tests. Recognize the occasional need to take a desperately ill patient immediately to the operating theatre. This is nearly always because of calamitous bleeding or the development of a complication that is threatening a vital function. At such times keep calm and in control of yourself. The other participants will take their lead from you and the injection of an atmosphere of drama blurs common sense.

If the patient's life is not immediately threatened, try to make the best judgement of when the intervention should take place and what can be done to improve his condition. A distinguished American surgeon recently stated 'The second most difficult decision a surgeon has to make is when to operate—the most difficult decision is when to reoperate'. Make every effort to localize and identify the complication. Having done so, make preliminary plans for the procedure and contingency plans if the expected cause is not encountered. Do not hesitate to discuss the problem with colleagues or read up the possible manoeuvres in the library. Cancel, defer or delegate other pressing commitments.

Reopen the old incision in most cases. After 'scrubbing up', wear two pairs of gloves. Prepare the skin and apply sterile towels. Ask for a kidney dish containing stitch-cutting scissors, toothed forceps and a single gauze swab. Remove the skin sutures and place them together with the instruments in the dish, discarding it. Remove the outer pair of gloves. Only rarely is there a new and unrelated cause at a distance that warrants a fresh approach. Carefully identify the true cause of the complication. Reoperative surgery requires considerable experience because it is easy to indict some relatively trivial abnormality and miss the important one. Many changes are seen following a recent operation and they can be misinterpreted by the inexperienced operator, particularly the volumes of fluid or blood-stained exudate lying in cavities, the presence of adhesions and the rather 'meaty' oedematous appearance of a recently operated upon bowel.

Control haemorrhage, leaking bowel content, and release a strangulating band. As soon as possible thoroughly inspect the whole area of the previous operation and all the contents of the cavity that had been entered to exclude associated complications or even abnormalities that were missed at the first operation.

Now decide the best course of action, taking into consideration the patient's age, condition, the primary pathological lesion, and the severity of the complication. As a rule select the least demanding procedure that will fully relieve the complication. The choice is critical and not subject to any scientific logistical analysis. Attempt to 'follow through' each possibility. Will the favoured procedure control the complication? What if it does not? How severe a procedure is it for the patient to survive? What if he does not—will you wish that you had chosen a lesser procedure? If so, why are you not employing it now?

Plan to correct the complication only, not to restore the patient to normal. The restoration can be accomplished later. Remember the American aphorism 'A living problem is better than a dead certainty'. Do not be carried away by over-ambitious 'once for all' procedures.

Having made a decision, carry it out as carefully and completely as possible. Time is rarely a consideration. With modern anaesthesia you can take as long as reasonably necessary, provided you are gentle, and guard against ischaemia, tension and imperfections in accomplishing the aim of the corrective operation.

At the end check the procedure, recheck the other contents to make sure that there are no other worthwhile manoeuvres to prevent further complications, such as inserting drains, extra stitches, covering a repair with omentum, peritoneum or pleura, and defunctioning the repaired segment by creating proximal and distal stomata, or by intubating them.

Determine to monitor the patient carefully during the recovery period.

Further reading

Atkinson, M., Wulford, S. & Allison, S.P. (1979) Endoscopic insertion of fine-bone feeding tubes. *Lancet, ii*, 829.

Belghiti, J., Langonnet, F., Bourstyn, E. & Fekete, F. (1983) Surgical implications of malnutrition and immunodeficiency in patients with carcinoma of the oesophagus. *British Journal of Surgery, 70*, 339–341.

Cerra, F.B., Siegel, J.H. & Coleman, B. (1980) Septic autocannibalism: a failure of exogenous nutritional support. *Annals of Surgery, 192*, 570–574.

Couch, N.P., Tilney, N.L., Rayner, A.A. & Moore, F.D. (1981) The high cost of low-frequency events. The anatomy and economics of surgical mishaps. *New England Journal of Medicine, 304*, 634–637.

Daly, J.M., Massar, E., Giacco, G., Frazier, O.H., Mountain, C.F., Dudrick, S.J. & Copeland, E.M. (1982) Parenteral nutrition in esophageal cancer patients. *Annals of Surgery, 196*, 203–208.

Dudley, H. (Ed.) (1983) *Rob and Smith's Operative Surgery*, 4th Edn: *Alimentary Tract and Abdominal Wall*, Vol. 1. London: Butterworth.

Hardy, J.D. (Ed.) (1981) *Complications in Surgery and their Management*, 4th Edn. London: W.B. Saunders.

Karran, S. (1982) Who needs nutritional support? In Lumley, J.S.P. & Craven, J.L. (Eds) *Surgical Review*, Vol. 3, pp. 25–62. London: Pitman.

Kirk, R.M. (1978) *Basic Surgical Techniques*, 2nd Edn. Edinburgh: Churchill Livingstone.

Kirk, R.M. & Williamson, R.C.N. (1986) *General Surgical Operations*, 2nd Edn. Edinburgh: Churchill Livingstone.

Sagor, G., Mitchenere, P., Layfield, J., Prentice, H.G. & Kirk, R.M. (1983) Prolonged access to the venous system using the Hickman right atrial catheter. *Annals of the Royal College of Surgeons of England, 65*, 47–49.

Smith, J.A.R. (1985) *Complications of Surgery in General.* London: Baillière Tindall.

White, T.T. & Harrison, R.C. (1979) *Reoperative Gastrointestinal Surgery*, 2nd Edn. Boston: Little, Brown.

2 Local Complications

Bleeding

Following operations on the upper gastrointestinal tract bleeding may develop either into the tract or into the surrounding tissues of the chest, abdomen or the external wound.

Bleeding may occur at the time of the operation and not be recognized, or it may be recognized but not controlled. It may develop following the operation, especially when the blood pressure was low and has now been restored, so that a clot is forced out of the end of a vessel, and a similar phenomenon may occur in veins when straining causes a rise in venous pressure. It may develop later if infection causes digestion of the sealing clot.

Primary bleeding—at the time of operation
Reactionary bleeding—during recovery
Secondary bleeding—later, as an effect of infection

Bleeding may be overt or occult. It may result from technical failure at the operation site or develop as an incidental complication of the primary condition, the operation and the anaesthetic. The patient may have a known or unsuspected bleeding tendency.

Intra-abdominal bleeding: vessels, viscera, mesenteries, wound edges, drain wounds
Intraluminal bleeding: suture lines, ulcers, varices

Preoperative assessment
Check that the patient is not clinically anaemic and does not have any clinical cardiovascular or respiratory disability. Ask if there has been any tendency to bleeding after minor injury, tooth extraction or previous operation in the patient or immediate family. Make sure the patient is not taking drugs that may depress the bone marrow. Remember that Blacks, Mediterranean races, Indians and Arabs may have diseases and disorders of blood that increase the risk of operative bleeding, as do patients who are jaundiced or taking anticoagulant drugs.

The extent of investigation depends on the clinical condition of the patient and the severity of the operation. For a minor operation a mere check of the blood haemoglobin may be sufficient, but for more major procedures the red and white blood cells and platelet counts should be checked. Jaundiced patients and those suffering from liver disease require prothrombin time estimations. Tests for thalassaemia and sickle-cell disease must be made in appropriate patients. Check if the patient is taking anticoagulant drugs.

Exclude existing sepsis and bleeding. If sepsis is present, identify it, since major surgery in the presence of infection may provoke intravascular coagulation. If the patient is already bleeding and the operation is for its control, then take every measure to identify and localize the source of bleeding.

Prophylaxis If the patient is anaemic, when possible delay an elective operation until it is corrected by the oral or intramuscular administration of iron, or more urgently by blood transfusion. If the prothrombin time is extended, correct it before operation whenever possible, by giving injections of vitamin K analogue. If bleeding is already occurring and clotting is imperfect, obtain the advice of a haematologist whenever possible. Fresh frozen plasma contains all the clotting factors and may be given to gain control before an operation, especially when this is for the purpose of dealing with the bleeding source.

Bleeding—five major considerations
Anaemia
Bleeding tendency
Major operation
Already bleeding
Sepsis

Operation In most operations the surgeon controls bleeding satisfactorily, but often, without any warning, a patient bleeds more than average for a particular procedure and control is more difficult. The desire to complete the operation may lead the surgeon to accept a higher rate of bleeding than he would normally allow and to fail, at the end of the operation, to achieve perfect haemostasis. Such a patient is at risk of wound haematoma or wound sepsis following a minor operation and of continuing life threatening bleeding after a major procedure. For this reason haemostasis must be perfect at each step of the operation.

There are a number of well-known traps for the careless surgeon. If a blood vessel has been picked up using the tips of artery forceps, do not attempt to tie it. The ligature will inevitably drop off as the haemostat is removed. Instead place a second, horizontal forceps below the first, with tips projecting, so that a ligature can be safely tied to encircle the blood vessel at a distance below the end (Fig. 2.1). Do not gather a large bunch of tissue into a ligature because the bulk tends to push off, in a rolling action, the ligature from the end of the blood vessel (Fig. 2.2). This is reinforced if the structure is pulled upon, widening

Figure 2.1
(a) This ligature will slip off. (b) This ligature will not slip off.

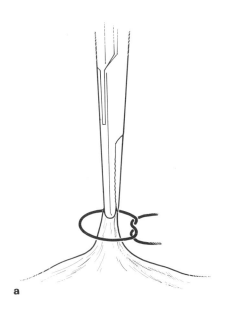

a

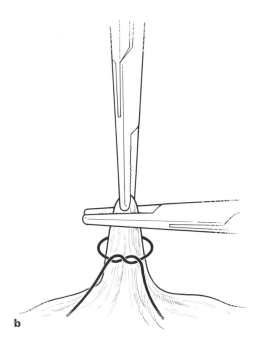

b

Figure 2.2
Bulky tissue within a
ligature tends to push
off the ligature.

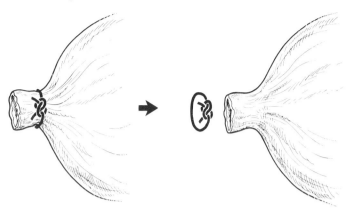

Figure 2.2
Bulky tissue within a
ligature tends to push
off the ligature.

the base of the bulky tissue (Fig. 2.3). An additional factor is the retraction of the cut blood vessel as it contracts, drawing it out of the grasp of the ligature (Fig. 2.4). This is a frequent cause of mesenteric haematoma when too much tissue is included, and it becomes difficult to find the vessel within the haematoma. Overtight ligatures on atheromatous vessels may fracture them: the calcified rigid walls are incapable of contracting and bleeding continues indefinitely.

The most feared bleeding may be venous oozing, welling up in the depths of a wound so that the bleeding vessels cannot be

Figure 2.3
The ligature is pushed
off if the base is
stretched.

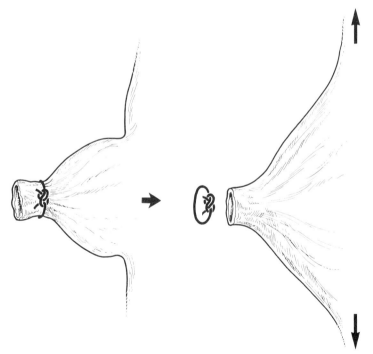

Figure 2.4
A vessel tied within
bulky tissue may
retract and continue
bleeding, producing a
haematoma within.

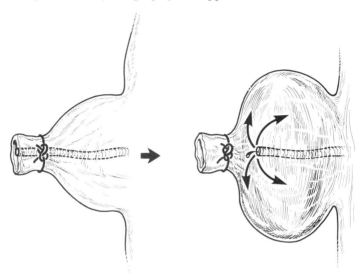

identified and isolated. As a rule it is best to pack the area for five minutes, timed by the clock, and then to withdraw the packs gently, in the hope that the bleeding has ceased or is so reduced that the vessel can be picked up and ligated or oversewn.

Occasionally during an operation that has been conducted with ease, all the raw tissues begin to ooze for no apparent reason. The anaesthetist is often blamed, but frequently there is no known cause. Stop the procedure at once and control the bleeding by concentrating on each area in turn, being willing to go back many times. Sometimes the use of warm saline packs or the application of absorbable gelatine sponge, absorbable hae-mostatic mesh (Fig. 2.5) or crushed muscle, reinforces the use of mattress sutures, ligatures, oversewing and diathermization.

A serious failure of haemostasis is when creating anastomoses, especially if non-crushing clamps are used to prevent spillage of bowel contents, thus compressing the blood vessels that would otherwise overtly bleed. The Connell stitch, often used on the anterior suture line of anastomoses, is notoriously not haemosta-tic, whereas the simple over-and-over continuous stitch carried from the posterior wall to the anterior wall has a good reputation for haemostasis (Fig. 2.6). If the Connell stitch is used, all the blood vessels must first be isolated, clamped and ligated with the non-crushing clamps released, to obtain complete haemostasis.

The most likely operations to produce bleeding as a complica-tion are those carried out to control bleeding. Either the source is not correctly identified or if it is, complete control is not achieved. Whenever possible always identify and localize the source of bleeding before operation. It is often extremely difficult to do so during the exploration. Whatever method is used to control the bleeding, make sure that it is effective by watching

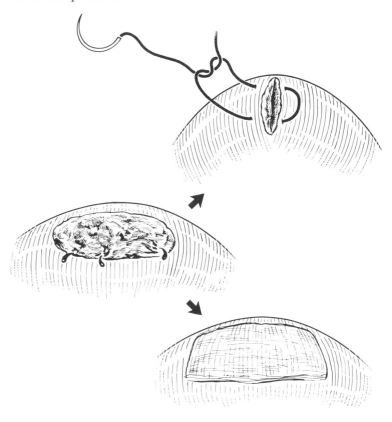

Figure 2.5
Preventing persistent bleeding from a raw area. It may be folded over with sutures or covered with haemostatic mesh or gauze.

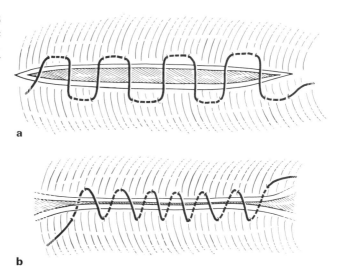

Figure 2.6
(a) Non-haemostatic Connell stitch.
(b) Over-and-over haemostatic bowel sutures.

and waiting while the anaesthetist restores the blood pressure to normal. Make sure that all the sources of bleeding are identified and controlled.

Why bleeding continues
1 Failure to identify cause
2 Treatment of incidental lesion
3 Imperfect control of cause

During the operation the anaesthetist monitors and controls the patient's general condition and advises the surgeon on the cardiovascular state. It is important that mutual confidence exists between surgeon and anaesthetist.

A major coagulopathy may develop during the operation, especially when this is for the control of bleeding or follows a major operation, trauma, and particularly in the presence of sepsis and liver disease. Bleeding is at first controllable, but then becomes unmanageable, with an absence of clots. Prompt infusion of fresh frozen plasma and fresh blood occasionally brings it under control. More usually the only hope for the patient is to firmly pack the wound (Fig. 2.7) and abort the operation until the coagulopathy can be controlled. Do not doggedly proceed with the operation. Stone and his colleagues (1983) recommend rapidly oversewing the ends of cut bowel, packing and closing the abdomen under pressure, until clotting power can be restored.

Intraoperative autotransfusion is rarely appropriate in surgery of the upper gastrointestinal tract because the most severe bleeding encountered is into the bowel. It may be valuable during

Figure 2.7
Packing a bleeding
cavity.

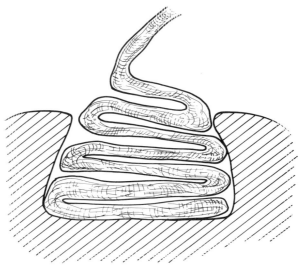

operations following associated liver or spleen injuries, or when unexpected bleeding develops during an elective operation.

Aftercare   Bleeding is usually the earliest of the serious postoperative complications presenting at any time from the completion of the operation. Regularly check the wound, drains, nasogastric and other tubes, the patient's colour and general condition, and if indicated, the abdominal girth at a marked level. Order a chest X-ray for signs of intrathoracic bleeding or elevation of the diaphragm in intra-abdominal bleeding. In particular monitor the pulse rate, blood pressure and urinary output for signs of hypovolaemic shock. In case of doubt insert a central venous catheter to measure the pressure.

If the wound shows signs of swelling or discharge of blood locally, remove some skin sutures. If possible secure bleeding superficial vessels or pack them. If the bleeding comes from deep within the wound in considerable quantity, arrange to return the patient to the operating theatre to explore deeply. Similarly explore bleeding from a drain site to determine if it is merely a subdermal vessel or if it demands exploration because the origin lies deeply. Intra-abdominal bleeding may be detected by inserting a plastic intravenous catheter through the abdominal wall, running in 500 ml of sterile physiological saline and allowing it to run out again after a few minutes to see if it is heavily bloodstained.

Intraluminal bleeding may produce blood in nasogastric tube aspirate, or vomiting of blood. If this is coffee ground in type, it suggests that the blood has been in contact with gastric acid, as in peptic ulceration. If it is dark and unchanged, it is more likely to be from the suture line or erosive bleeding. If the operation was for the control of bleeding, was the source definitely identified and confidently controlled?

Rapid intraluminal bleeding produces a laxative effect and blood may be passed rectally or be detected on the glove following rectal examination. Again blood that has been in contact with acid is black, tarry and has an unmistakable odour, distinguishing it from the dark unchanged blood from a bleeding suture line or erosions. In selected cases endoscopy, usually following intubation and washout of blood, may elucidate the cause. Inflate the bowel sparingly. Angiography may be helpful, especially in revealing undetected gastrointestinal bleeding—and on occasion embolization can be carried out to occlude the vessel.

In the presence of a rising pulse rate, falling blood pressure and low central venous pressure with low urinary output in a restless patient with peripheral vascular shutdown, consider intra-abdominal, intrathoracic or intraluminal bleeding in appropriate circumstances. Check the abdominal girth at a marked level for signs of expansion. Obtain a plain X-ray of the chest to note mediastinal and intrapleural shadowing or elevation of the diaphragm that suggests intra-abdominal bleeding. If a viscus such as the spleen or liver might have been damaged, ultrasonic scanning is useful, since physical signs are difficult to elicit and interpret. Try the effect of infusing 100 ml of blood or other intravenous fluid to note its effect on the central venous pressure. If this rises, only to sink slowly to its former level, this suggests hypovolaemia. Ensure that adequate supplies of cross-matched blood are available. Do not forget the possibility that the clotting mechanism may have been exhausted, especially if the operation was major, was for the control of bleeding or was carried out in a septic patient.

It is sometimes difficult in such patients, to distinguish hypovolaemia from septicaemic shock, since the deterioration resulting from overwhelming infection may present catastrophically. If sepsis is a possible or likely explanation, take blood for culture and administer versatile antibiotics intravenously, if necessary after obtaining advice from the microbiologist about the likely organism and most potent choice of treatment.

Searching for postoperative bleeding site
Wound
Drains
Nasogastric tube
Abdominal girth
Rectal examination
Chest X-ray
Endoscopy
Ultrasound
Angiography
Technetium scan

If the bleeding is chronic, isotope labelling of blood cells with subsequent scanning may be helpful. If these are not available, the patient may be asked to swallow a length of string which is subsequently withdrawn and tested along its length for evidence of bleeding. Barium meal X-ray is not popular nowadays for the diagnosis of gastrointestinal bleeding.

Reoperation   It is impossible to generalize about re-exploration in patients who bleed following upper gastrointestinal tract surgery. In most cases plan to re-explore the patient if bleeding continues following a single attempt at adequate correction of his general state and a check on clotting factors. If the bleeding is brisk or calamitous, re-exploration is mandatory without delay, while supplementary supplies of crossmatched blood are ordered.

When the bleeding is intraluminal following an upper gastrointestinal tract operation, many surgeons believe that endoscopy is contraindicated. I (RMK) try to perform endoscopy in the

Reoperative procedure for bleeding
Resuscitate
Full team
Endoscope available
Blood cross matched, serum to lab
Haematologist's help
Suction
Clotting—haemostatic foam or gauze
Large packs

anaesthetic room prior to reoperation, with adequate washout facilities available. It may be of vital help in revealing an unsuspected cause, such as variceal bleeding, a missed peptic ulcer or multiple erosions, or it may demonstrate that the previous operation to control bleeding has failed. Occasionally such generalized mucosal bleeding is seen that operation is deferred in the hope that it can be controlled conservatively, as by angiographic embolization.

Before commencing the operation ensure that the anaesthetist is satisfied that he has restored the patient's condition as close to normal as possible and that adequate supplies of replacement blood are available. Fully reopen the wound, controlling bleeding all the time. If the main cause of bleeding is encountered, control it completely. This usually entails evacuating blood and clot and identifying, if necessary by careful dissection, the exact vessel or vessels that are bleeding. Ligate medium and small vessels, repair damaged major ones. If there is general oozing from a raw area, control it with mattress sutures, appose the raw surfaces accurately with sutures, and apply haemostatic substances or sheets.

If you cannot see what is bleeding, there are two manoeuvres that may help. If there is a main feeding vessel, compress it between the fingers (Fig. 2.8); if the only available controlling vessel is the aorta, compress it against the vertebral column (Fig. 2.9). Remove all the blood that has collected. Have available a sucker tube and forceps. Do not use haemostatic forceps, which may irrevocably damage a vital structure, but use swab-holding forceps without the swab. These can be applied to provide just sufficient pressure to control bleeding without causing damage.

The second manoeuvre that may help is to pack the area. Use large gauze packs and press upon them with your hand or fist. Leave them in place for five minutes, timed by the clock, and then gently lift them off after arming yourself once again with a sucker and swab-holding forceps. As a rule the bleeding has stopped or is diminished so that the site of origin can be identified and controlled. On occasion the pack controls the bleeding but this recurs furiously when it is removed. When control cannot be achieved except with a pack, take a long roll of sterile gauze and

Figure 2.8
Compression of
vessels supplying a
bleeding structure.

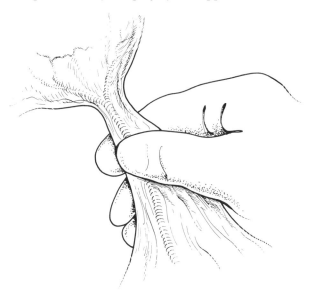

Figure 2.9
Compression of the
aorta against the
vertebral column.

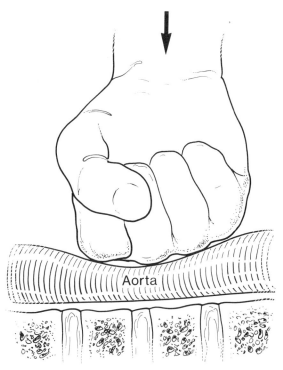

lay it in, back and forth like a jumping jack cracker, compressing
it until the bleeding is controlled by the pressure of the pack; then
bring the tail of the gauze out of the wound (Fig. 2.7). Close the
wound around the protruding gauze. Plan to reoperate on the

patient and reopen the wound in 24 to 48 hours, when the patient's general condition has been restored, and when clotting factors have been checked and if necessary corrected and blood is available for transfusion. As a rule when such precautions are taken the bleeding is found to have stopped when the gauze pack is gently removed.

If the bleeding is intraluminal, is there a suture line? If so, cut the stitches in the centre of the anterior suture line and unpick them until the whole anterior part of the anastomosis is separated and the ends of the threads are sufficiently long to tie to a fresh suture when the anastomosis is refashioned (Fig. 2.10). Do not, as is often recommended, make a fresh incision which prejudices the view, makes a corrective procedure difficult and potentially devascularizes a strip of viscus between the new incision and the anastomotic line.

Suture line bleeding is almost invariably from the anterior line and is obvious. Catch and ligate the bleeding points and resuture the edges using an over-and-over stitch, tying the unpicked ends to the new suture ends (Fig. 2.11).

If the intraluminal source has not been identified, do not hesitate to resort to endoscopy now, becoming unsterile to pass the endoscope and rescrubbing to continue the operation. Control of bleeding is exactly as at a primary operation and must be perfect.

Do not be impatient to close the bowel or the wound after controlling postoperative bleeding. When the anaesthetist reports that the patient is normotensive, check again that no further bleeding has developed.

After completing the operation, ensure that the patient is monitored, ideally in an intensive care unit, until it is certain that there is no recurrence of bleeding. Patients who have bled considerably risk other complications, in particular further bleeding, sometimes from fresh sites, infection, deep leg vein thrombosis, poor wound healing, delay in the return of gut function, and delayed convalescence. Those who have bled calamitously or have not had prompt or adequate correction and

Figure 2.10
Exploring an anastomosis. Cut the stitch in the centre of the anterior suture line and unpick the threads to open up the anastomosis.

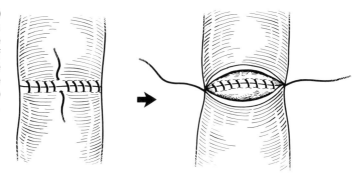

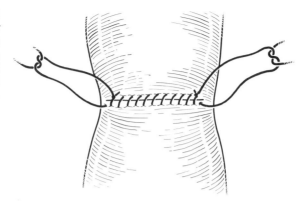

Figure 2.11
Reclosing the anterior suture line. Tie the newly inserted suture ends to the unpicked threads of the original suture.

blood volume replacement risk organ failure such as renal, cardiorespiratory and possibly permanent neurological damage.

Leakage

Whenever the bowel is opened and repaired or anastomosed, leakage may subsequently occur. This is likely if the suture line is under tension or will be under tension when the bowel contracts or is obstructed, if the arterial supply or venous drainage of the viscus is insufficient, or in the presence of infection, foreign body or neoplasm. Leaked bowel contents produce local necrosis, contamination and the risk of cellulitis and abscess formation, with possible tracking either to a body cavity or to the exterior, forming a fistula. The patient may remain stable for a day or two after operation, but then begins to deteriorate, either gradually or so suddenly that a cardiovascular calamity, such as cardiac infarct or pulmonary embolus, is diagnosed. Investigations such as electrocardiography may show changes compatible with the incorrect diagnosis and urgent action may be delayed, in which case the discovery of the true diagnosis may be made only at postmortem examination.

Surgery can be complicated by spontaneous perforation from unsuspected disease, misjudgement about the survival of damaged or ischaemic bowel, or complications, such as obstruction or failure of the blood supply, developing subsequently. This second type of complication is particularly dangerous because the surgeon does not expect it to happen; it sometimes develops away from the site of operation, and confuses the diagnosis.

Preoperative factors   Healing depends on many factors outside the surgeon's control, such as age, sex and malignancy. Patients taking cytotoxic, immunosuppressive or steroid drugs may have impaired healing. Anaemia, malnutrition, sepsis and jaundice may be corrected or alleviated before an elective operation and can be improved while preparations are made for an emergency operation.

Operation   Some surgeons rarely encounter leakage. This reflects their judgement in planning procedures and the technical skill with which they mobilize, open, close and unite the bowel. Leaks follow rough handling, too extensive mobilization, tension, obstruction, vascular damage, contamination from spillage of contents and casual stitching. Close defects with perfectly placed all-coats sutures that just appose the edges. If stitches are too tight they may cut out when postoperative oedema causes the bowel wall to swell. When forming anastomoses prefer to join matched stomata and avoid twists, tension and any potential ischaemia.

Of course it is all very well giving advice about tension and ischaemia, but in most cases the ability to bridge a gap following a resection cannot be judged until the bridging conduit is mobilized. What appears adequate before the resection may prove inadequate subsequently. If the ends cannot be brought together, the decision is already made. One possibility is to abandon the chosen conduit and employ another: for example, if the stomach or jejunum will not reach up to join to the cervical oesophagus, the colon may be used. A second choice is to bring each end to the surface separately as a stoma and plan to bridge the gap subsequently, or possibly interpose a free intestinal graft, employing microsurgical techniques to vascularize the graft. Most of these major resections are performed for cancer and if transection has not already been carried out, the surgeon may risk transecting too close to the tumour. If tumour is present in the cut end, there is a serious risk that the anastomosis will not heal. If it does heal, the unfortunate patient who has survived this major operation is usually doomed to develop malignant recurrence and obstruction subsequently.

The real dilemma comes when the ends meet—just! Perhaps the colour and tension are acceptable as suturing starts, but when the procedure is completed, one end is dusky. At the end of a long operation, possibly performed on a frail patient, the surgeon, who is himself tired and under pressure from his theatre colleagues and his own future commitments to close up, requires great strength of mind to resist.

Carefully investigate every possibility of gaining length and losing tension, perhaps by using an alternative pathway. Sometimes dividing a further main vessel, as in a jejunal Roux-en-Y loop, gives the extra length, while producing a plain line of demarcation at the end of the segment (Fig. 2.12), so that the anastomosis can be taken down, the ischaemic segment resected, and a sound anastomosis then constructed.

In case of doubt, cover the anastomosis with warm saline-soaked packs for five minutes by the clock. If there is no improvement, abandon the anastomosis. Occasionally it may be

Figure 2.12
Dividing further
vessels sometimes
gains length even
though further bowel
resection is necessary.

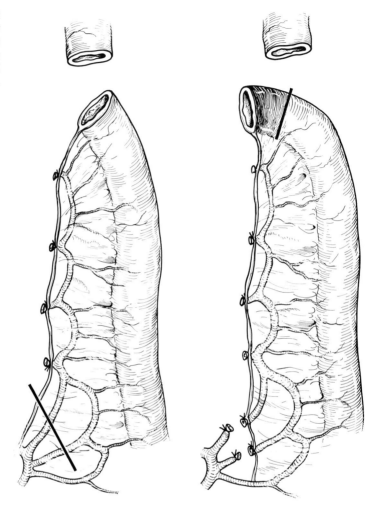

possible to bring the ends to the surface, wait a few days to determine if the bowel will survive, and subsequently unite them. Although this involves an extra procedure it is infinitely preferable to joining bowel ends that are suspect.

There are, of course, all shades of doubt. A minimally suspect anastomosis might be acceptable if it lies subcutaneously but not if it lies in the mediastinum, pleural cavity or abdomen. An anastomosis that can be securely wrapped with healthy omentum (Fig. 2.13), peritoneum or pleura can often be left, while the same anastomosis is uncertain if no wrapping is available.

The perfection with which the suturing is carried out is an important determinant of the outcome. Every stitch must pick up all the coats, and be placed so carefully that the two edges of bowel come together exactly. The sutures just appose the edges

Figure 2.13
Sometimes the
anastomosis can be
wrapped with a sheet
of omentum for extra
security.

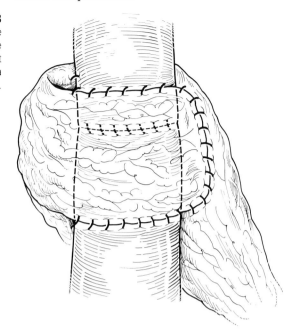

Figure 2.13
Sometimes the
anastomosis can be
wrapped with a sheet
of omentum for extra
security.

and do not constrict them or the inevitable postoperative oedema will cause them to cut out. In recent years excellent stapling devices have appeared to aid the construction of anastomoses and the closure of bowel. Do not expect them to compensate for technical deficiencies in mobilizing, arranging and apposing bowel segments.

Remember that an upper gastrointestinal leak is often a death sentence. Operating time, frailty of the patient, and failure to complete the intended procedure are secondary considerations. If you carry out upper gastrointestinal surgery, determine never to leave a doubtful anastomosis. Even with this degree of care you will have the occasional leak, hopefully of no clinical significance.

When possible defunction bowel that has been operated upon to allow it to heal and recover its function. This may be achieved by internal tube drainage, usually by nasoenteric tube. Some patients are intolerant of such tubes and certainly most patients cannot cough effectively with a tube in place. An alternative is to insert a pharyngostomy tube (Fig. 2.14). Pass a long curved Roberts' forceps through the mouth into one pyriform fossa. Push the forceps tip towards the surface anterior to the carotid sheath. It can be felt subcutaneously in the neck. Make a stab cut onto the tip of the forceps, push the tip through to grasp the end of a nasogastric tube and draw it into the mouth. Now pass the tip of the tube down the oesophagus as far as necessary, making sure that there is no kink in the pharynx. This tube is comfortable and can be left in situ without interfering with coughing.

Figure 2.14
Preparing to pass a
pharyngostomy tube.
Feel for the tips of
Roberts' forceps
pressed into the
pyriform fossa.

Endotracheal tube

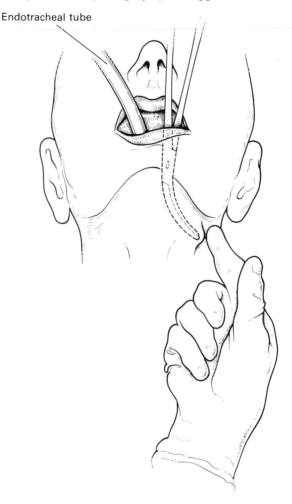

An alternative method of defunctioning the bowel is to pass a tube up from below. For example, a gastrostomy or jejunostomy allows tubes to be passed not only distally but also proximally to defunction an anastomosis.

As a rule it is not possible to defunction the upper gastrointestinal tract in the same manner as a defunctioning colostomy for the distal colon. Very rarely if this must be achieved, the cervical oesophagus can be mobilized and brought to the surface to create a stoma, thus defunctioning the bowel below.

The use of external drains is controversial. Since there is little to lose by inserting a soft drain down to a suture line, many surgeons do so, especially if they have doubts about the integrity of the closure. Of course no doubtful suture line should be left, and certainly the presence of a drain cannot be relied upon as a means of preventing or signalling a leak.

Features Careful monitoring of the patient does not always disclose a leak, which may be clinically silent. Indeed, small contained leaks probably occur more frequently than those that are detected.

Leaks reveal themselves later than bleeding, usually three to five days after operation. When the bowel begins to function again and to transmit fluid contents, mild, temporary and well-confined leaks may produce no features or merely an episode of discomfort, pyrexia or gastrointestinal hold-up. Occasionally, following an undetected leak, an abscess may discharge internally or externally after an interval, or the patient may become toxic and pyrexial, and tests reveal an abscess.

Serious leakage which floods the peritoneal or pleural cavities or the mediastinum often presents so catastrophically as to mimic a cardiorespiratory accident. The patient collapses, with thready pulse, low blood pressure, and peripheral vascular shut down, and becomes toxic and confused. Local physical signs are difficult to interpret, since the bowel is only now about to function and the paralysis that results when it is flooded with leaked fluid is missed. Tenderness, and the mass of adhering viscera, can occasionally be detected in the abdomen or rectally, but the postoperative wound tenderness may obscure the signs. Leakage into the chest may be difficult to separate clinically from postoperative pulmonary collapse or pleural effusion, except that the patient is more ill than would otherwise be expected. If a drain lies near the leak, bowel fluid may emerge but not reliably so. Fluid may appear between the wound stitches. If there is doubt about the nature of the fluid, some methylene blue may be swallowed by the patient to see if the emerging fluid is stained.

Features of leaks
3 to 5 days postoperative
Pyrexia
Loss of bowel function
Sometimes catastrophic collapse

Investigations The white blood cell count is raised. Electrocardiographic changes can be interpreted as confirming a cardiovascular accident. A plain radiograph of the chest may display mediastinal widening, pleural fluid or hydropneumothorax following leakage into the chest, or a raised diaphragm possibly with increased air beneath it, sometimes with a fluid level following leakage into the abdomen. Abdominal films show distended loops of bowel with fluid levels and apparent thickening of the bowel walls from fibrin deposition. Air is usually detected outside the bowel following operation, but if this increases a leak is likely (Fig. 2.15). If a fluid level is present, leakage is almost certain.

Figure 2.15
Gas under the right
diaphragm.

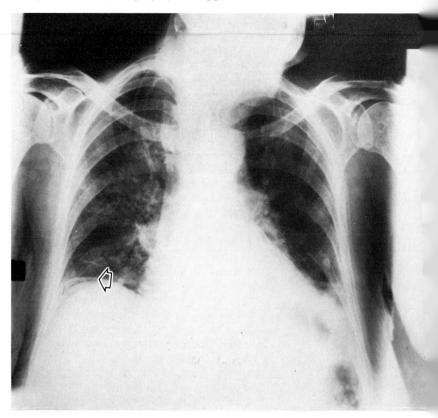

Radiography using water-soluble contrast medium is most valuable in demonstrating upper gastrointestinal leaks. Endoscopy is helpful, but use minimal air insufflation. Alternatively radio-opaque watery contrast medium may be infused into the sinus to determine if it enters the bowel when screened. Ultrasound and computed tomographic scans aid in the localization of leaked fluid.

Management   The diagnosis or suspicion of a leak cannot be ignored. Certain specific leaks can be treated conservatively but the majority of postoperative leaks must be treated surgically. Before taking direct corrective action the patient's general condition must be improved as much as possible. The time devoted to this varies according to the circumstances, and may take half an hour while the theatre is prepared, or several days or weeks while intensive parenteral nutritional correction is undertaken. An unfit patient should never be taken to the operating theatre without adequate resuscitation, fluid and electrolyte replacement, the ordering of blood for transfusion, and the start of a course of intravenous versatile antibiotics active against both aerobic and anaerobic organisms. However, if the leaked contents are retained within the abdomen, pleural cavity or mediastinum, the patient will rapidly deteriorate unless operation is urgently carried out.

If the leaked contents are already draining adequately through a well-established fistulous track when first seen, the patient is unlikely to be toxic or shocked and there is then no urgency. If the leak is discovered incidentally during radiological screening and is small and well localized, then it can be treated conservatively, continuing parenteral feeding and repeating the screening X-rays with water soluble medium after five to seven days.

Reoperation   At an emergency operation the primary intention is to drain the leaked contents. It is rarely possible or sagacious to repair the leak. The reason is that the breakdown results from a failure of the healing process, owing to ischaemia, infection or residual neoplasia, and the tissues soon become unable to heal because of the added infection that results from breakdown and leakage. This is in contradistinction to leaks caused by mechanical damage to previously healthy tissues. As a rule the best course is to defunction the segment either with intraluminal tubes or by creating a proximal stoma, and to arrange external drainage from the point of breakdown. This is most reliably achieved by bringing the proximal and distal ends of the bowel to the surface, assuming this is possible. If distal obstruction is discovered it should be relieved.

When leaked gastrointestinal contents drain completely and discretely to the surface collect the efflux while protecting the skin and feed the patient intravenously or into the gut below the leak. If the second method of feeding is selected, it is often possible to return the leaked fluid from the point of breakdown.

Once adequate drainage and replacement are achieved there is usually no hurry. The most important supportive measure once the leak is controlled and channelled is to maintain the patient's nutritional state. In some cases spontaneous healing occurs. If it does not, surgical repair should be carried out when the patient is in the best possible condition. This operation requires exceptional judgement to select the best procedure, great familiarity with the structures so that they can be recognized in spite of the effects of the leak, and skilful deliberate technique. Even so, if the patient is still catabolic, even the best technical operation will fail.

Reoperative procedure for leaks
Drain
Defunction
Arrange alternative feeding

Infection

Although many aspects of operative risk have been reduced, infection remains a serious danger. Occasionally, previously healthy patients having routine surgery develop severe infection with morbidity and even mortality. At particular risk are the elderly, those with severe cardiac, respiratory, diabetic and other generalized diseases, and those who have artificial heart valves.

The introduction of more versatile antibiotics has not diminished the problem because, especially in hospitals, antibiotic-resistant strains of micro-organisms have flourished as the sensitive competing organisms are killed. Methicillin-resistant strains of staphylococcus present a severe problem in many hospitals.

Pathology Whatever the source of infection, the mechanism is similar. The exotoxins and endotoxins produce a cellular effect. Local cellulitis develops and organisms may spread in tissue planes, body cavities, by lymphatics and into the blood stream. Many of the organisms encountered here are pyogenic so that abscess formation is frequent and the abscess often expands so that the pus spreads or bursts into other spaces or to the exterior. The systemic response to sepsis is metabolic, related to failure of oxygen utilization and appears to be independent of the responsible organism.

A dangerous and potent source of infection is bowel ischaemia. In gastro-oesophageal surgery bowel is often taken to bridge large gaps following resection and the blood supply may become attenuated, or subsequently compressed, undergo thrombosis or become insufficient because the patient's cardiorespiratory condition deteriorates, reducing the oxygenation of the bowel. The ischaemic or anoxic bowel fails to heal and function. Organisms flourish in the stagnant contents, and as the mucosa and subsequently the rest of the wall dies, they penetrate it. Eventually the gangrenous bowel ruptures, releasing its contents. The absorption of the toxic products of the virulent organisms produces profound septic shock.

Predisposing factors Obese, diabetic or jaundiced patients and those taking steroid, immunosuppressive or cytotoxic drugs have a higher than average rate of infection. Major, lengthy operations also predispose to infection. Contamination may occur from an external source away from the site of the operation on the patient, from the surgical team, from the operating theatre and its instruments, or from an endogenous source at the operation site, such as spilled gut contents or an existing infection.

Normally the rapid transit of contents through the smooth-lined oesophagus leaves it almost sterile. Gastric acid then kills off most micro-organisms and the duodenum and small bowel are virtually sterile. However, any stasis of the contents in the gut, or diverticula from it, allow organisms to flourish rapidly, as does mucosal disease including ulceration and neoplasia. The most frequently grown organisms in the upper gastrointestinal tract are streptococci, coliforms and some faecal anaerobes.

Predisposing factors for infection
Obesity
General diseases
Lengthy operation
Bowel contents spilled

Prophylaxis It is likely that any action that improves the patient's general condition increases his resistance to infection. Correction of nutritional deficiencies, unstable diabetes and anaemia are important, as is the reduction of obesity before a major elective operation. Foci of infection in the chest, paranasal sinuses and on the skin should be eradicated.

Preparation of the bowel includes the relief of upper gastrointestinal stasis using stomach or oesophageal tubes passed by mouth, with washouts using water until the effluent is clean. If the colon is to be opened or used, its contents may be sterilized using enemata, oral fluids such as mannitol 100 g in 3 litres of water and, less fashionably nowadays, non-absorbable antibiotics or gut sterilizing chemotherapeutic agents.

The use of prophylactic systemic antibiotics remains controversial. As a rule, ill, undernourished, jaundiced, obese patients and those at risk with cardiovascular or respiratory disease, a prosthetic heart valve or having a major prolonged operation should be given protection against possible infection. If the gut is to be opened and is likely to have organisms flourishing within it, or if the operation carries a high risk of contamination, give prophylactic antibiotics. The synergistic action of aerobes and anaerobes makes it important to give prophylaxis against both types of organisms if the lower bowel is to be opened. Aminoglycosides such as neomycin or kanamycin may be combined with metronidazole or erythromycin. Cephalosporins and mezlocillin are generally effective.

Operations may be classified as clean when the infection rate is below 5%, clean:contaminated when it is between 5% and 15%, and contaminated when it exceeds 25%. Prophylaxis implies that the antibiotic is present in the tissues as, or just after, contamination takes place. Therefore the first (and sometimes only) dose may be given by the anaesthetist as the operation begins. A single dose is usually effective and there is no reason to continue prophylactic, as opposed to therapeutic antibiotics beyond the day of operation. The appropriate versatile antibiotic must be given; in case of doubt, seek advice on the current best choice from the microbiologist.

Prophylactic antibiotics should be prescribed for:
The ill patient at risk
The patient with a prosthetic heart valve
Major, prolonged operation
Clean:contaminated or contaminated operation

If an infection already exists and cannot be eradicated, or the operation cannot be delayed, start effective treatment before operation and carry it on through and after the operation.

Be aware of the complications of each antibiotic, since the benefits carry risks also. In particular, they may cause hypersensitivity reactions and be toxic to the liver, kidney, ear and peripheral nerves.

Operation   Hypoxic tissues are at risk of infection. The anaesthetist assiduously maintains oxygenation and normal blood volume so that the tissues are fully perfused with oxygenated blood throughout the operation.

Trauma, ischaemia, and the insertion of foreign material render the tissues susceptible to infection so the surgeon must be gentle, and insert the minimum of foreign material. It is especially important that the blood supply is maintained to all the tissues, in particular when taking stomach, small bowel or colon long distances to bridge gaps following extensive gastro-oesophageal resections. Diathermization of bleeding points to coagulate vessels should be accurately applied for the minimum time and mass ligatures should be avoided.

When the bowel is to be opened, isolate the area with specially coloured towels—usually red for danger. Use non-crushing clamps and have a functioning sucker available to minimize spillage. Use the minimum number of instruments, keeping them separate from the remainder. When the bowel is reclosed discard the instruments, the towels, the sucker tube and your gloves, applying sterile gloves and taking fresh instruments to complete the operation. The theatre nurse usually remains sterile but any assistants who have participated in the manipulation of open bowel should also change their gloves.

A potent cause of infection is imperfect haemostasis. Blood and clot form an excellent culture medium. Ensure that the tissues are absolutely dry, and that all blood is mopped and sucked out. If infection is already present, take a swab for culture and determination of antibiotic sensitivities. Request the anaesthetist to administer a first dose of an appropriate and systemic antibiotic if he has not already done so. Arrange to drain the area. Of course leakage of bowel content contaminates the tissues so that in addition to taking great care in closing the bowel, attempt to divert or aspirate the contents until healing is certain. When unexpected contamination with bowel content occurs or infected material is encountered, the risk of wound infection is high. It may be advisable to leave the superficial part of the wound open for a few days and plan delayed primary closure. The use of local applications of antibiotic solutions is controversial. Some surgeons prefer simple washing with sterile saline solution, while others use antiseptic solutions, but the benefits are not certain. When generalized infection is encountered it may be advisable to leave the abdomen completely open, after laying sterile packs soaked in saline in the wound. The packs are changed daily or as often as necessary until the infection is controlled and the abdomen is then closed.

Drains are controversial. They usually provide a conduit for fluid already present but cannot be relied upon to guide infected fluid or pus to the surface in the future. Intraperitoneal and intrapleural drains become sealed off and isolated within two to three days and the efflux may then be merely fluid formed as a reaction to the foreign material. Closed systems of tube drains are now popular in contrast to open-guttered drains (Fig. 2.16). There are certain circumstances when drains are used conventionally, as when the biliary system has been entered or if a collection of fluid is encountered, and sometimes if a resection leaves an extensive raw area that cannot be closed. Continuous lavage may be used if infection is severe. Sterile physiological saline is run in through a small catheter and aspirated through a sump drain, placed in the pelvis (Fig. 2.17). It is usual to insert a tube drain, connected to an underwater sealed drain whenever the chest is opened, as prophylaxis against lung collapse rather than infection.

Figure 2.16
On the left is an open type of drain. On the right is a closed tubular drain.

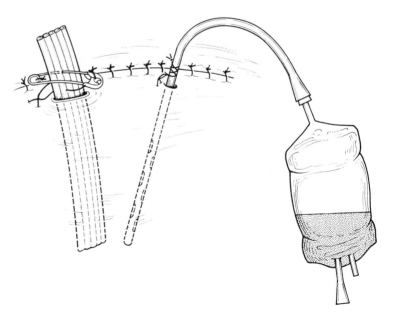

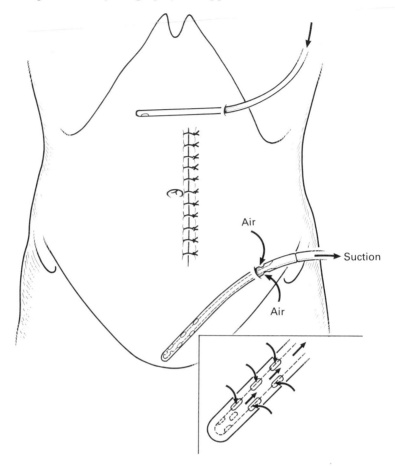

Figure 2.17
Through the upper catheter, sterile physiological saline is slowly infused into the peritoneal cavity. The lower system is a sump drain through which the fluid is removed.

Aftercare   The considerations that apply to the general care of the patient during operation are equally important in the postoperative period to prevent anoxia or poor tissue perfusion, which allow contamination to translate into infection. During the operation the highly trained anaesthetist constantly monitors the patient and this must be carried on by those in charge of the patient until he is fully recovered.

Apart from the operation site, stasis in the respiratory and urinary systems and the presence of intravenous catheters may allow infection to develop, which could spread elsewhere.

Features   At an early stage it is impossible to determine why a patient has developed a pyrexia or rigors, and whether it is related to the operation site or is generated elsewhere.

The wound should be inspected regularly if possible and it is usual to cover clean wounds with a transparent sheet or thin translucent tape so that swelling, redness and discharge can be detected early. Reflux from drain sites may indicate sepsis or leakage that will soon infect the tissues.

Early infection producing cellulitis with relatively little necrosis usually responds to the removal of the cause and systemic administration of an appropriate antibiotic. Once necrosis and abscess formation have occurred, drainage is usually necessary either surgically or by needle or catheter.

The signals of sepsis are rigors, swinging pyrexia, sometimes with confusion, a raised white cell count, rapid catabolism as demonstrated by weight loss, muscle wasting and power loss, and a negative protein nitrogen balance.

Exclude first by clinical means, wound sepsis, a pelvic collection, respiratory or urinary infection and infection around an intravenous catheter site. Send sputum, urine and blood to the laboratory for culture and order plain erect and supine abdominal films and a chest X-ray.

Intrathoracic infection is usually detected clinically and by observing mediastinal widening, air emphysema, and occasionally a visible fluid level on X-ray. Fluid within the pleural cavity appears as an opaque shadow rising higher in the axilla, or, if there is air or gas above it, there is a fluid level (see p. 54). The fluid can be tapped, inspected, submitted to biochemical analysis to exclude leaked bowel content, and cultured for organisms.

Intra-abdominal sepsis is notoriously difficult to detect in the postoperative period when wound tenderness, postoperative cessation of gut function and the effects of surgical defunctioning of the gut obscure clinical features. As a rule if good gut function has returned, it ceases again, but the brief period of function may be missed. The abdomen becomes distended, there may be localized tenderness and rectal examination reveals the boggy feel of pus collection. Bowel sounds are absent apart from the occasional slop as fluid splashes in time with respiratory movements.

Investigations Plain X-ray of the erect abdomen shows dilated bowel loops with fluid levels and the walls of the distended bowel may appear unusually thick (Fig. 2.18). This is called 'layering' and is thought to be from fibrin deposition between adjacent bowel loops. There is often air in the abdomen following operation. If this is increased, it usually signals a leak. If there is a fluid level in it, there is almost certainly an abscess. Sepsis just under the diaphragm often stimulates the production of a 'sympathetic' pleural effusion above it. The diaphragm may be raised above an abscess. If the diaphragm is screened while the patient breathes, its movement may be seen to be inhibited above a septic focus. Swallowed, or catheter-introduced, water soluble contrast medium may demonstrate communication between bowel and abscess cavities radiologically.

Scanning techniques are most valuable not in making the diagnosis of intra-abdominal sepsis but in localizing clinically

Figure 2.18
Ileus and layering—
thickening of
interfaces between
bowel loops. Both
small and large bowel
loops are dilated.

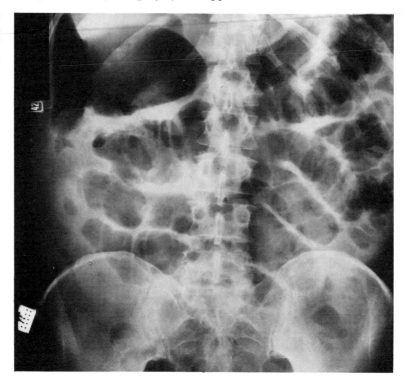

diagnosed infection and revealing loculated and multiple abscesses. Ultrasound is valuable (Fig. 2.19), and can be used to guide an exploratory needle into the abscess to obtain culture material, or to insert a catheter to drain a chronic, static collection. Diagnosis is difficult beneath a wound scar, which obscures the picture. Computed tomographic scanning (Fig. 2.20) may be more helpful in postoperative patients. Autologous radioactive labelling of leucocytes using gallium-67 citrate or indium-111 may give valuable localization of intra-abdominal pus. Indium is concentrated in the spleen and may be misinterpreted but can give a result within 24 hours (Fig. 2.21). Technetium-99 scans of liver or spleen may reveal filling defects, but other scans are usually preferable. Angiography may help to identify a filling defect suspected to be an abscess.

Septic shock
When infection develops a patient may gradually deteriorate (see *Complications of Surgery in General*) or suddenly collapse so that a major catastrophe is diagnosed. Respiration rate and pulse rate are raised and blood pressure falls. The patient may have rigors, oliguria and mild jaundice and is restless and may be confused. The extremities are often warm and cyanosed at least initially. Occasionally skin rashes, or embolic skin abscesses, are seen.

Figure 2.19
Intra-abdominal
abscess cavity (in the
upper part of the
photograph)
demonstrated by
ultrasound scan.

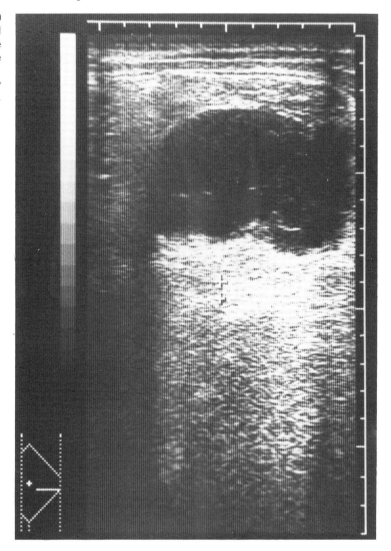

Positive blood cultures are found in less than 40% of patients. Organ failure of the heart, lungs and/or kidneys may develop and gastrointestinal bleeding sometimes complicates the picture. Secondary infection becomes evident and intravascular coagulation disorders are seen, sometimes progressing to disseminated intravascular coagulation (DIC).

Monitoring Severely ill patients are best managed in an intensive care unit. Apart from monitoring pulse rate, respiration rate and temperature, it is wise to insert a central venous catheter to estimate venous return to the heart. The skin and core temperature should be monitored, since a difference of more than 2°C implies poor

Figure 2.20
(a) Abscess in left
iliac fossa, and
(b) abscess being
drained by
percutaneous
cannula,
demonstrated by
computed
tomography.

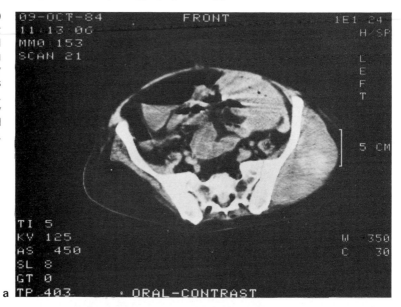

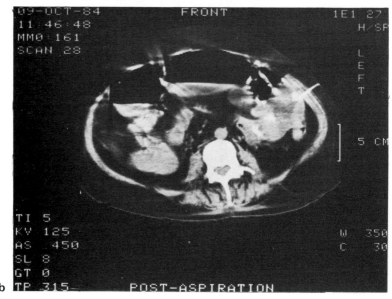

Figure 2.20 (a) Abscess in left iliac fossa, and (b) abscess being drained by percutaneous cannula, demonstrated by computed tomography.

peripheral perfusion. A blood count may show low haemoglobin, increased white cells of the granulocyte series with a shift to the left. The C-reactive protein is raised. Send blood for culture.

Urine volume should exceed 40 ml in each hour. Blood urea should not exceed 6.5 mmol/litre. The urine osmolality/plasma osmolality ratio normally exceeds 1.5:1. A ratio of 1.2–1.4:1 suggests impaired renal perfusion, while a ratio below 1.2:1

Figure 2.21
Indium-111 leucocyte
labelling followed by
scanning to display a
subhepatic and right
paracolic abscess,
producing a 'tail'
below the right liver
edge.

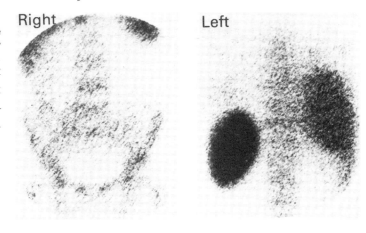

Right   Left

Anterior   Posterior

suggests acute renal failure. Serum electrolytes should be checked, especially to detect falling potassium. Blood glucose may rise and diabetes should be excluded. Serum albumin usually falls in septic patients.

Blood gas analysis may demonstrate hypoxia, and low PCO_2 in response to metabolic acidosis. In severe septic shock the blood may show hypercoagulability or DIC. In DIC bleeding may develop from previously normal sites, in addition to the operation area. The thrombin time, kaolin partial thromboplastin time, fibrinogen level and platelets should all be checked. In some patients it is difficult to evaluate the haemodynamic state and it may be advisable to insert a Swan–Ganz catheter into the pulmonary artery to measure right atrial pressure, pulmonary arterial pressure, pulmonary capillary wedge pressure and cardiac output.

Monitor:
Temperature—Core: peripheral difference
Pulse
Respiration
Full blood count
Blood culture
Blood pressure
Central venous pressure
Urinary volume, blood urea
Urine/plasma osmolality ratio
Blood glucose
Serum albumin
Serum electrolytes
Blood gases and acid/base
Clotting screen

Management   It is of paramount importance to gain cardiorespiratory control. If the patient is anoxic and delivery of oxygen with a face mask fails to raise the PaO_2 above 8.7 kPa, then intubate and ventilate the patient. Correct any hypovolaemia to maintain a systolic blood pressure of above 100 mmHg, a central venous pressure of up to 8 cmH$_2$O, and a urinary output of above 40 ml in each hour. Correct any deficiency in albumin, electrolytes, acid/base, glucose, clotting and haemoglobin.

Having taken local swabs and blood for culture, administer an antibiotic intravenously, the choice being based on the likely source of infection. If Gram-negative sepsis is likely, a cephalosporin with metronidazole may be used, but do not hesitate to take advice from the microbiologist since the position is constantly changing.

When infection is clinically evident and located in the wound, the removal of sutures and drainage bring about rapid resolution. Send culture swabs to the laboratory. If pus oozes between deep stitches or emerges from a drain site, reopen the wound in theatre. Respiratory, urinary and other infections can be dealt with, by giving appropriate management and antibiotics; if a central venous catheter is suspect, replace it and send the tip for culture (see *Complications of Surgery in General*).

Sepsis at the operation site causing rapid deterioration requires vigorous treatment. The patient may be severely· shocked, requiring restoration of circulating blood volume through an intravenous catheter. A versatile antibiotic should be administered systemically, and if one is already being used, solicit the advice of the microbiologist, who may suggest a change to a more effective agent. If the source of the infection has not been isolated but extrinsic infection has been eliminated, plan to re-explore the operation area as soon as the patient's condition has been improved as much as possible.

At operation, reopen the original wound and explore the whole extent of the original exposure. Of course if a localized cause, such as a leak, is found, with a well localized abscess, do not proceed, since this will only spread the infection. Take swabs for culture. Drain the abscess thoroughly. Plan to defunction the bowel at the site of the leak and aspirate the contents. Decide how best to feed the patient by intravenous catheter, by distal enteral feeding, or by a combination of both.

In a desperately ill patient with intra-abdominal sepsis it is sometimes justifiable to leave the abdomen open, packing it with sterile gauze packs that are changed regularly, allowing a free discharge of pus, planning to close the abdomen when the sepsis is overcome. I (RMK) have occasionally opened the whole wound in the ward, with or without local anaesthesia, to allow pus to discharge freely in this manner.

In some cases pus can be localized accurately clinically or by the various scanning aids, and can be drained directly by surgical means. There is some controversy at present about the place of surgical versus percutaneous drainage of intra-abdominal abscesses. These should be explored surgically if there is evidence of multiple abscesses, as occurs when there has been generalized sepsis, or if the patient remains toxic, suggesting that the cause, such as a leak, is still present, if the pus has solid material within it as demonstrated on the scan, or if percutaneous aspiration or catheterization has failed. I ask the radiologist to insert a large needle to aspirate a solitary static abscess in a reasonably fit patient, provided the contents are sufficiently fluid, and to repeat this if necessary, or to insert a pigtailed catheter.

Indications for percutaneous drainage
Single abscess on scan
Fluid contents
Cause apparently ceased to act
Patient not deteriorating
Drainage successful

Rapid deterioration in the patient's nutritional state demands urgent action and close monitoring. Many septic patients are intolerant of glucose and exogenous insulin may not correct this. Equally, the patient may not tolerate triglycerides or many of the standard amino acid preparations. Only vigorous control of sepsis restores the metabolic activity to normal.

Obstruction

Causes   Whenever the bowel is opened and repaired or anastomosed the repair or anastomosis may be the subsequent site of obstruction. Initially inversion of the edges may be too great, or subsequent oedema or submucosal haematoma can temporarily obstruct the lumen (Fig. 2.22). An obstructing tumour may have been missed or incompletely removed. The stoma may have been fashioned too small. Occasionally the lumen is inadvertently closed with stitches. Later, obstruction develops if the mucosal edges are not apposed, or following stitch ulceration of non-absorbable suture material eroding through the mucosa or the recurrence or failure to heal of a peptic ulcer: wound contracture narrows the lumen. A tumour may recur, producing obstruction and failure to heal, or there may be recurrence of ulceration, producing stenosis from contraction.

External pressure develops following leakage, abscess formation and compression from too tightly sutured passages through the mesenteries or the diaphragm (Fig. 2.23). Following any operation fibrinous adhesions may form between bowel loops or between the bowel and the parietes. The fibrin may later become organized to fibrous tissue. Talc or starch powder from the

Figure 2.22
Obstruction at an
anastomosis from
excessive
invagination and
oedema.

Oedema

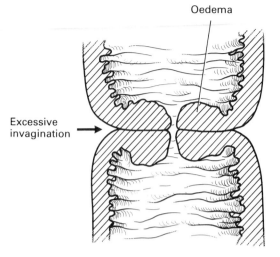

Excessive
invagination

Figure 2.23
Bowel obstructed at
diaphragm or
mesentery.

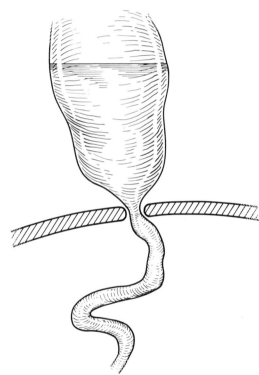

operator's gloves may produce granulomata and adhesions. At any stage adhesions can obstruct the bowel. Bowel may herniate through internal gaps from imperfectly closed holes or tears in completely sutured gaps (Fig. 2.24), or externally into wound gaps or hernial rings.

Figure 2.24
Bowel herniating
through diaphragm or
hole in mesentery.

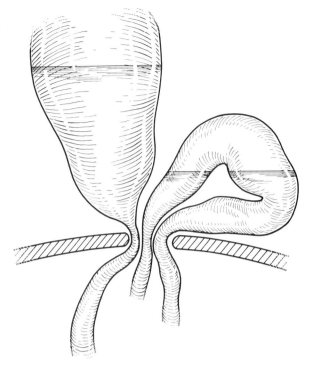

The bowel undergoes volvulus or kinking spontaneously or as a result of adhesions. It may develop intussusception from undiscovered or imperfectly removed polyps, oedematous or prolapsed mucosa. Following operations in which the metering action of the pylorus is destroyed or bypassed, large food boluses may pass into the small bowel and cause obstruction in the narrower terminal ileum.

Adynamic ileus normally follows the handling at operation. Continuing paralysis results if the bowel is in contact with leaked content or pus, or from general conditions such as uraemia or electrolyte imbalance. Vagotomy produces an adynamic state in a minority of patients. Acute gastric dilatation is a form of paralytic ileus, usually from unknown cause. It is of paramount importance that unrelieved obstruction passes imperceptibly into paralysis.

Mechanical obstruction of the bowel lumen may obstruct blood vessels, often the veins first and subsequently the arteries. The blood supply may be prejudiced at operation. Thrombosis can develop spontaneously in mesenteric blood vessels or spread from ligated blood vessels. The bowel becomes adynamic before turning gangrenous.

Prevention Even with the greatest care it is not possible to absolutely ensure against postoperative obstruction. Always carefully wash glove powder from gloves before opening the chest or abdomen. Certain principles must be observed at all times when mobilizing, resecting, suturing and anastomosing bowel in the upper gastrointestinal tract. The mobilization must be gentle, the blood supply must be preserved with the greatest care, tension must be avoided. If an anastomosis is performed, the holes should be matched carefully. Whatever method of suturing is used it should be meticulously performed, including an all-coats stitch. Whenever bowel passes through mesenteries or the diaphragm, ensure that the hole is either left wide open or carefully closed without tension.

At the end of the operation always thoroughly check all places where the bowel has been opened and repaired. Occasionally a surgeon inadvertently sutures an anastomosis so that the lumen is blocked. Ensure that the bowel wall can be invaginated on a finger through the anastomosis (Fig. 2.25)—and ask your assistant to check.

Features
Early obstruction is usually signalled by the aspiration of large volumes of fluid if there is a nasogastric tube in place. In the absence of a tube, vomiting occurs early in upper gastrointestinal tract obstruction. The vomitus contains bile if the obstruction is below the ampulla of Vater, although bile may reflux through a partial obstruction. Whenever bile stagnates organisms flourish in it so that it appears and smells faeculent: this is often mistakenly considered to represent low bowel obstruction.

Colic may be missed because of the background of wound pain and can soon disappear as paralytic ileus supervenes. Distension develops unless nasogastric aspiration is carried out. Neither flatus nor faeces are passed per anus. In partial obstruction, however, watery diarrhoea may occur. The pulse rate rises.

Figure 2.25
Test the patency of the anastomosis.

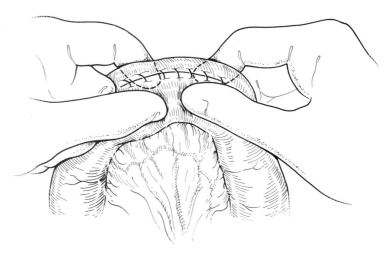

Tenderness is sometimes elicited over the site of the obstruction, but may be disguised by wound tenderness.

It is not possible to distinguish strangulation from postoperative simple obstruction with any confidence, but the patient becomes toxic and confused, with a rapidly rising pulse rate, falling blood pressure and eventual collapse.

Paralytic ileus presents no features initially, but the expected bowel sounds are delayed and nasogastric tube aspirate remains high. Abdominal distension develops. If there is a localized cause, then tenderness may be elicited.

Investigations   Obstruction within reach of the endoscope can be studied after passing a tube to aspirate the contents. In some cases the obstruction can be relieved by endoscopic techniques. Plain X-

Figure 2.26
Plain erect X-ray
showing small bowel
fluid levels.

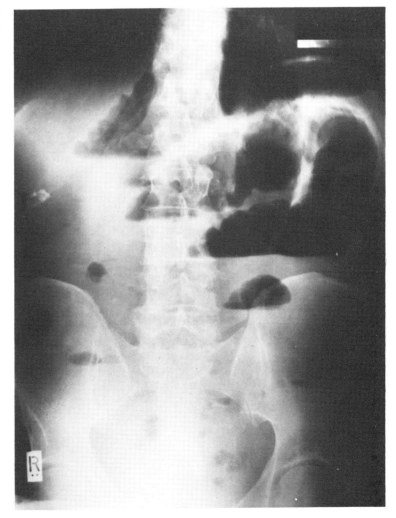

rays of the abdomen with the patient in erect and supine positions provide much information (Fig. 2.26). Gastric dilatation with a fluid level can be distinguished if there is a pyloroduodenal obstruction. Small bowel dilatation produces not only fluid levels but the ladder pattern so typical of small bowel, while large bowel dilatation produces haustrations.

Other investigations may suggest the cause of the dilatation; for example, if there is any inflammation, the white cell count is usually raised and a leak should be sought using water soluble radio-opaque medium and screening the patient. Carefully exclude uraemia and electrolyte disturbances by ordering blood analysis.

Management   Perhaps in no other complication is the aphorism 'Look and see, not wait and see', so appropriate. Since it is so difficult to distinguish postoperative simple obstruction from strangulation or ileus caused by a complication, the only safe course when in doubt is to re-explore the operation area.

It is of primary importance to restore the fluid, electrolyte and acid–base balance of the blood. As soon as the patient's condition is stabilized, proceed to operation. Simple adhesive obstruction can be freed. Decompress grossly distended bowel using a sucker tube (Fig. 2.27). If the bowel cannot be freed without transecting

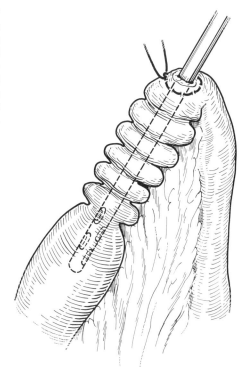

Figure 2.27
A sucker tube is inserted through a stab wound and secured by a purse-string suture. The bowel is drawn like a concertina over the sucker.

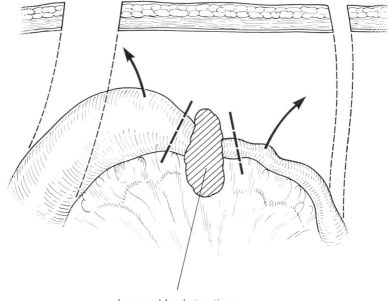

Figure 2.28
After transecting the obstructed bowel bring both ends to the surface.

Immovable obstruction

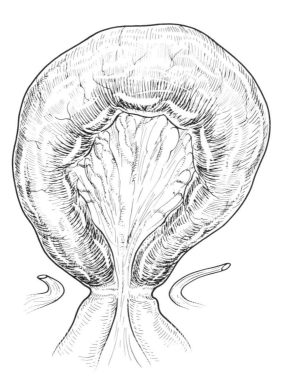

Figure 2.29
The congested plum-coloured loop may often be confidently pronounced viable. It is the white constriction ring that should in such cases be critically inspected.

it, the simplest and safest technique may be to bring the two ends to the surface for future repair (Fig. 2.28). If gangrenous bowel is found, excise it, again preferably bringing the two cut ends to the surface. Always check the trapped segments of strangulated bowel (Fig. 2.29).

No cause may be found for adynamic ileus, but this is no detriment to the patient who can now be confidently treated expectantly, since general causes have already been excluded. On the other hand, if a cause is found and corrected, recovery will soon follow.

Since enteral feeding has been delayed and will be further postponed, arrange for parenteral feeding. In some cases enteral feeding is still possible distal to the site of obstruction.

Early Complications Following Upper Gastrointestinal Surgery

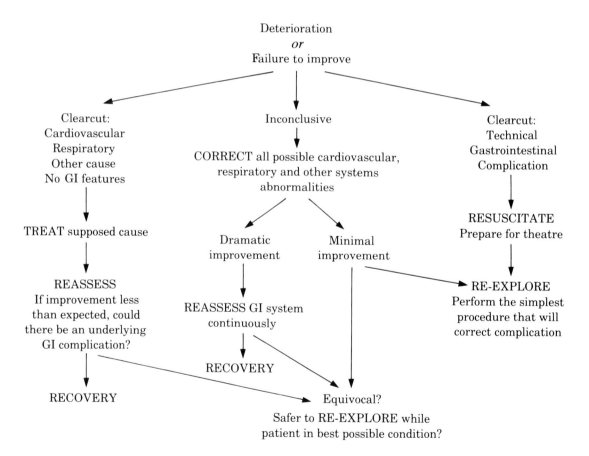

It is better to look and see than to wait and see.

Late Complications

The condition for which the operation was originally performed, such as ulceration or neoplasia, may recur. If the bowel has been operated upon, stricture formation may develop or adhesions and bands may provoke mechanical obstruction. Following some operations, such as those for peptic ulcer, well-recognized late sequelae may develop from the mechanical and functional effects of the operation.

Persisting Controversies

- Influence of sutured versus stapled anastomoses in various sites to prevent leakage.
- Value of single dose versus short or long course of antibiotic prophylaxis against infection.
- Value of drainage in general and type of drain in particular to prevent fluid collections or signal their presence.
- Role of percutaneous as opposed to open drainage of abscesses.

Further reading

Glass, C.A. & Cohn, L., Jr (1984) Drainage of intra-abdominal abscesses. A comparison of surgical and computerized tomography guided catheter drainage. *American Journal of Surgery*, *147*, 315–317.

Duff, J.H. & Mofat, J. (1981) Abdominal sepsis managed by leaving the abdomen open. *Surgery*, *90*, 774–778.

Gerzoe, S.G., Robbins, A.H., Johnson, W.C., Birkett, D.H. & Nabseth, D.C. (1981) Percutaneous catheter drainage of abdominal abscesses. *New England Journal of Medicine*, *305*, 653–657.

Glick, P.L., Pellegrini, C.A., Stein, S. & Way, L.W. (1983) Abdominal abscess. A surgical strategy. *Archives of Surgery*, *118*, 646–650.

Greenall, M.J., Atkinson, J.E., Evans, M. & Pollock, A.V. (1981) Single-dose antibiotic prophylaxis of surgical wound sepsis: which route of administration is best? *Journal of Antimicrobial Chemotherapy*, *7*, 223–227.

Kirk, R.M. (1978) *Basic Surgical Techniques*, 2nd Edn. Edinburgh: Churchill Livingstone.

Kirk, R.M. & Williamson, R.C.N. (1986) *General Surgical Operations*, 2nd Edn. Edinburgh: Churchill Livingstone.

Segal, A.W., Arnot, R.N., Thakur, M.L. & Lavender, J.P. (1976) Indium-111-labelled leukocytes for localization of abscesses. *Lancet*, *i*, 1056–1058.

Stephen, M. & Loewenthal, J. (1979) Continuing peritoneal lavage in high risk peritonitis. *Surgery*, *85*, 603–606.

Stone, H.H., Haney, B.B., Kolb, L.D., Geheber, C.E. & Hooper, C.A. (1979) Prophylactic and preventive antibiotic therapy. Timing, duration and economics. *Annals of Surgery*, *189*, 691–699.

Stone, H.H., Strom, P.R. & Mullins, R.J. (1983) Management of the major coagulopathy with onset during laparotomy. *Annals of Surgery*, *197*, 532–535.

3 Chest Complications

Causes   Many patients with oesophageal disease already have respiratory problems. In addition, oesophageal obstruction causes 'spillover' with aspiration pneumonia and eventual pulmonary fibrosis. Upper abdominal and oesophageal operations or endoscopic procedures are particularly likely to result in chest complications. Premedication reduces bronchial secretions but makes them viscous and difficult to clear. Surgery produces pain in the respiratory muscles of the chest, diaphragm and upper abdomen, reducing respiratory function. Most systemic analgesics depress respiration. The presence of a nasogastric tube makes coughing difficult. A thoracic or thoracoabdominal operation may be followed by pneumothorax, pleural effusion or both (see *Complications of Cardiopulmonary Surgery*).

Following endoscopy and instrumentation, aspiration may occur, especially if there is any mechanical or functional hold up in swallowing.

Assessment   Before operation check the patient's colour, the respiratory movements and the clinical signs in the chest at rest and following exercise. Sputum should be cultured and an appropriate antibiotic selected if necessary. Respiratory function tests are indicated for patients about to be submitted to major oesophageal or gastric resections if they already have impaired function. Order chest X-ray and measure vital capacity, peak expiratory flow and forced expiratory volume.

Smokers should stop. Breathing exercises can be taught by physiotherapists. Existing infections are improved using antibiotics and bronchospasm relaxants.

When carrying out endoscopy the minimum sedation should be used. If a painful manoeuvre must be carried out, it is safer to do it under a properly conducted general anaesthetic than in an oversedated patient. Following upper gastrointestinal endoscopy make sure that the patient lies on his side, without a pillow, face turned towards the mattress, under constant observation. As soon as he recovers he should sit up and be encouraged to breathe deeply and cough.

Following upper gastrointestinal surgery the anaesthetist ensures that the bronchi are carefully aspirated. Following major resections and especially after transthoracic oesophageal surgery it is customary in most units to ventilate the patient overnight in the intensive care ward. This provides the opportunity to stabilize fluid balance, since overloading with fluid produces pulmonary oedema. Before the cuffed endotracheal tube is removed, the bronchi are thoroughly aspirated and as soon as the patient recovers from sedation he is given analgesics, followed by active physiotherapy.

If there has been an anastomosis to the oesophagus or if there is any oesophageal obstruction, sit the patient up as soon as possible to avoid aspiration into the trachea, which can occur even when a cuffed endotracheal tube is in place. Remove the nasogastric tube as soon as possible because it makes coughing difficult. Sometimes an alternative method of draining the upper gastrointestinal tract, such as pharyngostomy or gastrostomy, is possible to avoid the presence of a nasal tube. It is important to decompress the bowel or aspiration is likely to occur and any abdominal distension pushes up the diaphragm and restricts respiratory movement.

All surgical patients are at risk from deep venous thrombosis and possible pulmonary embolism (see *Complications of Surgery in General*). In particular those who have had previous episodes following surgery for thrombosis or embolism, those having major operations for cancer, and elderly patients should be given prophylactic low-dose heparin over the operative period. Before elective operations, women taking the contraceptive pill, or oestrogens for menopausal symptoms, should stop treatment for at least one month before, and in an emergency they should be given low-dose heparin subcutaneously.

The special problems of throracoabdominal and transthoracic procedures are discussed in Chapter 5.

Atelectasis and Collapse

This is the most frequent complication, from bronchial obstruction followed by absorption of the air distal to the block. The collapsed lung is liable to infection. If collapse is massive, blood passing through it fails to be oxygenated, so the patient becomes anoxic.

Features   There are three cardinal signs, even before the patient is seen:

1 Pulse rate
2 Temperature
3 Respiratory rate

All of these rise simultaneously.

Movement of the chest on the affected side is reduced, there is a dull percussion note, with reduced breath sounds. The trachea and apex beat are displaced towards the affected side only if the collapse is considerable, and the patient may then appear distressed.

Investigations   Chest X-ray shows the opaque collapsed lung (Fig. 3.1), to be distinguished from embolic opacification and pleural fluid—which often coexists. Order a lateral view to determine the exact

Figure 3.1
Left basal collapse

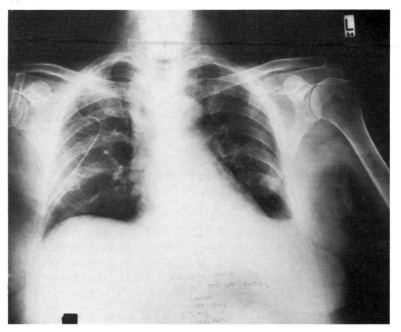

site. Send sputum for culture. If the collapse is extensive and the patient shows respiratory distress, check the blood gases.

Management Vigorous treatment with analgesics followed by physiotherapy, mucolytics and antibiotics usually clear the mucus plug responsible for the collapse. If these measures fail, carry out bronchoscopy to aspirate the blocked secretions. The fibreoptic instrument, passed under local anaesthesia, may not have adequate suction facilities and the passage of a rigid instrument in the unanaesthetized patient requires expertise. Intubation, or tracheostomy, allows the passage of catheters and 'bagging'— inflation by compressing an anaesthetic bag attached to the endotracheal tube.

Once the condition is corrected do not let it recur. Although the patient is exhausted by the necessary procedures, it is important not to lose valuable ground, so continue vigorous physiotherapy.

Pleural Effusion

Following transthoracic oesophageal operations, and upper abdominal surgery, fluid collects in the costophrenic angle. It may be simple reaction fluid, but if oesophageal perforation or leakage occurs, then gastrointestinal fluid collects, although air usually leaks as well, forming a hydropneumothorax. The underlying lung collapses.

Features The fluid is dull to percussion and breath sounds are reduced. Chest X-ray (Fig. 3.2) reveals a shadow in the costophrenic angle, appearing to rise towards the axilla. It may be difficult even on lateral films to determine if the diaphragm is raised, perhaps above an intra-abdominal collection or a distended abdomen.

Management Aspirate a sample of fluid using a size 1 needle attached to a 20 ml syringe, inserted through a bleb of local anaesthetic, passing the needle just above a rib in the posterior axillary line. Send a specimen for culture. If the collection is considerable, aspirate it after attaching a three-way tap between needle and syringe.

Institute physiotherapy to allow the collapsed lung to re-expand. If the fluid recollects, insert an underwater sealed drain (see p. 59).

If this is a gastrointestinal leak urgent surgical treatment is required. When the diaphragm is raised, investigate the possibility of an intra-abdominal complication with subdiaphragmatic irritation.

Figure 3.2
Left pleural effusion

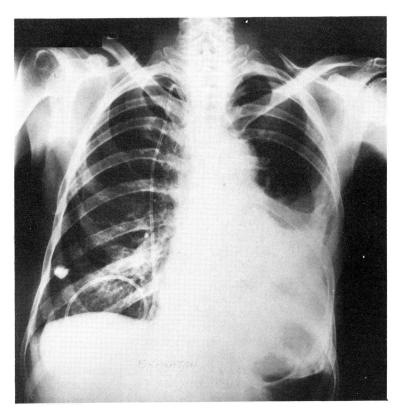

Pneumothorax

<table>
<tr>
<td>Causes and
prevention</td>
<td>This can occur following perforation of the oesophagus and pleura during endoscopic procedures, especially when air is insufflated through a fibreoptic instrument.</td>
</tr>
</table>

Causes and prevention

This can occur following perforation of the oesophagus and pleura during endoscopic procedures, especially when air is insufflated through a fibreoptic instrument.

Following upper abdominal surgery around the hiatus it is possible to perforate the pleura inadvertently. Pneumothorax most frequently follows thoracic, abdominothoracic or cervicothoracic procedures. The pleura may be inadvertently breached when attempting extrapleural procedures.

During transpleural surgery the opposite pleura may be breached without it being noticed or the lung can be damaged and leak subsequently. Pleural drains must be inserted correctly so that there are no holes near the surface and fixed securely so that they cannot be accidentally pulled out (see p. 59).

When in doubt always have a chest X-ray before moving the patient from the operating table.

Features

The patient's respiratory rate rises and he may become distressed. If there is tension, the mediastinum and hence the trachea are pushed to the opposite side. The chest is hyperresonant and breath sounds are absent. Chest X-ray shows a cavity with no lung markings, but the edge of the collapsed lung can usually be seen (Fig. 3.3). If fluid is present, it forms a horizontal level (Fig. 3.4).

Management

Without delay, using local anaesthesia, insert a chest drain anteriorly in the mid-clavicular line above the third rib, using a trocar point. In females the mid-axillary line may be preferred. Connect the tube to an underwater sealed drain and fix the tube firmly with stitches. Air will bubble out. Confirm the reexpansion with X-rays and institute chest physiotherapy.

Empyema

Infection within the pleural cavity following surgery on the upper gastrointestinal tract is most frequently the result of leakage (Fig. 3.5). The patient is usually ill and air is often present in the pleural cavity. Aspiration often reveals bile-stained fluid. If this follows a missed perforation at endoscopy, there may be a collection of saliva. Send this fluid for culture but institute systemic antibiotic treatment against gastrointestinal organisms.

Resuscitate the patient, explore the chest, deal with the cause, then thoroughly drain the chest using underwater sealed drains (see p. 59).

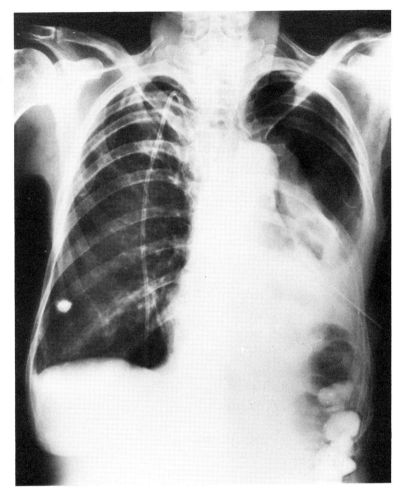

Figure 3.3
Left pneumothorax.
The collapsed lung
can be seen next to
the cardiac shadow.
Note the absence of
lung markings on the
left periphery.

Acute Respiratory Insufficiency

Causes   Respiratory insufficiency may develop from a number of causes. There may be pre-existing disease, the effects of aspiration, sepsis, postoperative pulmonary collapse, consolidation (Fig. 3.6), effusion and empyema, overloading with fluid, and left ventricular failure, all of which prejudice pulmonary function.

Management   In a weak, and sometimes septic, patient there is insufficient reserve and unless the causes are corrected he will succumb. The degree of failure is reflected by blood gases showing oxygen below 10 kPa and carbon dioxide above 7 kPa. The advice and help of the Intensive Therapy team is essential. Intubation, sedation and ventilation are usually necessary. It is important to correct blood urea, electrolyte and acid/base balance. Anti-

Figure 3.4
Left
hydropneumothorax.
The apex of the left
chest shows no lung
markings. There is a
horizontal fluid level.
The gas shadows in
the left chest are from
bowel taken up for
anastomosis.

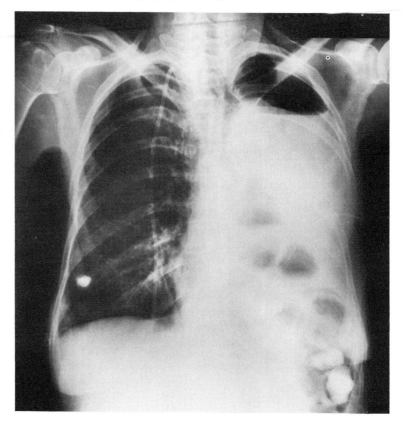

biotics may be required, together with nutritional replacement and if necessary, blood, plasma proteins, vitamins and trace elements.

Complications of Thoracotomy

Pulmonary complications

Whenever the chest is opened, and especially if the lung is collapsed during operation, it may not re-expand. Collapse (see p. 51) is better prevented than corrected. This starts with the anaesthetist ensuring at the end of the operation that the lung is aerated and the bronchi patent by sucking out the retained mucus. The surgeon checks the lung carefully to exclude any surface damage that might allow leakage, inserting fine catgut stitches to repair the lung. He carefully checks that as the anaesthetist reinflates the lung, no fresh leaks develop.

An important surgical contribution is the insertion of chest drains (see p. 59), followed by secure closing of the chest.

A chest X-ray is taken as soon after an operation as possible to check that the lung is fully expanded without collapse, consolida-

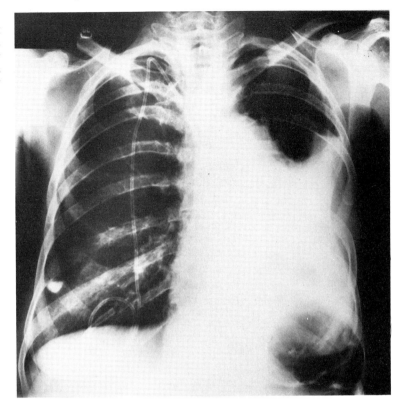

Figure 3.5 Empyema. The left lower chest is opaque. Initially aspirated fluid was clear; it is now purulent.

tion, widening of the mediastinum, air emphysema, pleural effusion or pneumothorax.

It is now common practice to maintain the patient on assisted ventilation overnight following transthoracic oesophageal operations, but it is important to ensure that the lung remains fully expanded. The bronchi are regularly aspirated through the cuffed endotracheal tube. As soon as the tube is removed and the sedation reduced the patient should be given intensive physiotherapy to actively clear the bronchi. Chest X-rays are taken as often as necessary to elucidate any clinical changes and in addition blood gases can be checked. Send sputum for culture and to determine antibiotic sensitivities. If liquid or air re-accumulates in the pleural cavity, aspirate it and be willing to insert further underwater sealed drains if it persists.

If the patient cannot cough the bronchi clear, and collapse develops, bronchoscopy should be carried out without delay. A skilled operator can pass a rigid bronchoscope using minimal sedation and aspirate the sticky mucus. It is possible to pass a fibreoptic bronchoscope with ease, but its suction capability is limited.

Inevitably some fluid forms in the pleural cavity and it is wise to aspirate this with a simple syringe, needle and three-way tap.

Figure 3.6
Combination of
consolidation with
collapse. The collapse
can be deduced
because the tracheal
shadow is drawn to
the patient's left side.

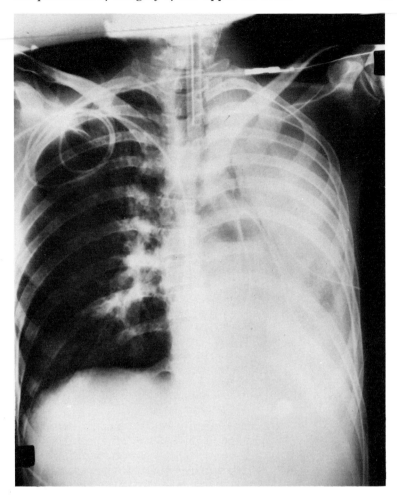

If collapse is allowed to persist, patchy bronchopneumonia develops, becoming confluent. The pneumonia will not usually clear up until the bronchus is unblocked by physiotherapy or suction. Give a systemic versatile antibiotic such as ampicillin while awaiting sputum culture and sensitivity determinations.

Preventing collapse
Underwater sealed drains
Aspiration of secretions
Physiotherapy
Bronchoscopy
Chest aspiration

Aspiration pneumonia
A serious problem following oesophagectomy with oesophago-gastric or oesophagoenteric anastomosis is regurgitation of gastric or intestinal fluid into the oesophagus and then into the trachea. This occurs even in the presence of a cuffed endotracheal tube and regurgitated acid gastric contents provoke severe bronchospasm. For this reason, if for no other, it is valuable to keep a nasogastric or nasoenteric tube in place and regularly aspirated to prevent reflux, particularly if the patient must lay flat or even head down. As soon as he is able to sit and lie more upright, the tube can be removed if its presence makes coughing difficult.

Mediastinitis
Leakage rather than contamination at operation is the usual cause of mediastinitis. Following thoracotomy and incision of the mediastinal pleura, the patient may develop a pleural effusion. If the mediastinal pleura has resealed, or has not been breached, as following oesophagectomy without thoracotomy, then air and fluid remain in the mediastinum and set up an intense cellulitis which may progress to an abscess which remains here or bursts into the pleural cavity.

The classic presentation of severe substernal pain, worse on swallowing, is absent following surgery. The patient is toxic, with tachycardia and pyrexia, but may have no localizing features. X-rays show pneumomediastinum and increased width if the pleura remains intact or has resealed but otherwise may show only pleural effusion or hydropneumothorax.

The patient should be urgently resuscitated and returned to the operating theatre to deal with the leakage (see p. 101).

Chylothorax
The thoracic duct may be damaged during radical surgery of the oesophagus, especially from the right side in the upper chest. It lies between the aorta, on its left, and the azygos vein, on its right, on the anterior vertebral ligament. At the fifth thoracic vertebra it veers to the left to lie on the left side of the oesophagus.

Chyle drains from the chest drain or is aspirated from the chest when an effusion is tapped. Unless it rapidly stops draining, re-explore the lower right chest, identify and ligate the duct.

Chest Drains

Whenever the chest is opened at least insert a basal drain and if an intrathoracic procedure has been carried out that could result in pulmonary collapse or the collection of fluid in the pleural cavity, preferably insert basal and apical drains. If the chest is not opened, try to have a chest X-ray available to see the diaphragmatic height. Basal drains are usually inserted in the posterior axillary line, apical drains through the anterior chest wall in the mid-clavicular line above the third or fourth rib. Insert a 20–24 F drain just above a rib under fully sterile conditions.

If the patient is not anaesthetized, raise a bleb of local anaesthetic in the skin just above a rib, and infiltrate through the chest wall to the pleura with local anaesthetic. Make a skin incision through the bleb. Insert the drain, mounted on a trocar, holding them firmly half a centimetre from the skin, while pushing, until the gripping fingers meet the chest wall. Take a second grip half a centimetre from the skin and repeat the manoeuvre until the slight 'give' is felt, indicating that the tip is in the pleural cavity, confirmed by the fact that the drain can be advanced into the chest while holding the trocar still. Withdraw the trocar slightly and advance the tube to make sure the end is well within the pleural cavity and the side holes are not near the chest wall. Insert a skin stitch, tie it loosely, then take a number of turns around the tube and knot the ligature securely.

Pinch off the tube while withdrawing the trocar and then connect it to an underwater seal (Fig. 3.7). The bottle stands on the floor and the fluid in the bottom exerts a negative pressure. If the tube becomes blocked, air or liquids can collect in the pleural cavity and the lung collapses. If the tube slips, a hole may lie in the chest wall and produce air emphysema. If the hole slips outside the chest, air leaks in and allows the lung to collapse.

An incorrectly sited or clumsily inserted drain may injure subdiaphragmatic viscera, the lungs, heart or great vessels. If placed closely beneath a rib, it may traumatize the intercostal vessels and cause bleeding, or damage the nerve. If any injury is suspected, order an X-ray and be prepared to explore the track of the drain.

Diaphragmatic Dehiscence

This is a rare complication of thoracoabdominal surgery. Abdominal distension places a great strain on the diaphragmatic repair and occasionally it gives way. The abdominal contents herniate into the chest, resulting in pulmonary collapse, and mediastinal shift to the opposite side, with cardiorespiratory distress.

The best safeguard against diaphragmatic rupture is to carefully insert horizontal mattress sutures of non-absorbable material (Fig. 3.8) and avoid distension within the abdomen after operation. Provide effective regular nasogastric or nasoenteric aspiration. Gross distension suggests obstruction or adynamic ileus and in each case operative intervention is urgently required to relieve the cause.

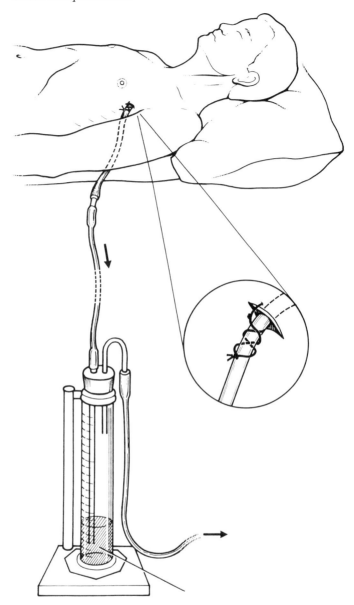

Figure 3.7
Underwater sealed
chest drain.

Chest Wall Disruption

Fortunately this is a rare complication of thoracotomy. Especially if there is infection or leakage in a previously malnourished patient, healing is prejudiced. When closing the chest, catgut sutures are no longer relied upon. There are two methods of opening the chest, each requiring careful closure.

Figure 3.8
Horizontal mattress
suture used for
repairing diaphragm.

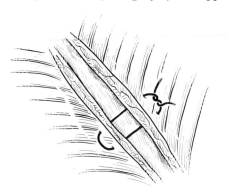

In a young patient with reasonably flexible ribs, sufficient exposure is possible without excising a rib. Incise the periosteum between the upper and lower borders and strip the upper half from the rib (Fig. 3.9). Open the chest through the posterior layer of periosteum. If necessary a small segment of rib can be removed posteriorly. When closing this wound, use a rib approximator or insert two pericostal stitches of strong non-absorbable material just above the next higher rib and through a hole made with an awl midway between the upper and lower edges of the lower rib to avoid damage to the neurovascular bundle. Pass both stitches, then tie them just tight enough to allow unabsorbable stitches to be inserted between the periosteum of the upper cut edge and the intercostal muscles and periosteum at the lower edge of the rib (Fig. 3.10).

The ribs of elderly patients are often rigid and fragile, so it may be best to remove a rib by incising the periosteum over it midway between its upper and lower borders. Strip the periosteum from the rib along its length using Price Thomas' and Doyen's rib strippers. Cut through the rib anteriorly and posteriorly and remove it. Open the chest through the middle of the exposed inner periosteum. When the chest is closed, there is strong periosteum above and below which holds stitches well (Fig. 3.10).

If dehiscence does occur, it is obvious. The lung may not collapse if it has adhered to the wound. An underlying cause may be overlooked. If there is a gush of fluid from the wound, could it represent a leak? Examine the last chest X-ray and if possible obtain another for comparison.

Return the patient to theatre and under general anaesthesia, with a cuffed endotracheal tube in place, re-explore the wound. If there is any possibility of a complication such as a leak, re-explore the chest. Assuming that there is no visceral complication, insert pericostal stitches of strong non-absorbable material and re-repair the chest wall.

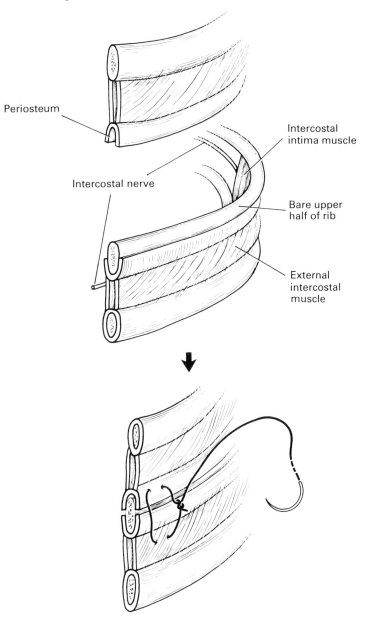

Figure 3.9
The chest has been opened without removing a rib. The upper half of the rib periosteum is stripped and the incision is made through it. The wound is closed using horizontal mattress sutures inserted into the periosteum above and the fibrous origin of the external intercostal muscles below.

Periosteum

Intercostal nerve

Intercostal intima muscle

Bare upper half of rib

External intercostal muscle

Chest Wall Pain

Thoracotomy entails injury to the respiratory muscles and the possibility of injury to the intercostal nerves, producing immediate postoperative pain. This prejudices postoperative breathing and coughing, increasing the risk of pulmonary collapse and

Figure 3.10
Closing the chest wall
after excising the rib.
The sutures pick up
the periosteum on
each side.

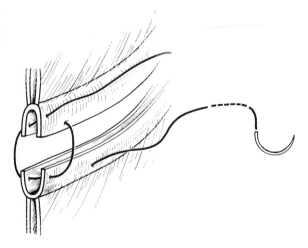

consequent infection. Subsequently the patient may develop chronic pain related to the wound, presumably from involvement of the nerve in scar tissue.

The surgeon may reduce the likelihood of pain by dissecting out and transecting the nerve at the neck of the rib at the level of the thoracotomy. The nerves above and below may be divided or blocked by injecting long-acting local anaesthetic, such as bupivacaine 0.5%, or better, 6% aqueous phenol solution. It is possible to block the nerves with a cryosurgical appliance if this is available. Epidural anaesthesia reduces postoperative pain.

When inserting pericostal stitches it is important to avoid including the intercostal nerves.

If pain continues chronically, inject bupivacaine just below the neck of the rib, and if this relieves the pain, inject 6% aqueous phenol solution to permanently block the intercostal nerve.

Persisting Controversies

- Necessity of inserting an underwater sealed drain after exploration of the chest in the absence of any intrathoracic procedure.
- Value of tracheostomy, as opposed to soft-cuffed endotracheal tubes, in postoperative chest complications.

Further reading
Campbell, D. & Spence, A.A. (1978) *Norris and Campbell's Anaesthetics, Resuscitation and Intensive Care*, 5th Edn. Edinburgh: Churchill Livingstone.
Simon, G. (1978) *Principles of Chest X-ray Diagnosis*, 4th Edn. London: Butterworth.
Smith, G.H. (1984) *Complications of Cardiopulmonary Surgery*. London: Baillière Tindall.
Webb, W.R. & Moulder P.V. (1981) Postoperative pulmonary complications. In: Hardy, H.J. (Ed.) *Complications in Surgery and their Management*, 4th Edn. London: W.B. Saunders.

4 Oesophagus— Endoscopic Procedures

Instruments

Whenever possible prefer to use the flexible rather than the rigid endoscope, especially if you are inexperienced. For the same reason, remember that a sedated patient can respond if you injure him but a fully anaesthetized patient can not.

The modern flexible, end-viewing fibreoptic endoscope is extremely versatile. Brushings can be taken for cytology. It does have some limitations, however. The biopsy forceps bite only ahead (Fig. 4.1) and not to the side, so it is difficult or impossible to obtain a biopsy specimen from within a stricture. Brock's side-biting forceps (Fig. 4.2), on the other hand, are excellent for obtaining specimens from within a stricture through a rigid instrument. In addition these forceps can obtain a deeper bite, which sometimes reveals pathological changes not visible on the small superficial specimens obtained through a flexible instrument. The rigid instrument is valuable for dilatating strictures when a guide-wire cannot be passed beyond the stricture (Fig. 4.3). Graded sizes of gum elastic bougies can be passed under vision into the stricture, often revealing the obstruction or angulation beyond (Fig. 4.4). Finally, the rigid instrument is invaluable for removing some foreign bodies, since the grasping forceps can be controlled easily. A sharp foreign body can often be withdrawn within the instrument for safe removal (Fig. 4.5).

Rigid instrument only for:
Biopsies within a stricture
Deep biopsies
Dilatating difficult strictures
Removing sharp foreign bodies

Bleeding

Predisposing causes   The mucosa of the oesophagus is fragile but does not bleed excessively when traumatized and considerable bleeding follow-

Figure 4.1
Flexible end-biting
biopsy forceps.

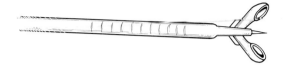

Figure 4.2
Brock's rigid side-
biting biopsy forceps.

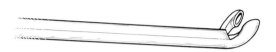

Figure 4.3
Eder–Puestow flexible
guide-wire cannot be
manoeuvred through
an irregular angulated
stricture.

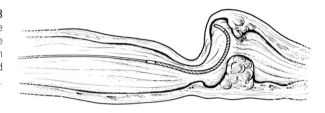

Figure 4.4
Dilatation of proximal
part of an irregular
stricture with bougies
under direct vision
through a rigid
endoscope allows the
distal track to be
identified.

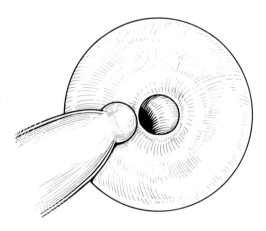

Figure 4.5
Sharp foreign body
drawn into a rigid
oesophagoscope for
safe removal.

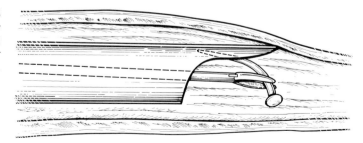

ing endoscopy suggests a lesion such as varices or an ulcer eroding large blood vessels. Occasionally an aortic aneurysm ruptures into the oesophagus during or following endoscopy or an oesophageal tumour invades the aorta. Sometimes a vascular polyp bleeds following biopsy or attempted removal. Infrequently severe oesophagitis produces bleeding after traumatization. Bleeding infrequently follows perforation or splitting of the oesophagus during instrumentation or intubation.

Prevention   Be cautious in carrying out instrumental procedures in the presence of varices or other vascular lesions. Make sure that every manoeuvre possible is carried out under vision, or if this is not possible, inspect the area immediately afterwards. Examine the whole gastrointestinal tract visible through the endoscope to exclude other possible sources of bleeding.

Recognition   A danger of unrecognized bleeding in a heavily sedated or unconscious patient is that the blood may be inhaled and cause respiratory obstruction. Always aspirate all blood from the oesophagus as the endoscope is withdrawn and recheck if a source of bleeding is seen.

Following endoscopy the patient may vomit fresh or altered blood and may pass melaena, since blood in the bowel acts as a laxative.

Treatment   The management depends on the severity of the bleeding. An anaesthetized patient should lie on the one side, the pillow is removed, the bed is angled with 20° of Trendelenburg tilt and the face is turned towards the bed, so that any blood runs easily out of the mouth. The patient should not be given any further sedation, but should be reassured. As soon as he has fully recovered he should sit up so that any blood will be passed into the stomach.

Severe or continuing bleeding demands urgent arrangements to correct hypovolaemia with transfused crossmatched blood. Monitor the patient's blood pressure, pulse rate, respiration and general condition. As a rule the endoscopist will have recognized the lesion that produced the bleeding, but if not, stabilize the patient's condition as rapidly as possible and repeat the endoscopy with the patient sedated as little as possible. Use a fibreoptic endoscope with a large suction channel and have available a rigid oesophagoscope. Have an anaesthetist standing by who could anaesthetize the patient so the rigid endoscope can be passed. Aspirate the blood from within the oesophagus and identify the cause. If no cause is seen, the blood may be regurgitated from a missed source in the stomach or beyond, so examine the upper gastrointestinal tract to the limits of the instrument.

It may be possible to diathermize a vascular polyp or point source of bleeding using a flexible lead passed through the biopsy channel of a fibreoptic endoscope or a rigid lead passed through a rigid oesophagoscope. Argon laser-beam coagulation and the spraying of coagulation inducing substances are under trial. Using a rigid instrument it is possible to apply local pressure with a small swab dipped in 1:1000 adrenaline solution to localized lesions. It is rare for bleeding other than from varices to be uncontrollable by local treatment. Occasionally thoracotomy is necessary to discover and deal with a vessel bleeding into the oesophageal lumen. In such a case carefully note the level and side of the lesion (see p. 92).

If bleeding has recurred following injection of varices, a further injection, accompanied by pressure from the tip of a rigid oesophagoscope for five minutes may stop it (but see p. 170). Bleeding may be controlled by passing a Sengstaken tube into the stomach, inflating the gastric balloon and exerting traction on the tube. This technique can be combined with variceal injection. If this fails and general measures such as injection of vasopressin do not control the bleeding, other urgent methods of treatment, such as oesophageal transection and percutaneous transhepatic embolization of the varices, must be considered. Emergency portal-systemic shunt operations have not found favour in Britain but are used in some American centres.

Perforation

Sites A frequent site for perforation of the oesophagus is at the cricopharyngeal sphincter, where there is narrowing and where osteophytes may project forwards from cervical osteoarthritis and press against the tip of a rigid instrument. Another frequent site is at the oesophagogastric junction, where the oesophagus angles forward and to the left: this is also the site of the majority of oesophageal lesions. Perforation may occur at any site within the oesophagus, especially at or just above an obstruction (Fig. 4.6).

Upper thoracic perforations often extend into the right pleural cavity; perforations of the lower thoracic oesophagus frequently extend into the left pleural cavity. Lower oesophageal perforations may extend into the abdominal cavity.

Predisposing factors There is a greater risk of perforation when using the rigid as opposed to the flexible instrument. Although figures vary, a routine flexible endoscopy is about one-tenth as likely to result in perforation as rigid oesophagoscopy, in spite of the fact that the former is often performed by junior and inexperienced operators. The fact that the flexible instrument is slimmer and bends before an obstruction makes it safer. Of equal importance is that it can be passed under sedation rather than requiring an anaesthetic, and therefore the patient can complain if injury is caused. Perforation does not usually occur at an examination but when a manoeuvre is carried out such as the dilatation of a stricture

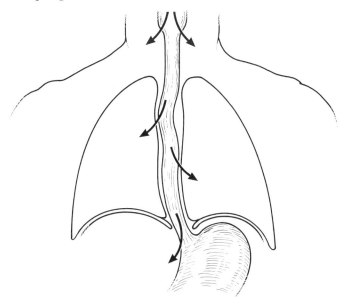

Figure 4.6
Instrumental
perforation of the
oesophagus.

(Fig. 4.7), the insertion by pulsation of a tube through a stricture, and the hydrostatic dilatation of an achalasic lower segment or stricture of oesophagus (Fig. 4.8). Foreign bodies often do not penetrate the oesophageal wall when they are swallowed, but they may do so during roughly performed endoscopic removal. The rigid instrument may be safer than the flexible instrument in this circumstance, because sharp objects can be withdrawn within the tube of the endoscope. Perforation is much more

Figure 4.7
Oesophageal
perforation during
dilatation for an
irregular stricture.

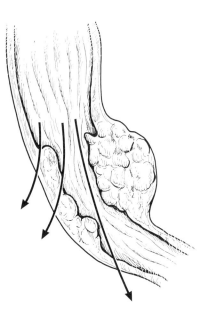

Figure 4.8
(a) An X-ray of a hydrostatic balloon distended within the oesophagus. (b) A subsequent X-ray showing radio-opaque medium leaking out of the oesophagus through a split.

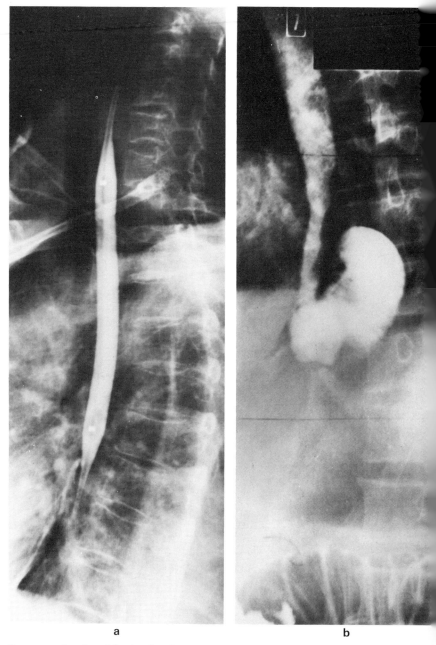

a   b

frequent in the elderly, in the presence of carcinoma, and when the operator is inexperienced.

Pathology The oesophageal wall is thin but flexible. The mucosa alone may be split, leaving the outer wall intact, or the split may extend through the full thickness of the wall. At the inlet the whole thickness of the wall may be crushed between a rigid instrument and the osteophytes of the cervical spine. Elsewhere it is usually diseased oesophagus that gives way during instrumentation, but the wall will rupture anywhere if the procedure is roughly performed. Leakage of oesophageal contents, including fluid refluxed from the stomach, produces an acute cellulitis. If the leak is into the cervical tissues, fluid may also track into the superior mediastinum. Leakage within the mediastinum produces a diffuse inflammation and air emphysema opens up the tissues, allowing leaked contents to track. If the mediastinal pleura is breached, fluid collects in the pleural cavity and a hydropneumothorax develops. Continuing leakage is inevitably followed by infection, initially as cellulitis, with subsequent necrosis and abscess formation. Mortality is related to the site and extent of the leak. It is usually low for minor perforations in the neck but may rise to 80% following thoracic perforations through the mediastinal pleura.

Prevention   Before carrying out a potentially difficult manoeuvre order radiological studies and carefully examine the films to determine the anatomy.

Whenever possible use the flexible rather than the rigid instrument. As a rule perforations occur not with simple endoscopic examinations but during such procedures as dilatation, intubation and the removal of foreign bodies or biopsy specimens. Be especially gentle when passing the cricopharyngeal sphincter.

Many dilatations are carried out using the Eder–Puestow flexible guide-wire and dilators, or Celestin's stepped dilators. Never use a kinked guide-wire, since the friction it produces reduces the 'feel' as the dilator passes over it. Although the guide-wire is passed under vision, the dilators are passed 'blind'. When pushing the dilators, ensure that they slide easily over the guide-wire lubricated with water-soluble jelly, and extend the neck at the atlanto-occipital joint to straighten the passage and thus give the greatest 'feel'. If an obstruction is met, stop pushing, withdraw the bougie slightly, and ensure that the guide-wire still slides freely within the bougie. If this manoeuvre is overlooked, the guide-wire may kink at the lower end of the bougie which then angles away from the line of the wire and can perforate the wall (Fig. 4.9). The same precaution must be taken when inserting a pulsion tube.

When passing a rigid endoscope, manoeuvre the patient so that the tip lies as far as possible in the centre of the lumen. Do not use leverage against the teeth or vertebral column. Pass bougies under vision. If a distal block is felt, do not persist but try a thinner flexible bougie or try feeling gently with closed alligator forceps. This sometimes clarifies the anatomical situation. If the forceps negotiate the stricture, gently open the blades while withdrawing the forceps, allowing the length, elasticity and surface to be assessed (Fig. 4.10).

Always try to inspect the oesophagus following any instrumentation. If a rigid oesophagoscope has been passed, it is usually easy to insert through it a paediatric flexible endoscope to see within and beyond a newly dilated stricture. It can also be passed through an oesophageal splinting tube inserted by pulsion, to ensure that it is properly sited and that there is no damage to the oesophageal or gastric walls.

Small oesophageal tears are often unrecognized, especially if there is a split in a dilated stricture through which the instrument cannot easily pass. If a tear is seen during examination, note its distance from the incisor teeth and carefully inspect it to estimate the amount of damage. Rarely the tip of the instrument passes through into the mediastinum or pleural cavity, to be recognized by the operator.

For small tears pass a nasogastric tube with multiple side holes so that the holes lie equally above and below the tear. Arrange for parenteral feeding and administer a course of antibiotics. Order an immediate chest X-ray, and look for mediastinal emphysema, which is most commonly seen after using a flexible endoscope with insufflation of air. Look for pneumothorax, indicating a breach of the pleura. Provided that there are minimal mediastinal signs, with no pneumothorax, plan to maintain continuous gentle suction on the naso-oesophageal tube and to feed the patient parenterally. Administer a versatile systemic antibiotic. Provided that the patient's general condition and the chest X-ray show no deterioration, plan to carry out a radiological examination using a water-soluble contrast medium after five to seven days. If this is satisfactory, remove the tube and commence oral fluids, followed by solid foods. If it is not, continue the conservative management for a further five days and repeat the X-rays.

Major tears may be obvious or declare themselves later. Through the endoscope the tear may look extensive, or the mediastinal or pleural contents can be recognized. The chest X-

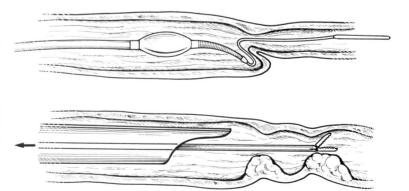

Figure 4.9
Eder–Puestow flexible guide-wire kinked so that the tip of the dilator deviates from the lumen.

Figure 4.10
Using alligator forceps to explore a complex stricture.

ray taken after an apparently trivial injury may demonstrate gross distension of the mediastinum or pneumothorax, or a patient being treated for an apparently trivial injury may deteriorate and contrast X-ray films show unexpected gross leakage. These patients require urgent exploration.

Drain a recognized major cervical tear of the oesophagus, and attempt repair. Immediately arrange for the operation to continue under sterile conditions (see p. 101). Start treatment with antibiotics and feed the patient parenterally for four to five days, then check radiologically that the oesophagus has healed, using a water-soluble iodinated medium. If this is satisfactory, the patient may restart oral feeding, first with fluids, progressing to semi-solids and solids.

The most frequent cause of serious perforation at endoscopy is during the attempted dilatation and intubation of carcinomatous strictures. As the dilator or tube is passed through there is a sudden giving way of the oesophageal wall. This is best managed by impacting a tube of the Mousseau–Barbin, Celestin or Atkinson type across the split. It may be possible to do this by the pulsion technique (Fig. 4.11). If this cannot be achieved, do not force a tube through and compound the damage. Have the patient anaesthetized and under sterile conditions explore the upper abdomen, perform gastrotomy, and pass upwards from below a gum elastic bougie. Ask the anaesthetist to recover the bougie tip and attach to it a Mousseau–Barbin or Celestin tube (Fig. 4.12). The tube is then pulled through from below, correctly sited, and the excess is cut off (Fig. 4.13). The gastrotomy is then closed. The patient should subsequently be treated for a few days with antibiotics and intravenous feeding.

If an intrathoracic split occurs in the absence of a malignant stricture, measure the site of perforation using the endoscope markings. Minor tears can be successfully managed using a correctly sited endo-oesophageal tube with multiple side holes placed at, above, and below the tear, maintained on suction, with parenteral feeding and systemic antibiotics. In my experience it is difficult to know how extensive is the damage, so I favour the more conventional approach of immediate repair and drainage. Plan to explore the chest under full anaesthesia with endotracheal intubation. Perforations in the upper oesophagus are best explored through the right chest, with ligation and division of the vena azygos if necessary. Perforations in the lower oesopha-

Figure 4.11
Impacting Atkinson pulsion tube through stricture to seal tear in oesophageal wall.

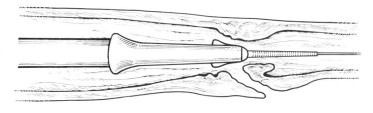

Figure 4.12
A bougie has been
passed up through a
gastrotomy, the end is
drawn out of the
mouth by the
anaesthetist in order
to attach the tube
leader to it.

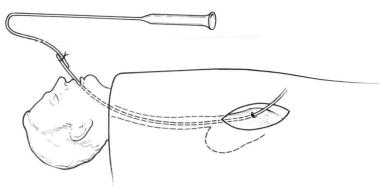

Figure 4.13
Mousseau–Barbin
tube drawn through a
gastrotomy. The
excess will be cut off
and the gastrotomy
will be closed.

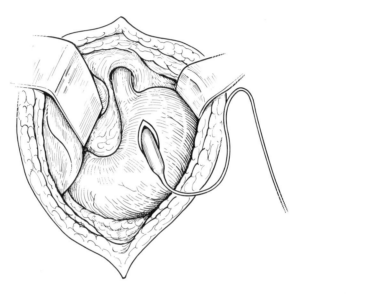

gus are best explored through the left chest. Recent perforations
in the absence of malignancy are often capable of immediate
repair, with subsequent closure of the chest and insertion of a
drainage tube connected to an underwater system. The techniques are described in Chapter 5.

Perforations of the abdominal oesophagus may best be
approached through the abdomen (see p. 86) or through a left
thoracoabdominal incision in the line of the upper border of the
sixth or seventh rib. If the tear cannot be sutured, it is possible to
utilize the Thal gastric fundic patch (see p. 81). The repair can be
reinforced using mediastinal pleura or a mobilized strip of
muscular diaphragmatic crus.

In some cases the degree of disruption prevents adequate
closure. The oesophagus can be drained and isolated by creating
a cervical oesophagostomy above and a gastrostomy or jejunostomy below (see p. 83).

Features It is best to make the diagnosis of endoscopically ruptured oesophagus before clinical signs develop, either at the time of endoscopy or subsequently. Whenever a difficult dilatation or intubation is carried out, perform chest X-ray as soon as the patient recovers from sedation or anaesthetic, preferably within three hours. Look for evidence of air emphysema in the neck and mediastinum. Sometimes a double line can be seen at the mediastinal pleura, indicating that the mediastinal pleura has separated from the arch (Fig. 4.14). If the pleura has been breached, pneumothorax is present. If the peritoneum is entered, subdiaphragmatic air is seen. Air is more prominently seen in the tissues and in cavities following fibreoptic endoscopy than following rigid endoscopy since air is insufflated with the flexible instrument. If there is any evidence of leak or if the patient complains of pain, immediately carry out a radiologically monitored swallow using water-soluble contrast to determine the site and extent of the leak.

A cervical perforation produces pain in the neck, often made worse by movement, phonation and swallowing. There may be accompanying hoarseness of the voice. The neck is tender, especially on moving the larynx or hyoid bone. Nearly always there is some air emphysema which produces crepitus, and

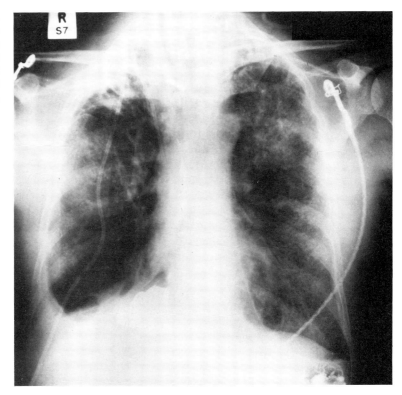

Figure 4.14
Chest X-ray demonstrates a double line along the left edge of the heart from air emphysema in the mediastinum.

eventually there may be swelling in the neck. Soft tissue X-ray confirms the presence of air emphysema.

Intrathoracic perforation often produces well-localized pain, mainly substernal but sometimes passing through to the back. In the presence of a hydropneumothorax, there may be dyspnoea. As a rule there are no specific clinical features of intrathoracic perforation except if there is already a large collection of air, fluid or both in the pleural cavity. Chest X-ray shows widening of the mediastinum, with air emphysema in some cases or hydro-pneumothorax if the mediastinal pleura has been breached.

Perforation into the abdominal cavity may produce severe upper abdominal pain. Tenderness and guarding suggest an abdominal catastrophe. Plain X-ray films of the erect abdomen often reveal subdiaphragmatic gas.

Endoscopy at this stage is usually of little value in determining the severity of the leak. In all cases assess the site and extent of the leak radiologically after giving the patient water-soluble radio-opaque contrast medium.

The patient soon develops pyrexia. A major intrathoracic perforation produces signs of surgical shock, with thready rapid pulse, hypotension, peripheral vascular shut-down and cold, pale extremities. There is mental confusion and the patient may be oliguric. Extensive or ignored leakage into the pleural cavity with pneumothorax, hydropneumothorax, pulmonary collapse and mediastinal shift causes respiratory distress.

Treatment   Small perforations detected soon after instrumentation can usually be treated conservatively, applying continuous suction through a naso-oesophageal tube, with multiple side holes placed across the leak. The patient is given prophylactic antibiotics and parenteral feeding is instituted for four to five days to give the perforation time to seal. Provided there is no distal obstruction, this is usually successful. Explore major leaks or those that were missed immediately following instrumentation. Drain and possibly repair the oesophagus.

Intrathoracic perforation should be explored conventionally. However, good results are reported if the leak is discovered within the first few hours, following intubation with a nasoenteric tube with multiple side holes, placed so that the holes lie above and below the leak, and kept on continuous gentle suction. The patient is given parenteral feeding until radiology demonstrates that the leak has sealed.

Nearly all leaks to the pleural cavity must be treated surgically. Approach upper thoracic perforations through a right thoracotomy. Explore lower oesophageal perforations through a left thoracotomy (see p. 105).

A number of patients with malignant or even benign strictures, in whom a leak is discovered following attempted dilatation and intubation of the intrathoracic oesophagus, are not suitable for major procedures. It is often preferable to attempt intubation with a Celestin or Mousseau–Barbin type of tube to impact the tube across the perforation. The chest is then drained with an underwater sealed chest drain.

On occasion late or severe disruption occurs that cannot be suitably closed or simply drained. A possibility that I (RMK) have personally not used is to isolate the oesophageal disruption temporarily, by performing a cervical oesophagostomy above and a gastrostomy below and occluding the oesophageal lumen with tapes (see p. 84).

When extensive disruption has occurred, especially in a neoplasm, excision of the disrupted segment, including the primary disease, is usually the best treatment. Continuity is achieved immediately or subsequently using stomach, jejunum or colon.

Persisting Controversy

● There is as yet no unanimity about the correct procedure after the discovery of a rupture following an endoscopic procedure. Conventionally all leaks are explored. Most surgeons do not explore as a routine splits resulting from attempts to dilate and intubate inoperable malignant oesophageal strictures, preferring to impact a tube across the split. Most surgeons do not as a rule explore cervical tears discovered early. All agree that in patients with a reasonable prognosis tears into either pleural cavity must be managed surgically.

Operations for Instrumental Perforation

Cervical perforation

Although controversy exists about the necessity for surgical drainage following perforation of the oesophagus in the neck, if there is anything more than a trivial local injury it is always better to err on the side of caution and drain it. It is often difficult at the time of endoscopy to estimate the degree of damage and the likelihood of leaked contents tracking into the mediastinum. If an unsuspected leak is discovered later, a radiographic study should be performed to determine the extent and severity of the leak.

If surgery is to be carried out, the sooner it is performed the better, before serious contamination occurs. If endoscopy was performed in the operating theatre, the patient should, ideally, be immediately anaesthetized and the operation carried out under sterile conditions. Otherwise, the patient should be transferred to the theatre as soon as possible.

The anaesthetized patient is given a parenteral dose of versatile antibiotic. The anaesthetist will have inserted a cuffed endotracheal tube and should also perform central venous catheterization, since the patient will be fed parenterally for several days following the operation.

Prepare the skin of the neck and wrap the head in sterile towels so that the neck can be extended and turned fully to the right. Drape the rest of the wound and arrange for the whole table to be angled so that the patient is in the head-up position to prevent venous congestion in the neck.

Make an incision along the anterior border of the left sternomastoid muscle, through skin, subcutaneous fascia, platysma muscle and the deep cervical fascia just anterior to the sternomastoid, thus entering the space between the sternomastoid and carotid sheath laterally and the central column of the trachea, thyroid gland and pharyngo-oesophagus (Fig. 4.15). There are three structures crossing the space, which may need to be divided if they interfere with the exposure (Fig. 4.16). The lower belly of omohyoid muscle almost certainly will be divided, and probably also the middle thyroid vein. The inferior thyroid artery can usually be preserved, but if it is divided, it should be divided between two ligatures placed well laterally to avoid damaging the recurrent laryngeal nerve.

Aspirate any leaked fluid. Gently rotate the central column of trachea and oesophagus and attached structures towards the right so that the circumference of the pharynx and oesophagus can be inspected and palpated to recognize and assess the

Figure 4.15
Diagram of approach to left side of cervical oesophagus. The omohyoid muscle, middle thyroid vein and inferior thyroid artery are not shown.

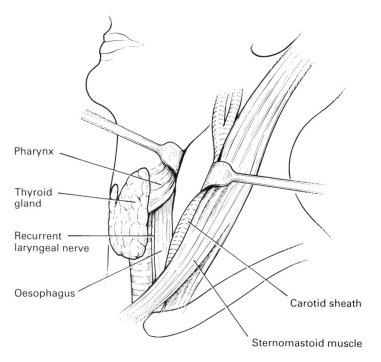

Pharynx

Thyroid gland

Recurrent laryngeal nerve

Oesophagus

Carotid sheath

Sternomastoid muscle

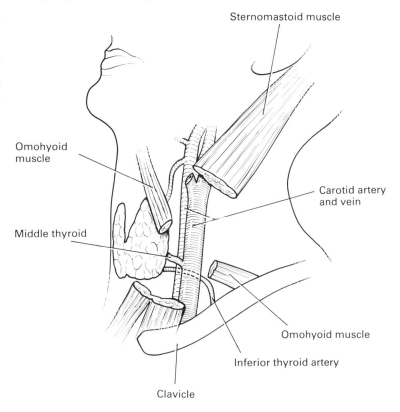

Figure 4.16
Diagram of approach to left side of cervical oesophagus. A segment is shown removed from the sternomastoid and omohyoid muscles.

Sternomastoid muscle

Omohyoid muscle

Carotid artery and vein

Middle thyroid

Omohyoid muscle

Inferior thyroid artery

Clavicle

damage. Ask the anaesthetist to pass a naso-oesophageal tube down and guide it past the damaged segment.

Now repair the injury, inserting all-coats sutures of 2/0 catgut on eyeless needles. The blood supply is excellent, so a perfect repair should be possible.

Insert a tubular suction drain through a separate stab wound and close the deep fascia and skin.

Feed the patient parenterally for five to seven days, then screen him while he swallows water-soluble contrast medium.

Intrathoracic perforation

Controversy exists about the need to explore simple perforations within the mediastinum that are discovered early. Of course malignant strictures that perforate during intubation are treated by impacting a tube across the damaged segment. Many endoscopists would, provided—and only provided—that the leak is discovered in the first few hours, pass a tube with many side holes to lie at the site of a perforation. The tube is maintained on continuous suction while the patient is fed parenterally for five to seven days and given antibiotic cover. There is unanimous agreement that if the perforation extends into the pleural cavity, operation is mandatory. Whenever there is doubt, always prefer to explore intrathoracic perforations and do so as early as possible.

Carefully note the level of the perforation. Start the patient on a course of versatile antibiotics. The anaesthetist will pass a double lumen tube so that either lung can be collapsed. Place the patient on his side with the lower leg flexed at knee and hip, upper leg straight. The arms are brought in front of the face as though the patient is performing the hornpipe dance. If a thoracoabdominal approach will be needed, the patient is allowed to fall back 30° and is fixed with supports and non-stretch adhesive tape. If the perforation is in the upper chest, plan to have the patient on his left side, opening the chest along the upper border of the right fifth or sixth rib. If the perforation is in the lower chest, turn the patient on his right side and open the chest above the left sixth or seventh rib. If the tear is very low, it may be necessary to convert this into a thoracoabdominal incision.

On the right side the lung is turned forwards, the mediastinal pleura is incised, and the vena azygos is divided between ligatures above the lung root to expose the oesophagus (Fig. 4.17). On the left side divide the pulmonary ligament, lift the lung forward and incise the mediastinal pleura. Gently mobilize the oesophagus and examine the tear (Fig. 4.18).

Assess the tear carefully but do not mobilize the oesophagus more than necessary. Have the anaesthetist pass a naso-oesophageal tube and guide the tip past the tear. Now carefully repair the oesophagus using all-coats catgut stitches, making sure that the submucosa and mucosa do not slip away from the needle. If necessary insert all the stitches before tying them so that the inner layers can be exposed throughout. It may be possible to raise a flap of mediastinal pleura, which is sewn over the tear to

Figure 4.17
Diagram of approach to the oesophagus through the right chest.

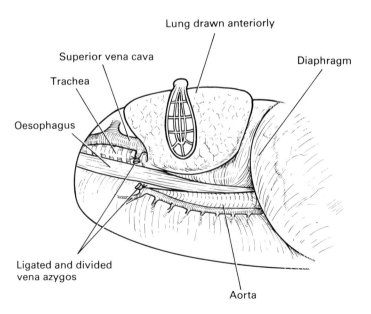

Lung drawn anteriorly

Superior vena cava

Diaphragm

Trachea

Oesophagus

Ligated and divided vena azygos

Aorta

Figure 4.18
Diagram of approach
to the oesophagus
through the left chest.

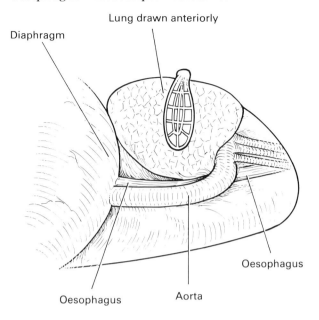

reinforce the repair. In the lower oesophagus a strip of diaphragmatic muscle can be raised to cover it. Severe disruption of the lower oesophagus may not be amenable to simple repair. The method of Thal may be useful (Fig. 4.19). The gastric fundus is first mobilized. This entails freeing the cardia by enlarging the hiatus and dividing the phreno-oesophageal ligament, and dividing the upper short gastric vessels between double ligatures. If necessary, the fundus may be freed through an incision in the tendinous portion of the left diaphragm or even by extending the

Figure 4.19
Thal patch of gastric
fundus to repair lower
oesophagus.

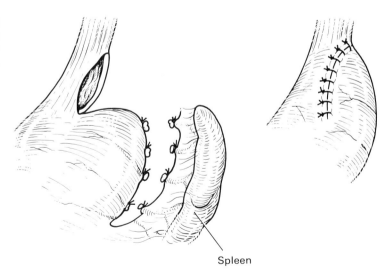

incision into a thoracoabdominal approach. The freed gastric fundus is now used as a patch to repair the lower oesophagus, being sewn to the margins of the defect so that a part of the oesophageal lining is formed by gastric fundic seromuscularis.

Sometimes there is a previously unrecognized obstructing carcinoma. If it is obviously unresectable or if the patient is unfit, one option is to impact a tube through it, although the presence of the double lumen endotracheal tube makes the passage through the pharynx and thoracic inlet difficult. An assistant can pass a guide while the operator ensures its onward passage. A pulsion tube can then be gently inserted while the thoracic operator checks that no further damage is done. I (RMK) prefer to draw a tube through by traction. This could mean making a fresh upper abdominal incision to perform a gastrotomy, but most such tears occur in the lower third of the thoracic oesophagus and the upper stomach may be approached through the tendinous part of the diaphragm or through the oesophageal hiatus. A small upper gastrotomy is made. Through it, a bougie is passed from below upwards and the anaesthetist identifies it in the pharynx, draws it out of the mouth and attaches it to the leader of a Mousseau–Barbin or Celestin tube. The tube is gently drawn through until it is impacted across the tear, the excess is cut off and the gastrotomy is closed, followed by repair of the diaphragm. It may be possible to cover the tear with a fold of elevated mediastinal pleura, or diaphragmatic muscle if the tear is low down. An underwater sealed drain is inserted so that the end lies near the injured oesophagus, and the chest is closed.

In the presence of benign disease the oesophagus may be severely disrupted, making repair hazardous, or a carcinoma may be present that is resectable in an otherwise fit patient. Exceptionally, primary resection and anastomosis of the carcinoma may be a possibility. As a rule, however, the safest course is to excise the thoracic oesophagus (Fig. 4.20). First take steps to occlude the disrupted lumen using stitches or wrap the mobilized segment with a swab or sterile glove. Gently mobilize the oesophagus. Transect the lower end at the level of the diaphragm after placing an occluding ligature above the line of division. Securely close the lower cut end with sutures. Gently dissect out the damaged segment and continue right up to the root of the neck, separating the oesophagus from the back of the trachea without damaging the thin membranous posterior wall of the trachea, which bulges where the endotracheal tube lies within it. If the oesophagus is very bulky, heavily contaminated or has crumbling surface neoplasm, tie two occluding ligatures as high as possible and remove the specimen; otherwise the freed thoracic oesophagus will be drawn up into the neck and resected there. Close the chest after inserting one underwater sealed drain to the site of contamination and another apical drain.

Have the patient placed supine. Now explore the neck through an incision along the anterior border of the left sternomastoid muscle (see p. 78). Identify the cervical oesophagus with the recurrent laryngeal nerve lying in the tracheo-oesophageal groove and taking care not to injure the nerve, and gently separate the oesophagus from the trachea, carrying the dissection down to the root of the neck, keeping strictly to the oesophageal wall. The mobilized thoracic oesophagus or its stump can now be drawn into the neck. Transect the cervical oesophagus low down, since it rapidly shortens, so that it can be sutured to the skin at the lower end of the incision as a stoma (Fig. 4.21). Insert all-coats stitches through the cut end of oesophagus and suture it to the skin edges. Close the neck and apply a plastic stoma bag over the oesophagostomy.

Now make a left upper abdominal incision and create a jejunostomy (see p. 4). The patient should then be allowed to recover and achieve nutritional balance.

At a second operation the abdomen is explored through an upper midline incision. The stomach is mobilized on the right gastric and right gastro-epiploic vessels. The lowest part of the oesophagus is freed in the hiatus. Kocher's duodenal mobilization is fully carried out and the pylorus is checked to be free of stenosis by ensuring that the anterior gastric antral wall can be invaginated through the pylorus on an index finger. The gastric

Figure 4.20 Resection of disrupted thoracic oesophagus. The fundus of the stomach will be brought up now or later to be joined to the cervical oesophagus.

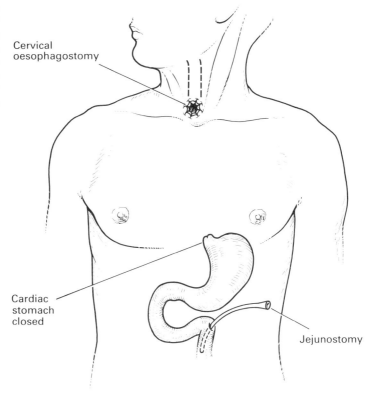

Cervical oesophagostomy

Cardiac stomach closed

Jejunostomy

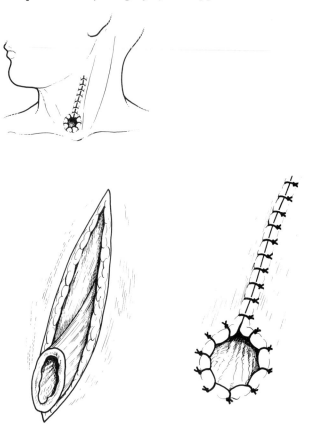

fundus is taken up to the neck for anastomosis to the freed cervical oesophagus after dissecting it free of the skin (Fig. 4.22). The stomach may be taken through the posterior mediastinum, but this may be adherent and it is better to take it through the substernal route after incising the xiphoid slips of the diaphragm and gently inserting a hand through the anterior mediastinum, keeping strictly against the sternum. Alternatively the stomach may be taken subcutaneously; this produces a swelling, but it becomes less prominent with the passage of time. Exceptionally, immediate reconstruction could be carried out, but this is running an unnecessary risk in a patient who already has suffered from oesophageal disruption followed by a major resection.

A method that I have not used is to isolate the damaged oesophagus (Fig. 4.23). The anaesthetized patient lies supine, with sterile head towel, neck extended and rotated to the right. The rupture is repaired through the chest and drained. The cervical oesophagus is approached through an incision along the anterior border of the sternomastoid muscle (see p. 78), mobilized, and drawn to the surface. A side hole is created and

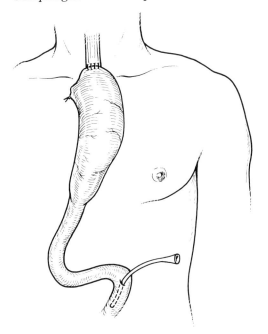

Figure 4.22
The stomach is brought to the neck subcutaneously, substernally or through the posterior mediastinum for anastomosis to the cervical oesophagus.

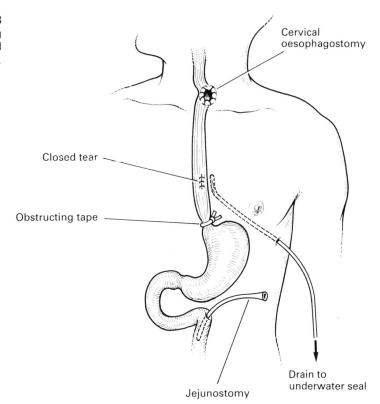

Figure 4.23
Method of isolating disrupted oesophagus.

Cervical oesophagostomy

Closed tear

Obstructing tape

Drain to underwater seal

Jejunostomy

through this a sucker tube is inserted to empty the oesophagus of contents. The margins of the side hole are sutured to the skin as a cervical oesophagostomy. The abdominal oesophagus is now approached through an upper midline abdominal incision. A plastic occluding tape of Teflon or Silastic is tied around it. A jejunostomy is created and the abdomen is closed. When the patient has fully recovered, the abdomen is re-explored, the occluding tape removed, the cervical oesophagostomy closed and the jejunostomy discontinued.

Intra-abdominal perforation

Endoscopically-induced perforation of the abdominal oesophagus cannot be satisfactorily repaired through the abdomen except in a very thin patient. Unless it is a perforated carcinoma through which a tube can be impacted, preferably by traction, it is best to approach a perforation through a left thoracoabdominal incision. Benign conditions resulting in perforation can usually be repaired with sutures, if necessary reinforcing the repair with a mobilized strip of pleura, diaphragmatic muscle or the mobilized gastric fundus. If simple repair is not possible, then the Thal patch of gastric fundus can be sutured into the margins of the defect. Drain the upper abdomen and insert underwater sealed chest drains.

If there is a perforation of a lower oesophageal or cardiac stomach carcinoma, primary resection and anastomosis may be performed in a fit patient.

Abscess

The cellulitis which develops following perforation of the oesophagus may progress to abscess formation and this can track within the mediastinum, the neck (Fig. 4.24) or from the neck into the mediastinum. The patient develops typical features of sepsis, often with pain, fever and toxic shock. If the abscess develops in the neck, a swelling can be seen and felt. In the mediastinum the swelling produces widening of the shadow on an X-ray, and if the abscess forms within the pleural cavity, an empyema is seen on plain anteroposterior films. Subphrenic abscess may develop following perforation of the lower oesophagus and as a rule can be seen on diaphragmatic screening.

Ultrasound computed tomography and radioactive gallium scans may help to identify and localize abscesses that cannot be discovered by simpler methods. Operative drainage should be instituted. Following exposure of intrathoracic abscesses an underwater sealed drain should be inserted through an appropriate intercostal space. Subphrenic abscesses are nowadays sometimes treated by aspiration or insertion of a percutaneous drain under ultrasonic or computed tomographic scan control (see p. 36).

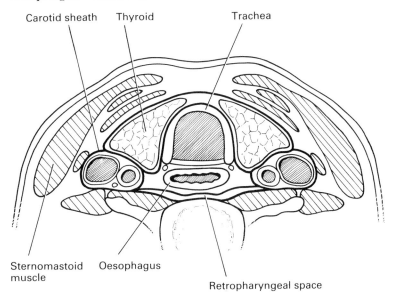

Figure 4.24
Tissue planes within
the neck. Perforation
of the oesophagus
results in separation
of the fascial layers
and may extend into
the mediastinum.

Carotid sheath   Thyroid   Trachea

Sternomastoid   Oesophagus
muscle

Retropharyngeal space

Fistulae

External fistulae may develop following spontaneous or surgical drainage of fluid collections or abscesses following leakage. They always heal provided that there is no distal obstruction.

Tracheal and bronchial fistulae to the oesophagus develop spontaneously from the breakdown of growths, from trauma during instrumentation, or more commonly from the continuous pressure of the tube used to splint malignant strictures (Fig. 4.25). In a few patients it is possible to resect the oesophagus and an alternative is to isolate the segment of oesophagus involved in the fistula, resecting the remainder and closing each end of the isolated oesophagus. Mobilized stomach or colon is then taken up to the upper oesophagus. Some of these patients are amenable to intubation and radiotherapy.

Obstruction

If the endoscopy was carried out for the detection and treatment of obstruction, treatment may not have been attempted, or may have been unsuccessful. In suitable cases a further attempt at endoscopic dilatation may succeed where the first attempt failed. If the dilatation was partially successful, the patient may have been over-optimistic and swallowed food such as meat, fruit or lumps of bread that have impacted. Mucolytic agents are sometimes helpful. The patient should be advised on the need to cut up food finely, to chew it well, to swallow solid food with a

Figure 4.25
Oesophagotracheal
fistula. A splinting
tube is positioned in
the oesophagus.
Swallowed contrast
medium has leaked
into the trachea
producing a
bronchogram
anteriorly (to the right
side).

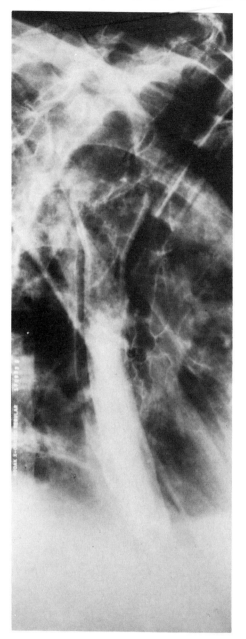

little fluid, and to drink half a glass of water containing half a
level teaspoonful of sodium bicarbonate half an hour before
meals (to wash through some of the accumulated mucus).

If after endoscopy the patient develops sudden dysphagia, the
endoscopy should be repeated and the impacted food removed
with forceps. Sometimes it can be pushed through the stricture.

Following endoscopic intubation, obstruction may develop initially because the tube has become blocked with food, or the end is resting against the wall of the oesophagus or stomach (Fig. 4.26). This can be checked radiologically using a radio-opaque fluid medium. If the tube is imperfectly sited, it may not completely traverse the stricture or may already have slipped proximally, especially if there is no cuff or lip to prevent it (Fig. 4.27). It must then be resited. This is usually best performed with the patient under general anaesthesia. Sometimes the upper lip of the tube can be grasped through a flexible or rigid oesophagoscope, and the endoscope, forceps and tube withdrawn together, prior to attempting to resite the tube. Occasionally it is impossible to grip the tube. It is then necessary to open the abdomen under sterile conditions, perform gastrotomy, grasp the tube from below with long-handled forceps and reposition it. Rarely the tube must be pushed up from below, and removed by the anaesthetist. A bougie is then passed from below into the pharynx. The anaesthetist attaches the leader of a new tube to the bougie and the tube is drawn down. The end is cut off, and the gastrotomy and abdominal wounds closed.

Later obstruction may be the result of the tube slipping or because the patient has blocked the tube with food. Gradual blockage may signify that tumour is overgrowing the top of the

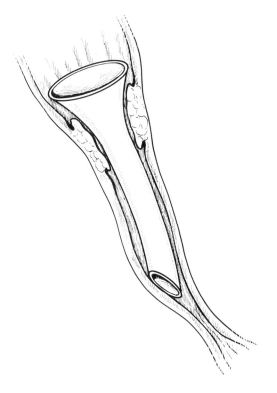

Figure 4.26
End of endo-oesophageal tube pressing against the wall, blocking the passage of food.

Figure 4.27
The endo-
oesophageal tube has
slipped proximally
above the narrowing
so that the
obstruction has
recurred.

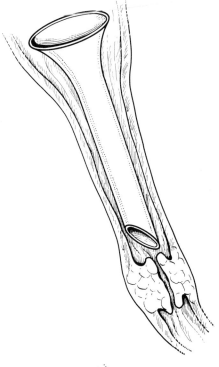

Figure 4.28
Growth has extended
up over the lip of the
endo-oesophageal
tube obstructing the
lumen.

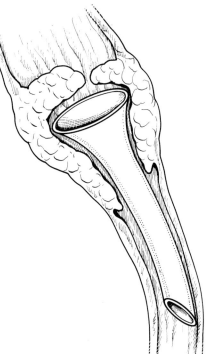

tube (Fig. 4.28). Radiography or endoscopy identifies the cause and the tube is unblocked or resited.

Persisting Controversies

- Management of instrumental leaks discovered early.
- Operative management of major introthoracic instrumental leaks.

Further reading
Dawson, J. & Cockel, R. (1981) Oesophageal perforation at fibreoptic gastroscopy. *British Medical Journal, 283*, 583.
Katz, D. (1967) Morbidity and mortality in standard and flexible gastrointestinal endoscopy. *Gastrointestinal Endoscopy, 14*, 134–137.
Kirk, R.M. (1983) Oesophagoscopy. In Dudley, H., Pories, W.J. & Carter, D.C. (Eds) *Rob and Smith's Operative Surgery*, 4th Edn. *Alimentary Tract and Abdominal Wall 1*, pp. 8–16. London: Butterworth.
Lancet (1984) Instrumental perforation of the oesophagus. *Lancet, i*: 1279.
Mengoli, L.R. & Klassen, K.P. (1965) Conservative management of esophageal perforation. *Archives of Surgery, 91*, 238–240.
Sandrasaga, F.A., English, T.A.H. & Milstein, B.B. (1978) The management and prognosis of oesophageal perforation. *British Journal of Surgery, 65*, 629–632.
Thal, A.P. (1968) A unified approach to surgical problems of the esophagogastric junction. *Annals of Surgery, 168*, 542–550.
Tytgat, G.N. & den Hartog Jager, F.C.A. (1977) Non-surgical treatment of cardioesophageal obstruction—role of endoscopy. *Endoscopy, 9*, 211–215.
Wesdorp, I.C.E., Bartelsman, J.F.W.M., Huibregtse K., den Hartog Jager F.C.A. & Tytgat, G.N. (1984) Treatment of instrumental oesophageal perforation. *Gut, 25*, 398–404.

5 Major Oesophageal Procedures Including Resection

Early Complications

Bleeding

Following oesophagectomy and anastomosis bleeding may occur into the gut, and if a nasal tube has been passed through the anastomosis, blood is aspirated. If bleeding occurs into the chest, then it passes out through the chest drains, but mediastinal bleeding causes cardiac irregularities and widening of the mediastinum on chest X-ray if the mediastinal pleura has not been breached or if it has resealed. Bleeding may also occur in the abdomen and into the neck. Neck bleeding produces swelling and dyspnoea and the blood may track down into the superior mediastinum.

The patient displays signs of hypovolaemic shock. Exclude a clotting defect that could account for the bleeding, by engaging the help of the haematologists. If transfusion with blood does not quickly restore the patient's general condition or if the condition improves and then deteriorates in spite of the transfusion, the patient must be re-explored to find the site of bleeding and to control it. Initially the general condition should be restored as much as possible. If it is not already in place, a central venous catheter should be inserted to allow the blood volume changes to be monitored, and the blood should be crossmatched in readiness. A course of antibiotics should be started, since these patients are prone to secondary infection. Ensure that the theatre staff have adequate equipment available, including vascular clamps and sutures that might be required for the repair of a major intrathoracic blood vessel.

Reopen the wound. Seek the bleeding site. Control it by simple means (see p. 10). Wait while the anaesthetist restores the patient's general condition as much as possible before proceeding. Repair torn major vessels, clamp and ligate lesser vessels, and seal small vessels with diathermy current. If there is general oozing, try the effect of leaving warm gauze packs on the area for five minutes by the clock, or applying an artificial gauze patch such as haemostatic sponge.

We tend, when operating to control bleeding, to develop a sense of urgency. Control the desire to close the wound as rapidly as possible. When the bleeding appears to be stopped, gently lay large packs over the viscera and allow the anaesthetist to stabilize the blood pressure. Wait five or preferably ten minutes by the clock and then remove the pack and thoroughly reinspect the whole operation area. The reason for this delay is that following severe bleeding, previously dry areas may start to ooze because clotting factors have been used up and from the effects of the citrate in the large volumes of stored blood that may have been given.

When you are confident that there is no further bleeding, carefully close the wound, reinserting chest and other drains.

Anastomotic leak or disruption

Predisposing factors The oesophagus, through the pharyngeal constrictor muscles, is slung from the base of the skull (Fig. 5.1). Almost half its thickness is composed of powerful longitudinal muscle. Contraction of the muscle draws the lower end of a cut oesophagus upwards. In addition, the oesophagus appears to have a natural elasticity and is normally under some tension. As soon as it is cut, without the contraction of muscle, it shortens to about half its length when left in situ. Thus, when the oesophagus is transected, although it appears to be adequate in length for anastomosis, it rapidly retracts and requires considerable tension to bring it down to its previous extent. If an anastomosis is constructed under tension, the powerful contraction of the longitudinal muscle may disrupt it.

An additional disadvantage to the surgeon of the amount of longitudinal muscle is the fact that stitches placed in it tend to cut out between the fibres. Thus only about half the thickness of the oesophagus is able to take the longitudinal pull of stitches, namely the submucous coat and to some extent the squamous epithelial lining.

The transected and relaxed oesophagus usually has a lumen of about 1 cm in diameter. If it is sutured in this relaxed state, the sutures appear close together. However, the oesophagus is enormously distensible and when it is stretched transversely the stitches separate widely and may allow leakage between them.

It is usually stated that the blood supply to the oesophagus is tenuous, but there is no proof of this. Nevertheless, if the oesophagus is extensively mobilized for anastomosis, it is possible that the intramural blood supply may be attenuated.

Most of the bowel has a peritoneal coat that adheres whenever it is brought into apposition with peritoneum of bowel to which it is anastomosed. The oesophagus lacks this coat and the union does not seal so promptly.

The higher the resection, the greater the length that must be bridged by the conduit of stomach, jejunum or colon. Each of these has a fixed point of vascular supply unless a microvascular anastomosis is used to transfer the origin of the blood vessels higher. The longer the supplying vessels the greater the possibi-

Figure 5.1
The cardia hangs
from the base of the
skull.

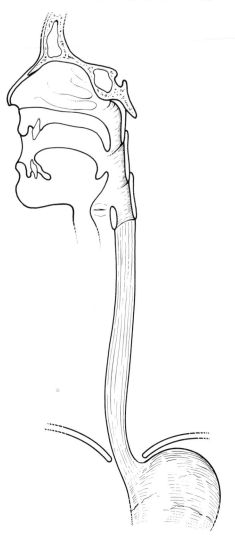

lity that the highest part of the conduit will be rendered ischaemic. Probably bypass is less at risk than resection and anastomosis. The oesophagus is fixed and the bypass conduit is thus not stretched. A side-to-side anastomosis can be made which is less likely to be distracted than an end-to-end union.

There is some evidence that healing in undernourished patients is impaired and this is a risk with carcinoma of the oesophagus, causing dysphagia and possible cachexia from the catabolic effects of the primary and any secondary tumour. This is certainly not of paramount importance. The cardinal determinant is technique, as attested by the outstanding results achieved by Chinese surgeons working without the facilities to correct nutritional deficiencies.

Prevention On theoretical grounds the patient's nutritional state should be restored to normal. If the patient can swallow, he should be given a normal diet supplemented if necessary with high-protein, high-calorie, vitamin-rich additions. When fluids only can be taken, a fully nutritious fluid diet can be made up, and if the patient finds difficulty in imbibing it, he can swallow a fine bore nasogastric tube and have it given by drip-feed.

If the patient cannot swallow, carry out endoscopy and dilate the structure to allow him to do so, being prepared to create a jejunostomy or to insert a Hickman central venous catheter if dilatation fails. I (RMK) prefer to create a jejunostomy (see p. 4). Properly managed it allows rapid restoration of nutritional state, as judged by weight gain, rising serum albumin, increased triceps skin fold thickness and muscle power measured by the grip testing apparatus. It can remain for postoperative feeding. Alternatively, the insertion of a Hickman cathether allows intravenous feeding to be instituted. There are a number of preparations that can be given, including proprietary mixtures, to restore the patient to a good nutritional state. Again, the catheter remains in situ for feeding after operation. Of course intravenous feeding can continue without a break, whereas jejunostomy feeding must await the recovery of the bowel.

Whenever there has been a hold-up in the upper gastrointestinal tract, organisms flourish that will prejudice the operation. It is important that any stagnant contents are emptied, if necessary by keeping an oesophageal tube on continuous suction before surgery. Prophylactic antibiotics should be started as the operation commences. It was usual to start a five-day course, but there is now evidence that if the blood levels are satisfactory over the period of the operation, this is unnecessary.

Operation The problems of anastomosing the oesophagus are similar to, but more critical than, anastomoses of any other tubular viscus. There must be no tension. The blood supply to each end must be perfect. As a rule a portion of the oesophagus cannot be removed with subsequent end-to-end anastomosis and as a result either stomach, jejunum or colon must be mobilized to be joined to the upper cut end of the oesophagus. The safest conduit to use to bridge the gap following oesophageal resection is stomach. It reliably survives on the right gastric and right gastroepiploic blood vessels (Fig. 5.2). The vessel stretched most when the fundus of the stomach is taken into the chest is the right gastroepiploic vein, so this must be guarded carefully. The gastrocolic omentum should be divided outside the gastroepiploic arch, which is preserved to carry the blood supply up to the fundus. Unless the stomach is scarred from gastric or duodenal ulceration, the fundus will usually stretch well into the neck, but unfortunately this cannot be assured until the stomach is fully mobilized. To resect an oesophageal carcinoma encroaching onto the lower third, the gastric cardia and glands along the lesser

Figure 5.2
Oesophagogastrostomy.
The right gastric and
right gastroepiploic
vessels must be
preserved to supply
the mobilized
stomach. There must
be no tension.

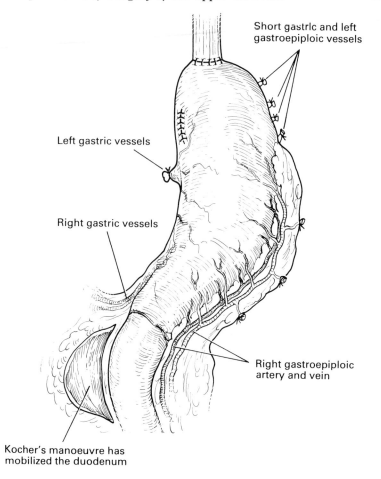

Short gastric and left
gastroepiploic vessels

Left gastric vessels

Right gastric vessels

Right gastroepiploic
artery and vein

Kocher's manoeuvre has
mobilized the duodenum

curve must be excised. It is important to close the gastric cardia longitudinally, without shortening the new lesser curve.

Colon is an alternative to stomach when the oesophagus is extensively resected, in particular when the stomach is scarred, short, or has already been resected (Fig. 5.3). The right colon is easy to mobilize on the middle colic vessels and the marginal vessels are usually reliable. When the caecum is swung upwards the colon drains isoperistaltically, but the caecum is rather bulky to take up into the neck—although it contracts during the next few months. The left colon can be swung upwards on the middle colic artery and will reach to the neck, but is antiperistaltic. Some surgeons have angiographic studies performed before using colon, but alternatively the vessels that will be divided can first be gently occluded with bulldog clamps to check the integrity of the marginal arteries. Belsey recommends using an isoperistaltic transverse and upper left colic segment based on the upper left colic vessels.

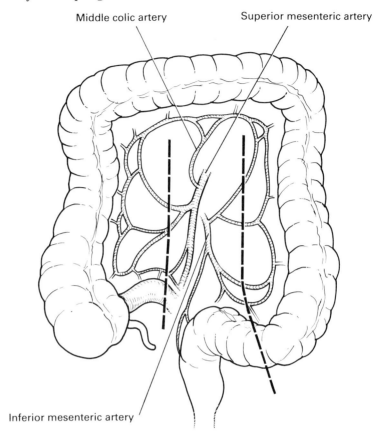

Figure 5.3
Mobilization of the
right or left colon on
the middle colic
vesels.

Middle colic artery

Superior mesenteric artery

Inferior mesenteric artery

Jejunum is the most capriciously supplied part of the bowel. A Roux-en-Y segment is suitable for short gaps, but since there is no marginal artery it is easy to run into difficulty (Fig. 5.4). Moreover, there is often much redundant jejunum because the bowel extends more easily than its blood supply. Allison and Da Silva (1953/54) recommended judicious stripping of the mesentery to leave the blood vessel loops free to gain length. It is the first choice to join to the middle or lower oesophagus when the stomach cannot be used or has been resected.

The blood supply to the oesophagus must also be good. As a rule do not mobilize more than 3–5 cm.

Whichever conduit is selected must, when mobilized, be capable of reaching the oesophagus without any tension, and remain a good colour. Unfortunately, until the surgeon has committed himself he has no way of ensuring that the conduit is sufficiently long and has an adequate arterial supply and venous drainage. Even when the conduit appears healthy and slack, leakage may occur because of the anatomical circumstances. The lack of a peritoneal coat on the oesophagus, except for the last

Figure 5.4
The difficulty of
creating a Roux-en-Y
loop arises because of
the variable blood
supply and absence
of a marginal artery.
The broken line
indicates the line of
transection.

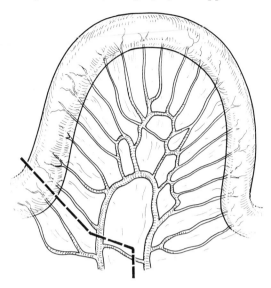

2 cm within the abdomen, prevents the rapid sealing that occurs
when intra-abdominal viscera are joined, so the anastomosis
must be constructed with extraordinary care. To allow for the
immense distension of the oesophagus when swallowing takes
place, it is advisable to slightly stretch the anastomosis with stay
sutures at each end while the stitches are being inserted (Fig.
5.5). The exact method of inserting the stitches and the type of
material used are less important than the perfection of the
technique. The sutures should be placed approximately 2 mm
apart and take all coats of the oesophagus and the viscus to be
joined to it, about 2 mm from the edge. The hole in the oesophagus
and the hole in the viscus must match perfectly. The tension in
the sutures must just appose the mucosal edges but not constrict
the enclosed tissue. The second layer of inverting stitches may be

Figure 5.5
The anastomosis is
stretched while the
closely placed all-
coats sutures are
inserted.

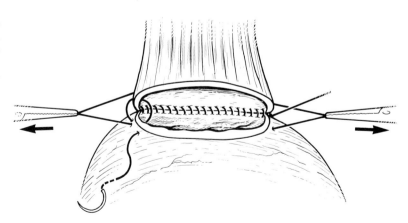

inserted at the surgeon's discretion. It is sometimes possible to reinforce the anastomosis by wrapping it with a healthy flap of omentum, or of mediastinal pleura.

Modern series, particularly from China and Japan, suggest that with good technique, anastomotic leaks should be very rare occurrences. Undoubtedly the best results are obtained by surgeons who regularly carry out these operations. Certainly this is not a field for the dilettante or occasional oesophagec-tomist. An alternative to suturing is the use of the circular stapling gun. It is often very useful but does not absolve the surgeon from the need to plan and accomplish the anastomosis with great care. In my experience thick-walled oesophagus may be crushed within the jaws of the stapling gun, so I favour sutured anastomoses, or use the gun after peeling back the thick muscle coat of the oesophagus, and then insert a musculo-seromuscular outer stitch to repair and seal the oesophageal muscularis to the conduit.

Whenever possible, reinforce the anastomosis with spare omentum, or pleura, wrapped around and tacked over to enclose the anastomosis. In the event of a minor leak this often localizes it.

If the anastomosis is safely achieved, it is not necessary to pass a nasoenteric tube, provided there will be no stasis. However, if there is any risk of early gastro-oesophageal reflux or bile reflux from a jejunal loop, it is wise to pass a tube for aspiration. Reflux through a high anastomosis is often the cause of aspiration, even when the patient is being ventilated with a cuffed endotracheal tube.

If a jejunostomy has not been performed or a Hickman catheter has not been inserted, it is wise to decide upon one or other now, especially in a malnourished patient. As previously mentioned, I prefer to create a jejunostomy for postoperative feeding. Before recommencing oral feeding, the integrity of the anastomosis is checked by X-ray screening of the patient after he has swallowed water-soluble radio-opaque medium, usually four to five days after operation.

The site of the anastomosis may be important in relation to leakage. The higher the anastomosis the more likely it is that the reconstructing viscus has a tenuous blood supply. However, if the anastomosis is made to the cervical oesophagus, any leakage is superficial and should not be a serious complication, although it may track into the mediastinum if the conduit passes through it. Leakage within the mediastinum or thorax is of serious import. Some surgeons site the anastomosis deliberately in the neck in the hope of preventing intrathoracic leakage.

Pathology   The consequence of leakage following surgical operation upon the oesophagus is quite different from that following sponta-neous leakage or leakage following endoscopic procedures: the local tissues have been disturbed and displaced. As a result, when leakage occurs the fluid tracks within the neck, mediastinum, thorax or into the abdomen. Even though the patient may have had no fluids by mouth, he swallows saliva, fluid regurgitates from below, and a large volume may collect rapidly and soon becomes infected.

Local cellulitis develops in the neck, mediastinum and thorax. Acute inflammatory reaction at the anastomosis may hasten phagocytic digestion of the sutures if they are absorbable so that disruption is increased. Possibly the inflammatory reaction overburdens a tenuous blood supply and ischaemic necrosis occurs in tissues that would otherwise have just survived.

Sometimes a small perforation occurs into closely adherent tissues so that it becomes sealed off and drains back into the oesophagus. Wrapping the anastomosis with omentum or pleura may effect a seal. This will usually gradually heal spontaneously.

If the oesophagus or the viscus that has been used for anastomosis was ischaemic or if the tension is great, then the whole anastomosis may be totally disrupted. The ischaemic end of the viscus will undergo necrosis and the two ends will separate. The disconnected oesophagus will contract and may lie several centimetres proximal to the original site of anastomosis so that the surrounding tissues are flooded with oesophageal contents and backflow from the conduit. This collection rapidly will become infected and form a spreading abscess.

Features Following oesophageal surgery the patient's condition may be stable initially, but within two to seven days, if leakage has occurred, the temperature rises and there is peripheral vascular shut-down, producing cold, pale extremities. The signs of septic shock may develop insidiously (see *Complications of Surgery in General*) or rapidly so that the blood pressure is unstable and requires repeated infusions of crystalloid and colloid solutions or blood to maintain it. The clinical presentation can vary widely from insidious deterioration to sudden collapse, which often misleads the clinician into believing that the patient has suffered either a coronary thrombosis or a pulmonary embolus.

Leakage into the neck produces a swelling, with subsequent breakdown of the skin. Initially it may be difficult to distinguish this from air within the viscus. Leakage into the mediastinum does not as a rule produce widening of the mediastinum because the fluid runs away into the pleural cavity. This may then drain through the underwater sealed intrapleural drains, but by the time leakage has occurred the drains may already be sealed off so nothing emerges, but signs of a pleural effusion develop.

Investigations Before commencing oral feeding, always order a radiological study using water-soluble contrast medium to study the integrity of the anastomosis, the ease and rapidity of passage, and the functional recovery of the conduit. Whenever a patient deteriorates following oesophageal surgery suspect leakage as a first diagnosis. Carefully performed endoscopy may help but does not reveal the extent of leakage and most surgeons are apprehensive about employing it in these circumstances.

The white blood cell count is usually raised. Electrocardiography is often misleading in suggesting cardiac infarction or pulmonary embolus: do not lightly accept these diagnoses until leakage has been excluded.

Fluid aspirated from the chest or draining from the chest drains may contain mucus, and usually grows bowel micro-organisms on culture. Order posteroanterior and lateral X-rays of the chest. Depending on the site of anastomosis and the operative approach, fluid can be seen to have collected in the mediastinum and pleural cavities. The mediastinum is not widened if the pleura on one or other side has been incised. Remember that the conduit, and its contents, will widen the mediastinum. Confirm leakage radiographically (Fig. 5.6) to localize it, determine how freely fluid escapes, and where it goes, and to judge the progress of the medium distally.

Management   If the leak is small and well localized, and the majority of the medium continues along the normal channel, it is safe to manage the patient conservatively. Using radiographic control, place a nasoenteric tube with multiple side holes so that the holes bridge the leak. Keep the tube aspirated and maintain the patient on jejunostomy or parenteral feeding for one week. Recheck the leak (Fig. 5.7). If it is static or diminished, it is safe to cautiously start oral fluid feeding.

If the opaque medium tracks to the surface along a well-defined path, and most of it passes on in the bowel, it is safe to try conservative management, provided that the patient's general condition does not deteriorate. As a rule the track will close, although the anastomosis may become stenosed and require dilatation or refashioning later.

Apart from these two exceptions, urgent surgical intervention is necessary following vigorous measures to improve the patient's general condition, especially the circulation and respiration. A central venous catheter is inserted to monitor the circulatory volume and if necessary infusions of blood or colloid solutions are given.

A course of intravenous antibiotic treatment is started, usually with a versatile cephalosporin and metronidazole. Cross-matched blood should be available. It is wise to plan the likely procedure before performing the operation since it is most unlikely that a simple repair of the anastomosis will be possible.

Reoperation   If the anastomosis was in the neck, then the skin sutures should be removed and a drain inserted. This may be performed on the ward if the anastomosis is superficial, and if the general condition of the patient is good, it is best not to re-explore the wound extensively for fear of breaking down adhesions that are

Figure 5.6
Water-soluble
contrast medium used
for radiological
screening five days
after
oesophagogastric
anastomosis. A small,
localized leak is
demonstrated.
(See also Fig. 5.7.)

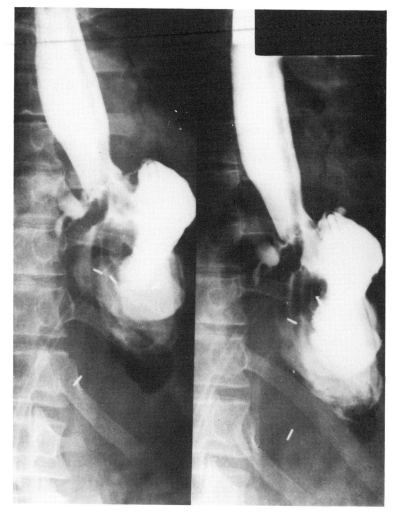

preventing drainage into the mediastinum. If the patient is ill, suggesting that pus has spread into the mediastinum, formal exploration will be required to assess the leak and drain it. If an anastomosis was previously made in the neck, reopen the wound. If this is an instrumental perforation (see p. 73), make an incision along the anterior border of sternomastoid muscle. Depending on the clinical features and radiological signs, explore on the appropriate side but on the left, take care not to injure the thoracic duct low down near the junction of the internal jugular and subclavian veins. Deepen the incision through the platysma muscle and deep fascia to reach the interval between the midline column of trachea, thyroid gland and oesophagus and the lateral bundle of carotid artery, jugular vein and vagus nerve. Three

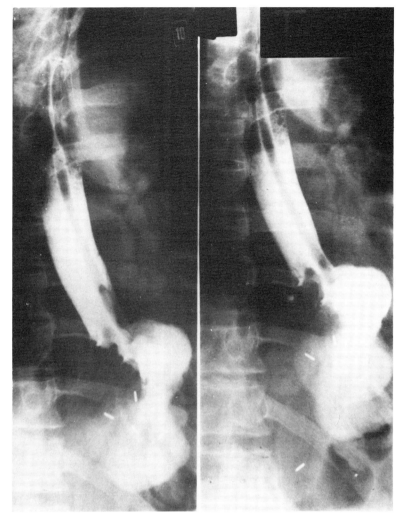

Figure 5.7
After one week of
conservative
management the leak
has sealed.
(See Fig. 5.6.)

structures cross the interval—the omohyoid muscle and middle thyroid vein superficially and the inferior thyroid artery more deeply (p. 78). Take swabs for culture and suck out all the debris and fluid. If this is an instrumental perforation, and the leak is small, repair it or merely drain it. If an anastomosis has leaked, do not attempt to repair it now, but drain it. The resulting fistula may be closed later using a skin or myocutaneous pectoralis flap. If the anastomosis is completely disrupted, disconnect it and bring the upper cut end of the oesophagus to the surface as a temporary stoma until reconstruction can be attempted at a later date. The method of dealing with the viscus that was joined on below depends on its accessibility. Preferably it should be temporarily closed with sutures, but if this cannot be achieved, insert a large tube, possibly held in with a purse-string suture, and bring the end of the tube to the surface (Fig. 5.8). Insert drainage tubes into the space into which leakage has occurred.

It will be necessary to institute alternate feeding through a central venous catheter, gastrostomy or jejunostomy. The central venous catheter should be kept well away from the site of leakage, on the opposite side from the leakage and drainage tubes. If the stomach is to be used to bridge the gap, prefer jejunostomy to gastrostomy for feeding. If necessary a stoma bag can be attached to the drain site so that first pus and later saliva are collected into it.

A small leak will seal spontaneously. Following a major leak or disruption, drained by the creation of a cervical oesophagostomy, reparative surgery can be attempted as soon as the patient has fully recovered, is nutritionally restored, and infection has been fully controlled. The stomach, colon or jejunum can be mobilized and brought up to the neck as a conduit. It is safer in the circumstances to bring the conduit subcutaneously. A segment of colon can be used to unite a cervical oesophagostomy and gastrostomy. Stomach or jejunum are less certain to reach subcutaneously to the neck.

Figure 5.8
Disruption of cervical anastomosis. Form a cervical oesophagostomy. Close or intubate the conduit and introduce an external drain.

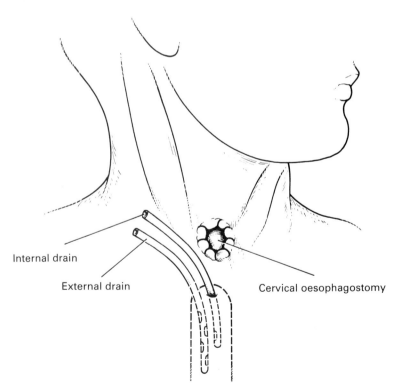

Internal drain

External drain

Cervical oesophagostomy

If the lower conduit was disconnected and drained following a leak, then it need not be resected, provided that it drains satisfactorily below. A drainage tube can be pulled out even after a track has formed; the track will soon close. The gap between this and the cervical oesophagus can often be bridged using a tube constructed of a myocutaneous flap, but consult a plastic surgical colleague to do this. Alternatively the gap can be bridged using a segment of jejunum, employing microvascular techniques to obtain a local blood supply.

Following an intrathoracic leak, explore the anastomosis through the original incision. If the leak occurred as a result of instrumentation, then explore the oesophagus from the side on which the leak was detected radiologically or endoscopically. It is usually possible to repair and drain the damage. As a rule upper intrathoracic leaks require right thoracotomy with division of the vena azygos and lower thoracic leaks require left thoracotomy or a thoracoabdominal incision (see p. 68).

It is rare to be able to salvage a leaked anastomosis because, assuming the original operation was competently performed, the leak has occurred as a result of ischaemia, infection, tension, or a combination of these, and simple resuture will be doomed. Occasionally the tissues are healthy and can be united without tension. Following oesophagogastrostomy, the stomach can sometimes be further mobilized, the leak repaired, and gastric fundus wrapped around it (Fig. 5.9).

A method that I have personally not used is to drain and defunction a leaked anastomosis. The technique can be used for an instrumental leak or following foreign body or spontaneous perforation. The leak is first drained transthoracically. A cervical oesophagostomy is then created after approaching it through an incision along the anterior border of sternomastoid, as described on p. 78. Carefully separate the oesophagus from the trachea, taking care to identify and safeguard the recurrent laryngeal nerve on the operated side, although the contralateral nerve is not seen. Draw the mobilized oesophagus to the surface. Make a longitudinal incision 2 cm long and sew the margins to the skin to create a cervical oesophagostomy (see p. 83). Create a gastrostomy or jejunostomy for the purpose of feeding the patient. Expose and encircle the abdominal oesophagus and tie a Teflon or similar tape around it to occlude the cardia. When the leak is sealed, the tapes are removed, restoring continuity. If the disruption was irrecoverable or the leak occurred from neoplastic oesophagus, it may be possible to resect it later and restore continuity.

Yet another possibility is to transect the cervical oesophagus and bring the upper cut end to the surface and to close the lower cut end with sutures before dropping it back. The leak can be drained through the chest and the oesophagus transected here or below the site, closing both ends. A gastrostomy or jejunostomy is fashioned and the gap between the cervical and abdominal

Figure 5.9
A minor leak can
sometimes be closed
and wrapped with lax
stomach.

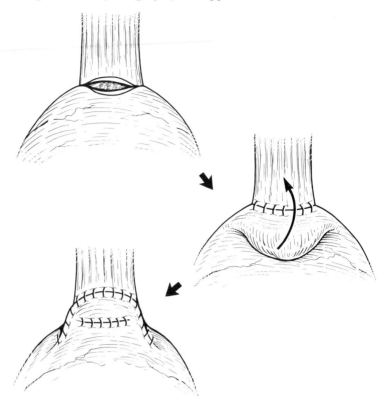

stomas bridged with stomach or bowel. The isolated oesophagus remains to form a mucocele, which causes no disability (Fig. 5.10).

Almost always the most effective procedure is to disconnect the anastomosis completely and resect the oesophagus above it to the neck. First mobilize the remaining thoracic oesophagus. Explore the neck as described (p. 78), identify and mobilize the cervical oesophagus, separating it from the trachea and drawing the thoracic remnant into the neck. Cut off the thoracic portion and suture the cut cervical oesophagus to the skin to form a stoma. The surviving viscus which was united to the oesophagus can be brought to the surface in the epigastrium for feeding purposes.

Wash out all the debris from the mediastinum and pleural cavity using sterile, warm saline solution. Insert large underwater sealed drains, with one lying at the site of the original anastomosis, before closing the chest.

As soon as the patient has fully recovered and is in a nutritionally good state plans can be made to bridge the gap between the cervical oesophagostomy and the stoma in the epigastrium, usually using colon placed subcutaneously or substernally.

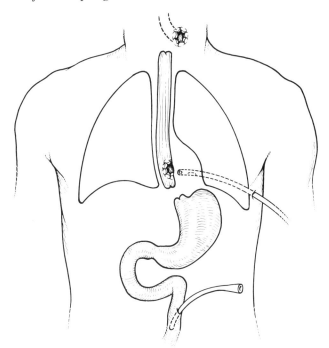

Figure 5.10
Oesophageal disruption treated by closure and isolation of the thoracic oesophagus. A cervical oesophagostomy and jejunostomy are created, and the repair is drained.

Infection

Predisposing factors

Oesophageal operations, involving as they frequently do exposure in the chest, abdomen and even the neck, leave large areas of raw tissue. The oozing which results makes an ideal site for infection to occur. If the oesophagus is ulcerated, or has been obstructed, then micro-organisms abound. When colon is brought up as a conduit, even though mechanical cleansing and prophylactic antibiotics have been instituted, contamination occurs. If there is any oesophageal obstruction, spill-over may have occurred into the respiratory tract and there may already be collapse and infection. The patient is often undernourished and may suffer from surgical shock, and is therefore susceptible to infection. The greatest liability to infection results from anastomotic leakage and from ischaemia of the viscera joined together.

Prevention

Before operation restore the patient as far as possible to a normal nutritional state. This may involve a preliminary period of feeding after dilatating a stricture, passing a fine nasal catheter through which highly nutritious fluid is constantly dripped, the creation of a preliminary feeding jejunostomy, or the insertion of a central venous feeding catheter (see Chapter 1).

Carry out adequate mechanical cleaning of the gut before operation. If there is any obstruction at the anastomosis, dilate it if possible, allowing the passage of food and also overcoming obstruction. If this is not possible, pass a naso-oesophageal tube to suck out the contents, aided by washing out with swallowed sterile water. This also protects the patient from aspirating the contents into the lungs. If colon is to be used as a conduit it should be emptied using repeated enemas or by giving oral mannitol solution to mechanically stimulate and empty it. In the past orally administered, non-absorbable antibiotics were routinely given before operation, but they are somewhat out of favour at present.

Prophylactic antibiotics may be given as a course starting after induction of anaesthetic, or as a single intravenous dose at this time.

At the time of operation the greatest care is taken to avoid leaving oozing areas and to avoid contamination from the bowel. Most important of all is to avoid the possibility of ischaemia and leakage, which are the most potent sources of infection.

Features Following major surgery a rise in temperature, signalling the increased metabolic activity, is usual, settling after about 48 hours. Almost all patients having nasoenteric tubes in place develop some pulmonary collapse following surgery, with a concomitant rise in pulse, respiratory rate and temperature. However, patients with serious infection following a major oesophageal operation have a high temperature, which develops during the first few days and is often accompanied by signs of septic shock, with unstable blood pressure, peripheral vascular shut-down producing cold extremities, and marked, rapid deterioration in general condition. The operation wound may display redness and swelling, and when a few stitches are removed, fluid or pus may be discharged.

Investigations The white cell blood count is raised. If there is any fluid discharging from the wound, or the chest or other drains, a sample should be sent for bacteriological culture, together with blood, sputum and urine samples. If there is a central venous catheter in place, replace it and send the tip for culture if no obvious cause is discovered elsewhere that has responded to active treatment.

Chest X-ray may reveal pulmonary signs of infection, or fluid within the chest which can be aspirated for bacteriological culture (Fig. 5.11). Whenever there is doubt, exclude leakage of the anastomosis by screening the patient while he swallows water-soluble radio-opaque medium. When no source of infection can be localized, ultrasonic, computed tomography and radioactive gallium scanning may help in localizing the site, and fluid may be aspirated for culture.

Management If the source of the infection is known, such as wound infection, it may be possible to treat it successfully by opening up the superficial part and allowing it to drain, without resorting to

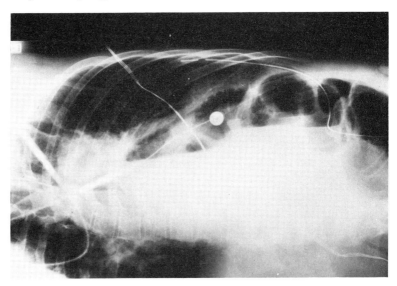

Figure 5.11
Following oesophagojejunostomy, the patient became toxic and pyrexial. Chest X-ray with the patient on his right side shows dilated loops with fluid levels, and the jejunal walls appear thickened. The Roux loop of jejunum was infarcted.

antibiotics. Similarly, vigorous physiotherapy may cure respiratory infection.

Serious infection demands the administration of a course of appropriate antibiotics, depending on the likely organisms. Initially intravenous cephalosporin and metronidazole may be started, to be changed if resistant organisms are discovered. A respiratory or urinary infection may be treated with appropriate antibiotics.

Deep-seated infection demands drainage. A static localized abscess can be drained by insertion of a needle or catheter if it is clinically evident, or under radiological or scanning control if it is not. If it does not respond to simple drainage, surgical exploration is demanded. If the patient remains septic in spite of an assiduous search for infection elsewhere, be prepared without delay to re-explore the operation site. The patient's general condition is restored as far as possible and then, with general anaesthesia, the wound is reopened in the operating theatre. A leaked anastomosis, ischaemic bowel, necrotic tissue or foreign body are identified and dealt with, followed by the institution of adequate drainage. Sometimes no active pathological lesion is discovered, but a relatively small collection of loculated pus is found. In a debilitated patient this is sufficient to delay recovery.

Throughout the management of sepsis following oesophageal resection, the patient requires the highest level of support. Sepsis in such circumstances produces a violent catabolic effect and every attempt must be made to restore the nitrogen balance with intravenous infusions of amino acids, protein-sparing calories in the form of glucose and emulsified lipid solutions, vitamins and trace elements. As soon as possible institute enteral feeding through a jejunostomy, gastrostomy, or through a nasal tube passed well beyond the anastomosis. Urinary, respiratory and cardiac function must be carefully monitored.

Chylothorax

I have not encountered this complication, but it is possible to damage the thoracic duct during oesophageal resection. As a result a milky pleural effusion develops and drains from the underwater sealed chest drain. If a drain is not in place, the patient develops an effusion, which when tapped proves to be milky chyle. Provided adequate drainage is instituted the condition can be watched for a day or two, but if it does not rapidly subside it is most important to re-explore the patient. Seek the cut thoracic duct and tie it off.

When the oesophagus is explored or anastomosed in the neck there is danger to the thoracic duct on the left side or to the lymph duct on the right side. McKeown (1978) elects to carry out cervical anastomoses on the right side, in the hope of avoiding damage to the thoracic duct on the left side.

Obstruction

Following oesophageal anastomosis there may be a temporary hold-up at the site of anastomosis from oedema. Continuing hold-up, however, suggests either leakage or ischaemia at the anastomosis, or a collection of fluid or pus outside that is compressing the anastomosis. In addition, obstruction or ischaemia of the viscus brought up to the oesophagus may cause hold-up. Obstruction may occur at other anastomoses and twisting of the bowel, with adhesions, may develop; prolapse of small bowel can occur through the diaphragm or mesenteric defects.

If a nasovisceral tube is in place, excessive volumes of aspirate are noted. In case of doubt order plain X-rays of the chest and abdomen. The patient should also be given a radiographic examination after water-soluble contrast medium has been swallowed or instilled through a tube passed through the nose into the bowel beyond to the anastomosis.

If obstruction is demonstrated, urgent re-exploration is called for as soon as the patient's condition has been restored to the optimum.

Retention

If the stomach is used as a conduit for anastomosis to the oesophagus, it is a vagotomized stomach. Some surgeons carry out pyloroplasty in the hope of improving gastric emptying, but Angorn (1975) showed that this was not necessary. I always invaginate the anterior antral wall through the pylorus to ensure that there is no stenosis or mucosal diaphragm and do not perform pyloroplasty unless there is narrowing.

Gastric retention may take days or weeks to settle and increases the risk of regurgitation of bile and acid through the anastomosis, with the fear of spill-over into the respiratory tract and consequent pulmonary collapse and aspiration pneumonia. Do not accept that the retention is physiological unless endoscopic and radiological investigations have excluded mechanical causes. If a mechanical cause is found, it is usually necessary to re-explore the patient and correct it.

When jejunum is brought up into the chest or neck, there is always redundant bowel, since the mesenteric vessels do not form a marginal supply. This forms a reservoir so that onward passage is delayed (Fig. 5.12). This can be minimized by excising the redundant bowel.

Colon can usually be safely mobilized because the marginal

Figure 5.12
As the mesenteric blood supply is shorter than the bowel, there is redundant bowel.

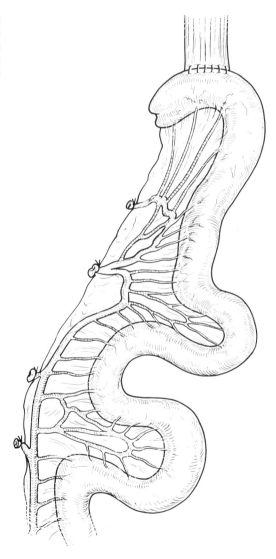

vessels are rarely deficient. If the right colon is mobilized on the middle colic vessels, the caecum can be swung proximally to join the oesophagus and the distal end anastomosed to the stomach, pylorus or jejunum below. The colon is thus isoperistaltic, and although the bowel is initially bulky, it shrinks later. The transverse colon can be used as an isoperistaltic conduit supplied by the upper left colic vessels. If the left colon is used, based on the middle colic vessels, the distal bowel is swung upwards and is thus anti-peristaltic (Fig. 5.13). Adaptation eventually occurs, but there may be considerable delay in the early weeks or even months following transposition of the left colon.

Late Complications

Recurrent stricture

Benign
Following oesophageal anastomosis stricture may develop. The earlier this occurs the more likely it is to be caused by some

Figure 5.13
If the left colon is swung up for anastomosis, it is antiperistaltic.

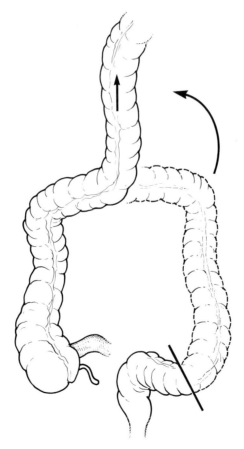

technical failure. The oesophagus or the conduit may be marginally ischaemic and undergo fibrosis. There may have been a small leak that has sealed spontaneously but which has provoked a fibrotic stricture. The stricture may also result from oesophagitis if the cardio-oesophageal reflux mechanism has been damaged or excised.

Suture material may cause inflammation and stenosis. Mechanically stapled anastomoses are not immune to late stricture formation. The oesophagus is not ideally suited to mechanical stapling because it is thick walled and often has a lumen that will accept only the smallest stapling head. The thick wall may produce too much bulk between the staple head and anvil. This causes crushing of the wall and occasionally the muscle wall is cut through. The result is possible leakage or subsequent fibrosis. If the oesophageal muscle wall is very thick, it is wise to dissect back the muscle cuff, carry out the anastomosis to the submucosal and mucosal coats, and then hand-suture the muscular coat to the seromuscularis as a second layer (Fig. 5.14).

Assess the stricture radiologically and endoscopically. A benign stricture can be managed conservatively. The Eder–Puestow guide-wire is passed through the stricture using a fibreoptic endoscope and the stricture is dilated using Eder–Puestow or Celestin dilators. However, following gastrectomy, it may not be possible to advance the guide-wire into the bowel

Figure 5.14
Oesophageal anastomosis with circular stapling device. If the oesophageal wall is thick, peel back the oesophageal muscle layer, staple the mucosa and submucosa to the bowel, and then suture the muscle to the seromuscularis of the bowel.

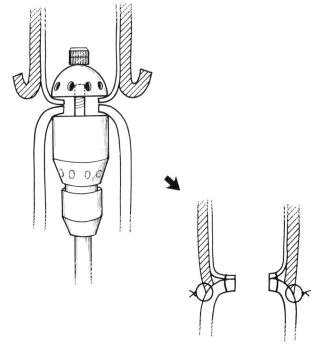

beyond. In this case it is safer to employ bougies passed under vision through a rigid endoscope (see p. 65). Immediately start the patient eating well-chewed solid food, since this is the safest oesophageal dilator. If the stricture recurs, repeat the dilatation.

Repeated stricture formation is best managed by teaching the patient to swallow Hurst's mercury-filled bougies. He sits in a chair, has his throat sprayed with lignocaine or sucks an amethocaine lozenge. The well-lubricated bougie is passed into the pharynx and the patient is asked to swallow it. If there is doubt about the success in passing the stricture, order a plain X-ray to demonstrate the level reached by the bougie. The stricture is initially dilated using the Eder–Puestow or Celestin dilators and the next day the largest Hurst's bougie that will pass is swallowed. The passage is repeated daily for a week, then every other day. The interval between passages is progressively increased. The patient rapidly learns the technique and can soon dispense with local anaesthetics.

If it is difficult to pass the Eder–Puestow guide-wire under vision, a guide-wire, over which a balloon dilator may be positioned across the stricture and inflated, may be passed under radiological control. Always check using water-soluble contrast medium that there is no split in the wall at the stricture subsequently.

Occasionally, recurring strictures are associated with stitch ulcers and the sutures protrude into the lumen. They can usually be pulled out using alligator forceps through either a flexible or rigid endoscope. Occasionally it is necessary to cut the loop using a fine scissors passed down the instrument.

If benign ulceration and stricture results from reflux and oesophagitis, it can usually be managed conservatively, as in patients who have had no previous operation.

Five rules to prevent reflux
Lose weight
Avoid tight clothing
Sleep propped up
Avoid stooping and bending
Take oral antacids and demulcents

Symptomatic improvement is usually best achieved by encouraging the patient to allow a tablet containing antacids and alginic acid, to dissolve spontaneously in the vestibule between the lower molar teeth and cheek, between meals and last thing at night.

Occasionally the reflux is caused by the mechanical arrangement, such as the anastomosis between oesophagus and distal stomach following excision of the cardia or an end-to-side anastomosis between the oesophagus and an intact loop of jejunum. Although nothing can be done following proximal gastrectomy, reflux of alkaline juice can be relieved following oesophagojejunostomy by using the 'Roux-19' technique (see p. 224). This can be carried out through the abdomen.

Malignant

This is nearly always an avoidable complication. It is well known that squamous carcinoma of the oesophagus and adenocarcinoma of the stomach spread extensively in the submucosa and the perivisceral lymphatics. Consequently it is useless to carry out the high-risk operation of resection unless the growth is given a clear margin on both sides; ideally this should be 12 cm, although this cannot be achieved routinely. Often the surgeon commits himself to a modest resection by, for example, trying to excise a carcinoma of the lower third of the oesophagus through a left thoraco-abdominal incision or a high middle third oesophageal carcinoma through a right thoracotomy. Lower third and low middle third oesophageal carcinomas are usually best excised using the Ivor Lewis technique, allowing a high resection and anastomosis through the right chest. However, for high middle, and upper third, tumours of the oesophagus a total thoracic oesophagectomy is necessary, with anastomosis of the cervical oesophagus to stomach, colon or jejunum.

When bypass is preferred the conduit should, if possible, widely bridge the unresected growth both longitudinally and laterally, otherwise it may be invaded and undergo malignant stenosis. This may be achieved using the subcutaneous or substernal route for the conduit.

If the patient experiences dysphagia following resection or bypass of a malignant tumour, obtain radiological, endoscopic and biopsy confirmation of the anatomy and pathology. Recurrent carcinoma must be treated on its merits in the same way as a primary tumour. If it appears to be localized and chest X-ray and CT scan do not reveal evidence of spread locally, to the glands or the liver, it may be worth re-exploring a fit patient. A further resection or wide bypass may be possible. If the tumour cannot be resected, mark its limits with metal clips, since it may respond to irradiation. Squamous oesophageal carcinoma is nearly always radio-sensitive and adenocarcinoma often responds also. If re-exploration is not contemplated, the CT scan allows the radiotherapist to plan treatment.

Unfortunately most patients with recurrent malignant dysphagia are not suitable for reoperation. Radiotherapy may be valuable, but meanwhile swallowing must be re-established. Endoscopically-controlled dilatation is usually possible, but the presence of a rigid and irregular tumour, or the absence of the capacious gastric reservoir beyond in some cases, may make the onward passage of a guide-wire difficult. This can sometimes be solved by passing bougies under direct vision through a rigid oesophagoscope. A decision must now be made as to whether to dilate the stricture only, or intubate it. If the stricture is easily passed but the walls are rigid, the hold-up is from failed peristalsis and the presence of a rigid plastic tube offers little relief. If the stricture is tight but elastic, dilate it and insert a tube. If the stricture splits under dilatation always impact a tube through it.

If it is impossible to dilate the stricture from above, perform gastrotomy or jejunostomy below the anastomosis through a high abdominal incision. Pass a bougie up from below. It is remarkable how effective and safe this usually is. If no other procedure is contemplated, have the anaesthetist recover the end of the bougie from the pharynx, draw it out to attach the leader of a Celestin or Mousseau–Barbin tube (see p. 73). Now draw the tube down to impact it in the stricture. Cut off the excess and close the incisions.

Very occasionally it is impossible to pass through the stricture either from above or below. In a terminal patient this can be accepted and he should be made comfortable for the last few days.

Figure 5.15
One end of a radio-opaque thread is swallowed, while the other end is attached to the cheek (a). When X-rays reveal the thread has reached the stomach—the small opacity in left upper quadrant of the abdomen (b), it is recovered and brought out through a temporary gastrostomy. It will be used to 'railroad' successively thicker threads through a previously impassable stricture so that finally a Mousseau–Barbin tube can, if necessary, be drawn through (c).

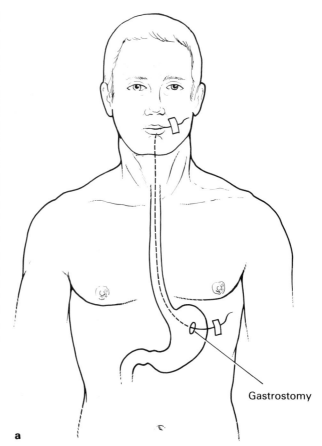

Gastrostomy

a

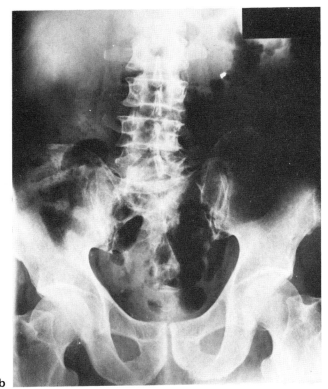

b

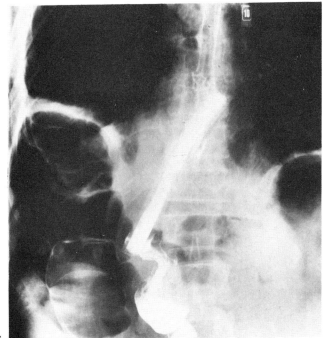

c

In a relatively fit patient the decision is agonizing. I (RMK) always give the patient a radio-opaque thread picked from a theatre swab, to one end of which is attached another thread of silk or linen which is strapped to the cheek. When X-rays demonstrate that the thread has negotiated the stricture, the lower end of the thread is recovered through the stomach or bowel. A temporary stoma is created and progressively thicker strings are attached to the upper end to be drawn through by 'railroading', while continuing to feed the patient through the stoma (Fig. 5.15). Subsequently the patient may be taken to the operating theatre and anaesthetized. The upper end of the thread is attached to the leader of a Mousseau–Barbin or Celestin tube, which is drawn through the stricture. The excess is cut off and the stoma is closed.

Many surgeons adamantly deprecate permanent gastrostomy or jejunostomy. Although I accept their arguments I cannot always set my face against the procedure. In the occasional previously vigorous patient who is starving to death in a distressful manner with the minimal intravenous fluid infusion, I have occasionally created a feeding stoma, after discussions with the patient and his relatives.

Nutritional
Patients who have had oesophagectomy, often with total or partial gastrectomy, may develop steatorrhoea, anaemia and macrocytosis. The steatorrhoea is not usually troublesome in the long term. Patients who have been subjected to oesophagectomy and anastomosis should be checked once a year with a blood count, blood haemoglobin, and serum calcium and phosphate levels, since they may also develop osteoporosis. If gastrectomy was performed, they should be given 1000 μg of vitamin B_{12}, short courses of iron tablets and, if indicated, have their calcium metabolism investigated (p. 242).

Persisting Controversies

- Best of many techniques for oesophageal resection.
- Best replacement conduit for oesophagus.
- Drainage and defunctioning of postoperative leak or complete resection and externalization?

Further reading
Akiyama, H., Tsurumaru, M., Watanabe, G., Ono, Y., Udagawa, H. & Suzuki, M. (1984) Development of surgery for carcinoma of the esophagus. *American Journal of Surgery*, *147*, 9–16.
Allison, P.R. & Da Silva, L.T. (1953/54) The Roux loop. *British Journal of Surgery*, *41*, 173–180.
Angorn, I.B. (1975) Oesophagectomy without a drainage procedure in oesophageal carcinoma. *British Journal of Surgery*, *62*, 601–604.

Cameron, J.L., Kieffer, R.F., Hendrix, T.R., Mehigan, D.G. & Baker, R.R. (1979) Selective nonoperative management of contained intrathoracic esophageal disruptions. *Annals of Thoracic Surgery*, *27*, 404–408.

Farndon, J.R. & Taylor, R.M.R. (1977) Cervical pharyngostomy. *Annals of the Royal College of Surgeons of England*, *59*, 507–510.

Kirk, R.M. (1981) A trial of total gastrectomy, combined with total thoracic oesophagectomy without formal thoracotomy, for·carcinoma at or near the cardia of the stomach. *British Journal of Surgery*, *68*, 577–579.

Kirk, R.M. (1983) Double indemnity in oesophageal carcinoma. *British Medical Journal*, *286*, 582–583.

Kirk, R.M. & Williamson, R.C.N. (1986) *General Surgical Operations*, 2nd Edn. Edinburgh: Churchill Livingstone.

Lancet (1977) The leaking oesophagus. *Lancet*, *ii*, 692–693.

McKeown, K.C. (1978) Carcinoma of the oesophagus. *Annals of the Royal College of Surgeons of England*, *60*, 301–303.

Ong, G.B. (1975) Unresectable carcinoma of the oesophagus. *Annals of the Royal College of Surgeons of England*, *56*, 3–14.

Postlethwait, R.W., Deaton, W.R. Jr, Bradshaw, H.H., Williams, R.W. & Winston-Salem, N.C. (1950) Esophageal anastomosis: types and methods of suture. *Surgery*, *28*, 537–542.

Thal, A.P. & Hatafuku, T. (1964) Improved operation for esophageal rupture. *Journal of the American Medical Association*, *188*, 826–828.

Thompson, W.R. & Goldstein, L.A. (1982) Esophageal perforations: a 15-year experience. *American Journal of Surgery*, *143*, 495–503.

Wu, Y.K. & Huang, K.C. (1979) Chinese experience in the surgical treatment of carcinoma of the esophagus. *Annals of Surgery*, *190*, 361–365.

6 Complications of Antireflux Surgery

There has been a major change in emphasis in the surgical treatment of gastro-oesophageal reflux over the past 25 years. Formerly hiatus hernia operations had two objectives: (i) to mobilize the hiatus hernia and return the stomach to the abdominal cavity; and (ii) to prevent redisplacement of the stomach back into the chest by suturing it to an intra-abdominal structure, such as the anterior abdominal wall, or to the undersurface, or median arcuate ligament of the diaphragm. In the mid 1950s it was realized that the principal barrier to gastro-oesophageal reflux was the lower oesophageal sphincter and that factors such as the angle of His, the phreno-oesophageal ligament and other tenuous peritoneal attachments in the area were less important. Operations are now designed to restore a high-pressure zone at the lower end of the oesophagus. This can be achieved by some form of 'fundoplication', whereby the fundus of the stomach is wrapped around, and anchored to the lower oesophagus. Most antireflux procedures now performed, whether through the chest or the abdomen, have three basic steps:

1 Re-establishment of a segment of intra-abdominal oesophagus
2 Reduction in size of the diaphragmatic hiatal defect by suturing the two margins of the right crus together
3 Fixation of the fundus of the stomach around the lower oesophagus—'the fundoplication'

Tethering operations such as anterior gastropexy have become less fashionable, for they do nothing to increase the pressure at the lower end of the oesophagus. The most recent addition to the surgeon's repertoire has been the use of a silicone Angelchik prosthesis. When this prosthesis is used the lower oesophagus is mobilized and then encircled by the silicone collar. This is held in position just above the gastro-oesophageal junction by tying and securely fastening the attached tapes. The device is not fixed directly to the oesophagus or the stomach. The technique is popular in North America and is currently on trial in a number of centres in the United Kingdom. Many surgeons believe that further strict evaluation is necessary before this prosthesis can be accepted as a satisfactory alternative to the conventional operations. Complications related to the use of the Angelchik prosthesis are described in a separate section in this chapter.

The adage 'prevention is better than cure' certainly applies to the complications of antireflux surgery. The operation is relatively straightforward and the incidence of complications can be reduced if attention is paid to the following details:

- Selection of patients for operation
- Choice of operation
- Operative technique

Selection of patients for operation
Careful selection of patients for operation is a major determinant of the success of the procedure. Ideally patients should have a good history of heartburn and regurgitation, evidence of oesophagitis on endoscopy and excessive acid reflux on 24 hour ambulatory intraoesophageal pH monitoring. They should not be smokers, not be overweight and have had a long trial of medical treatment which has failed to control their reflux symptoms. Neuromuscular disorders of the oesophagus, such as achalasia, must be excluded.

Patients frequently fail to fulfil all these criteria. Only 60% of patients with reflux oesophagitis have a typical history. Disabling symptoms can occur with little endoscopic evidence of macroscopic oesophagitis. Some patients have pancreaticobiliary reflux from duodenum to stomach and this material is then refluxed into the oesophagus. In this group of patients the 24 hour pH studies may not show any apparent abnormality using a conventional intraoesophageal pH recording technique. Smokers may not abstain from their habit and for some patients weight loss may be a desired, rather than an achieved goal. There is an overlap of symptoms in many upper gastrointestinal disorders which can make accurate diagnosis difficult. Two pathological conditions may occur simultaneously. Fifty per cent of duodenal ulcer patients have gastro-oesophageal reflux symptoms and one-third have endoscopic evidence of oesophagitis. Gastro-oesophageal reflux may not be the primary problem but may occur because of gastric outlet obstruction secondary to benign pyloric stenosis or an antral carcinoma.

Preoperative upper gastrointestinal endoscopy is necessary in all patients to confirm the presence of macroscopic oesophagitis whenever possible and to exclude other disorders, especially duodenal ulceration. Twenty-four hour intraoesophageal pH studies may be performed to quantitate the duration of abnormal reflux but are not mandatory in all patients. It is unlikely that pH studies would affect the management of a patient with reflux symptoms and severe oesophagitis who has failed to respond to medical treatment. However, pH studies are valuable in patients with typical reflux symptoms but no evidence of oesophagitis on endoscopy, when the surgeon wishes to compare the degree of reflux pre- and postoperatively, and when two methods of antireflux procedure are being compared in a clinical trial.

The principal indication for antireflux surgery is the failure of intensive medical treatment to control the patient's reflux symptoms. The patient generally has severe oesophagitis on endoscopy but no other upper gastrointestinal disorders. Abnormal pH studies will identify another group of patients with disabling reflux symptoms, but no oesophagitis endoscopically, who would benefit from surgery. Complications of reflux such as an oesophageal stricture, haemorrhage or a columnar-lined (Barrett's) oesophagus usually occur in patients with particularly severe reflux. The development of these complications in the young or middle-aged patient is an indication for antireflux surgery if there are no other contraindications to operation.

Choice of operation

A large number of different operations have been described for the treatment of gastro-oesophageal reflux. Modifications to original operations have been made. These are testimonies to the fact that there is no completely successful operation. Whichever operation is performed, perfection of operative technique is important. Many patients are suitable candidates for either a thoracic or an abdominal procedure and the choice of operation depends on the surgeon's individual preference.

Abdominal approach

The duration of operation and length of in-patient stay are less than after thoracotomy. Other intra-abdominal conditions such as cholelithiasis or duodenal ulceration may be present and can be treated appropriately during the same operation. Persistent pain in the wound is less frequent than after thoracotomy. However, it may be difficult to mobilize the lower oesophagus from the abdomen. This is particularly the case in the presence of severe perioesophagitis, acquired oesophageal shortening or when a sliding hiatus hernia more than 8 cm in length is present. Previous abdominal surgery may make a transabdominal approach difficult. If gastric or duodenal surgery has been performed, the stomach may be adherent to the under surface of the liver. Splenic damage is commoner after transabdominal antireflux surgery.

Thoracic approach

This allows a more thorough mobilization of the oesophagus under direct vision, which is valuable where there is perioesophagitis or a large hiatus hernia. If necessary all the intrathoracic oesophagus can be freed. However, thoracotomy is a more formidable operation than laparotomy for the patient and 10–15% will have persistent troublesome post-thoracotomy pain.

A surgeon who regularly undertakes antireflux surgery should be versatile and able to perform either a transthoracic or a transabdominal operation. I (CJS) favour an abdominal approach, reserving the transthoracic or a combined thoracoabdominal operation for patients with a large hiatus hernia and for some patients who have had a previous thoracotomy.

Operative technique

A transabdominal operation is facilitated by use of a sternal retractor to lift the sternum and costal margin upwards (Fig. 6.1). This improves access to the oesophageal hiatus and makes it unnecessary to divide the triangular ligament attaching the left lobe of the liver to the diaphragm. The hiatus can be seen

Figure 6.1
Sternal retractor used to facilitate transabdominal antireflux surgery.

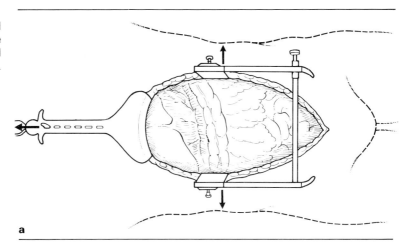

a

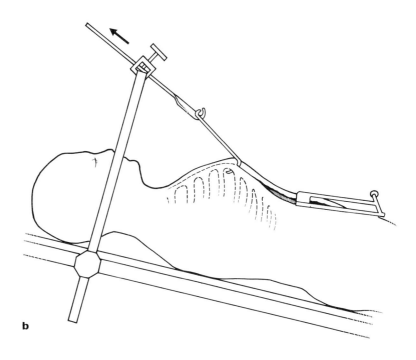

b

adequately by gently elevating the left lobe of the liver with a broad Kelly's retractor.

Oesophageal and fundal mobilization

Be careful and thorough in the mobilization of the lower oesophagus and the fundus of the stomach. Use sharp rather than blunt dissection with fingers or swabs. Cutting tissues causes less tissue damage and is less likely to produce local oedema. Cut blood vessels bleed readily and are more easy to identify for ligation or diathermy coagulation. This reduces the risk of a perioesophageal haematoma. With an abdominal approach first divide the peritoneum over the anterior surface of the oesophagus and continue the dissection on the left lateral side in the angle of His (Fig. 6.2). The oesophagus can then be lifted forwards easily for mobilization of its posterior and right lateral aspects. Be careful not to damage the vagus nerves. This is more likely to occur if the patient has had previous gastric surgery. Do not attempt to repair the right crus or begin the fundoplication before at least the lower 6 cm of the oesophagus has been mobilized. By gentle traction on the stomach the lower oesophageal vessels will become taut and can be easily seen or felt, diathermied and then divided. Mobilize the fundus by dividing the peritoneal reflection passing onto the under surface of the diaphragm. It is not necessary to divide the short gastric vessels, but be careful not to damage the superior short gastric artery as the peritoneal reflection is divided.

The same care is necessary when the oesophagus is mobilized during a transthoracic operation. Smaller oesophageal arteries may be diathermied and cut but the larger branches from the aorta should be ligated and divided. Do not damage the thoracic

Figure 6.2
Mobilization of the lower oesophagus and gastro-oesophageal junction by sharp dissection in the angle of His.

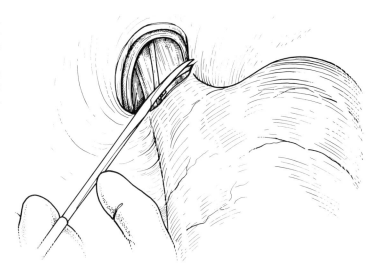

duct. This passes through the aortic opening in the diaphragm and ascends between the thoracic vertebrae and the right side of the descending aorta. It crosses behind the oesophagus at the level of the fifth thoracic vertebra and continues its ascent behind the subclavian artery at the left border of the oesophagus. Damage to the thoracic duct may occur anywhere along its course but is most frequent in the lower chest. Keep close to the oesophageal wall when mobilizing the oesophagus from the surrounding structures. Avoid damage to the ascending branch of the left gastric artery on the right lateral wall of the oesophagus.

Crural repair
Having mobilized the lower oesophagus assess the size of the oesophageal hiatus. If more than two fingers can be passed through the hiatus, approximate the margins of the right crus behind the oesophagus (Fig. 6.3). Two or three interrupted non-absorbable sutures of linen or silk are usually sufficient. When the approximation is complete it should be possible to insert the index finger comfortably through the hiatus alongside the oesophagus. If the hiatus will not admit a finger, the crural repair is too tight and the upper suture should be removed for fear of producing postoperative dysphagia.

The crural repair is performed for two reasons. First, it prevents displacement of the fundoplication into the mediastinum, which would result in compression of the body of the stomach by the diaphragm. Secondly, it reduces the chance of development of a postoperative paraoesophageal hernia containing either stomach or other abdominal structures such as transverse colon entering the chest. When an Angelchik prosthesis is used crural repair prevents its angulation and migration into the mediastinum.

Fundoplication
The fundoplication may involve encirclement of either the entire oesophageal circumference, e.g. a Nissen procedure or alternatively only 270–300° of the circumference, e.g. a Belsey or Lind procedure (Figs 6.4–6.6). Ideally the fundoplication should be approximately 3 cm in length and should be constructed without tension using non-absorbable sutures. We use 2/0 linen. When performing a total fundoplication (Nissen) have an F36 or F40 mercury weighted dilator positioned across the gastro-oesophageal junction as the fundoplication is constructed. This seems to be unnecessary with partial fundoplication. When the dilator is removed it should be possible to insert a finger between the oesophagus and the fundoplication (Fig. 6.7). If the wrap is too tight, it may be associated with persistent postoperative dysphagia, the gas bloat syndrome or even disruption with recurrence of reflux symptoms.

The sutures should pass through the seromuscular layer of the

Figure 6.3
Approximation of the
margins of the right
crus behind the
oesophagus.

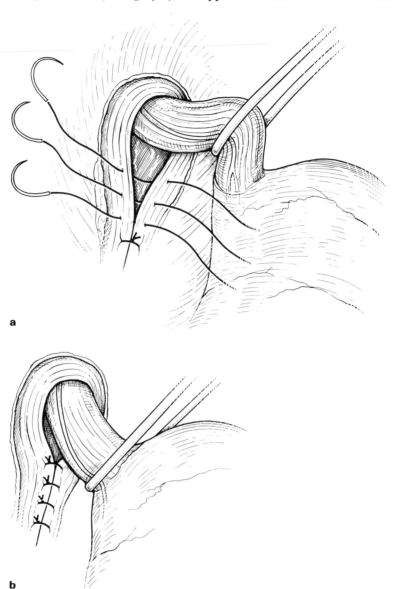

a

b

gastric wall but not the mucosa, for fear of causing either
bacterial contamination in the area, with development of a
subphrenic abscess, or a gastric fistula. Do not grasp the stomach
with Babcock's or Duval's forceps for fear of damaging the wall.
The sutures must also be attached to the superficial layers of the
oesophageal wall so that the wrap is firmly anchored in position
(Fig. 6.8). This prevents the gastro-oesophageal junction being
drawn through the fundoplication by the forceful contractions of

Figure 6.4
Nissen antireflux
procedure.

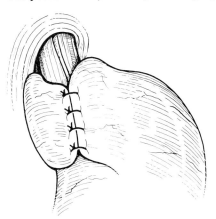

Figure 6.5
Belsey antireflux
procedure.

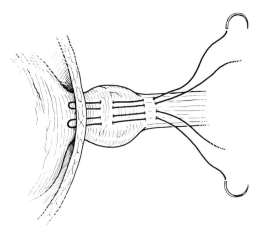

Figure 6.6
Lind antireflux
procedure.

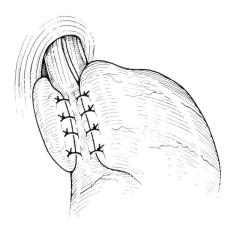

Figure 6.7
There should be room
to insert a finger
between the
oesophagus and
fundoplication.

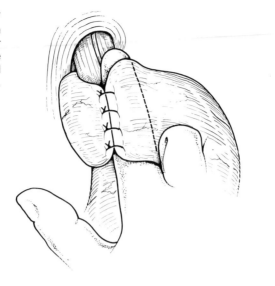

Figure 6.8
The fundoplication
sutures in the Nissen
procedure also pass
through the
oesophageal muscle.

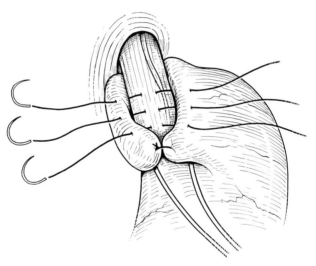

the longitudinal oesophageal muscle. Additional intra-abdominal fixation can be achieved by passing the upper suture of the fundoplication through the margin of the right crus of the diaphragm as it crosses the anterior surface of the oesophagus or by attaching the fundoplication to the undersurface of the diaphragm.

Care must be taken to identify the gastro-oesophageal junction accurately and to wrap the fundus around the oesophagus and not around the proximal stomach. If this error occurs, severe dysphagia results, for the fundus above the wrap is unable to generate enough pressure to overcome the extrinsic compression. Similarly, special care must be taken with the construction of the fundoplication when an antireflux procedure is performed after oesophagomyotomy, for achalasia or diffuse oesophageal spasm, or in a patient with scleroderma. These patients have poor (or absent) oesophageal peristalsis, and a standard fundoplication may produce postoperative dysphagia. A fundoplication in these patients should be no more than 2 cm in length, must not be at all 'tight' and preferably should be of the partial rather than the complete type.

Some patients may have coexistent duodenal ulceration and gastro-oesophageal reflux, both of which require surgical treatment. Reduction in acid secretion by vagotomy is insufficient to control the reflux symptoms. In this situation I believe that the best operation is a highly selective vagotomy combined with a partial fundoplication. Pyloroplasty or gastroenterostomy should be avoided because of pancreaticobiliary reflux and the possibility of subsequent biliary oesophagitis.

Postoperative Dysphagia

Dysphagia is a relatively common occurrence in the immediate postoperative period. It is more likely after total rather than partial fundoplication, and has been reported to occur in up to 50% of patients soon after a Nissen fundoplication. In most patients it is mild, transient and resolves within four weeks of operation. Six months postoperatively only 5–6% of patients still have dysphagia and by 1 year the figure has fallen further to between 2 and 3%.

Aetiology   Postoperative dysphagia may be due to:

- Local oedema
- Perioesophageal haematoma
- Excessive narrowing of the oesophageal hiatus
- Tight fundoplication
- Incorrectly placed fundoplication
- Displaced fundoplication
- Motility abnormality in the body of the oesophagus
- Persistent reflux and an oesophageal stricture
- Association with scleroderma or achalasia

In the immediate postoperative period any of these causes may be responsible for the dysphagia. The rapid resolution in the majority of patients suggests that local oedema, possibly associated with perioesophageal haematoma formation, is the commonest factor. Persistent dysphagia for more than two months is not due to oedema but to either a mechanical obstruction at the lower end of the oesophagus or a motility disturbance in the body of the oesophagus.

Investigation and treatment   The management of patients with postoperative dysphagia depends on the severity of symptoms and the time interval since operation. Mild dysphagia in the first ten days usually resolves without any treatment. There is no need for a barium swallow, endoscopy or oesophageal dilatation. Instruct the patient to avoid food such as meat, bread and potatoes until the symptoms subside as the perioesophageal oedema resolves. Reassurance that mild dysphagia generally resolves is good for the patient's morale.

Severe dysphagia which persists for more than 14 days after operation demands investigation. A plan of investigation is shown in Table 6.1. Perform a barium swallow using dilute barium to identify whether a mechanical obstruction is present and to give some indication of the size of the oesophageal lumen. Cine radiology will allow careful review of oesophageal motility. If narrowing is appreciable or there is considerable delay in the passage of the barium into the stomach, oesophageal dilatation is required after oesophageal lavage via a naso-oesophageal tube. Perform fibreoptic endoscopy before dilatation to determine

Table 6.1
Plan for the investigation of postoperative dysphagia following antireflux surgery.

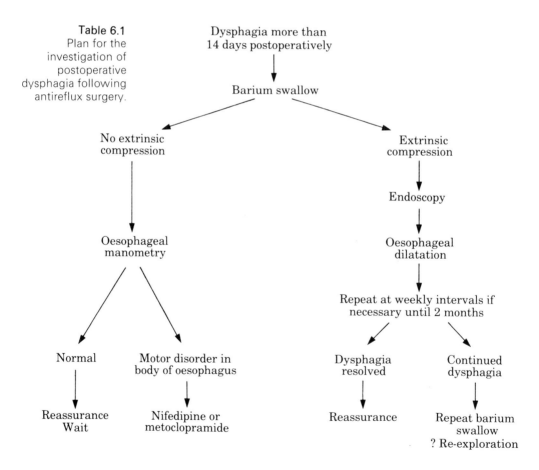

whether the dysphagia is due to (i) extrinsic compression from a tight crural repair or fundoplication, or (ii) persistent reflux with oesophagitis and an oesophageal stricture. Eder–Puestow's or Celestin's dilators may be used for the dilatation but our preference is for Maloney's or Hurst's mercury weighted dilators (Fig. 6.9). The patient sits upright, the pharynx is anaesthetized with 1% local anaesthetic spray, the bougie is placed in the pharynx and the patient is asked to swallow. Begin with a size F36 dilator and pass further bougies increasing in F6 increments until resistance to dilatation is first felt. The next bougie in the series should be passed and the dilatation terminated for that session. This procedure can be repeated in 48 hours and at weekly intervals thereafter until dysphagia disappears. Symptoms should improve after dilatation, but may recur.

If the dysphagia does not respond to dilatation and persists for more than two to three months, repeat the barium swallow, looking carefully at the site of obstruction. Try to determine whether the obstruction is due to compression by the right crus or fundoplication or whether the fundoplication was incorrectly wrapped around the stomach because of inadequate distal oesophageal mobilization. If there is extrinsic compression and the patient is losing weight or aspirating oesophageal contents, reoperation must be considered. Total dysphagia is an absolute indication for re-exploration, but with lesser degrees of oesophageal compression the decision to reoperate will depend on the degree of oesophageal narrowing, weight loss and the severity of respiratory problems.

Figure 6.9
(A) Maloney's and
(B) Hurst's mercury
weighted dilators.

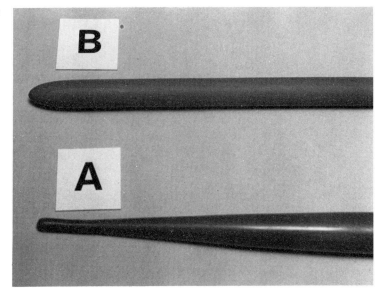

Dysphagia may be due to a motor abnormality in the body of the oesophagus rather than to mechanical obstruction. A motility disorder is responsible for dysphagia in more than half of the patients who are symptomatic one year after operation. Oesophageal manometry should be performed, looking particularly for repetitive, non-propulsive contractions or for aperistalsis in a patient with previously unsuspected scleroderma. Very rarely a diagnosis of achalasia may have been missed, the patient's preoperative dysphagia being incorrectly attributed to gastro-oesophageal reflux with a benign stricture. Patients with motility disorders do not have a lasting response to oesophageal dilatation. They may improve with nifedipine 10 mg. t.d.s. Metoclopramide or domperidone may be tried as alternatives.

Patients without a preoperative oesophageal stricture should not require dilatation more than one year after an antireflux procedure. If dilatation is necessary, then consider:

1 Was the initial diagnosis correct?
2 Does the patient have achalasia?
3 Does the patient have a motor abnormality?
4 Is re-exploration necessary?

Reoperation for
Dysphagia
Dysphagia is the commonest complication of fundoplication which requires reoperation. However, reoperation for dysphagia is necessary in less than 2% of patients who undergo antireflux surgery. Re-explore the patient through the original incision. Carefully separate the stomach from the undersurface of the diaphragm or the visceral pleura from the parietal pleura and lung. Inspect the diaphragmatic hiatus. Is the crural repair too tight? Will an index finger pass between the oesophagus and the margins of the right crus? If not, divide the last suture of the crural repair thus enlarging the hiatus.

If the crural repair is satisfactory, re-examine the fundoplication. Is the stomach correctly wrapped around the lower oesophagus? What is the length of the wrap and is it too tight? If the fundoplication is incorrectly placed or the patient has developed a 'slipped wrap', it must be dismantled and then reconstituted in the correct position. Be careful not to open the fundus, as this may result in a gastric fistula or subphrenic abscess. If the original fundoplication is more than 5 cm in length and no other abnormality can be found at the oesophageal hiatus, the fundoplication should be revised to one of 3 cm. Patients with a paraoesophageal hernia which develops after a previous antireflux procedure must have further surgery to reduce the hernia and effect a crural repair. There is considerable risk of strangulation and perforation of the herniated viscus if the abnormality is not corrected.

When significant postoperative dysphagia occurs in patients with either scleroderma or after oesophagomyotomy plus an antireflux procedure for achalasia, the symptom is unlikely to resolve without further surgery. Take down the original fundo-plication, and if surgical control of reflux is necessary, construct a lax partial fundoplication.

Intussusception Recurrence

This condition is due to the migration of the stomach through an intact fundoplication (Fig. 6.10) and occurs almost exclusively after a Nissen procedure. Because of the thickness of the gastric wall which herniates through the fundoplication, the lumen of the stomach is narrowed, producing obstruction. Dysphagia occurs, with accompanying weight loss, and there may be associated nausea and vomiting.

It may be difficult to differentiate an intussusception recur-rence from a tight repair, both symptomatically and radiologi-cally. However, the former develops some months or years after the initial operation, whereas the latter is usually evident immediately postoperatively. The risk of developing this compli-cation may be reduced by ensuring that the fundoplication sutures pass through the oesophageal wall as well as the fundus of the stomach (Fig. 6.8).

This condition may be difficult to diagnose. Solids added to the barium solution may aid radiological diagnosis. Manometry will exclude an oesophageal motor abnormality but will not confirm the diagnosis. The obstruction may not be recognized endoscopi-cally and oesophageal dilatation rarely improves the symptoms. Delayed onset dysphagia with radiological obstruction following a previous Nissen procedure are the warning signs. If the diagnosis is made, further surgery is required, for medical treatment will always fail. The previous fundoplication should be dismantled and a new one reconstructed in the correct position. The fundus must be securely fixed to the oesophagus to prevent a recurrence of the same problem.

Oesophageal Perforation

Predisposing causes

Perforation may occur during mobilization of the lower oesopha-gus. The risk is greatest with a transabdominal approach to a large hiatus hernia or when there is marked perioesophagitis from long-standing reflux. The perforation is usually on the posterior aspect of the oesophagus and is related to blunt oesophageal mobilization with the fingers rather than sharp dissection. Excessive force applied to a sling placed around the oesophagus just above the oesophagogastric junction may also damage the posterior wall of the oesophagus. Intraoperative dilatation of an oesophageal stricture in either an antegrade or a retrograde direction may result in perforation. Rarely, an oesophageal ulcer, which usually occurs in association with a columnar-lined oesophagus, may perforate as the oesophagus is freed.

Prevention   The lower oesophagus and cardia should be mobilized carefully, by sharp dissection, particularly in the situations described above. Do not apply excessive force to a sling placed around the oesophagus. After oesophageal mobilization always inspect its intra-abdominal portion, particularly the posterior wall, for signs of damage before proceeding to the crural repair or fundoplication.

Recognition   The oesophageal perforation may be one of three types:

1 A longitudinal tear
2 A circular or oval defect due to perforation of an ulcer
3 Severe disruption of a major part of the oesophageal circumference

With transthoracic procedures the perforation is usually longitudinal and easy to see intraoperatively. If a perforation is recognized during operation, note its site and length and perform an immediate closure. Ideally this should be in two layers: an inner continuous catgut and an outer layer of interrupted non-absorbable suture material. If it is difficult to perform a two-layer closure, use a single layer of interrupted non-absorbable sutures. Some tears situated just above the gastro-oesophageal junction do not cause any postoperative problems even if unrecognized and untreated, for the defect is covered by the fundoplication.

If the oesophageal perforation is above the level of the fundoplication and is not closed at the time of surgery, leakage of intraoesophageal contents will occur into the mediastinum. The symptoms of oesophageal perforation may be masked by regular postoperative narcotic analgesics. The postoperative symptoms and signs suggestive of oesophageal perforation are severe substernal pain exacerbated by swallowing, a persistent tachycardia and pyrexia, or subcutaneous emphysema in the supraclavicular fossae. Initially the mediastinitis is a chemical inflammation, but within a few hours bacterial contamination occurs and the patient may become septicaemic, with hypotension, tachycardia, peripheral vasoconstriction and oliguria.

When oesophageal perforation is suspected perform a penetrated posteroanterior chest X-ray. This may show mediastinal widening or emphysema. There may be a hydropneumothorax if there is communication with a pleural cavity (usually the left). The site and extent of the oesophageal perforation should be determined by contrast radiology using a water-soluble contrast medium such as Gastrografin.

Infrequently mediastinitis occurs from contamination at the time of surgery, without an oesophageal perforation. The patient

Figure 6.10
(a) X-ray, and
(b) Diagrammatic
illustration of an
intussusception
recurrence.

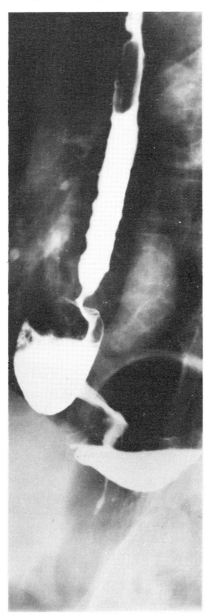

a

has a high swinging fever and tachycardia suggestive of infection, but surgical emphysema and a hydropneumothorax are absent. No perforation is seen on Gastrografin swallow, but there may be mediastinal widening on a chest X-ray. If a mediastinal abscess is suspected, the diagnosis may be confirmed by radionuclide scanning using gallium or radioactive-labelled leucocytes or alternatively by a computed tomography scan.

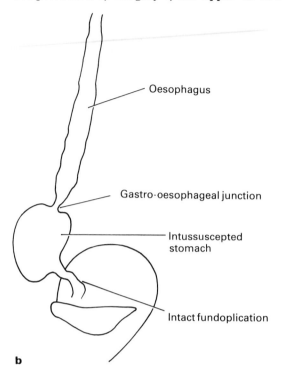

Oesophagus

Gastro-oesophageal junction

Intussuscepted stomach

Intact fundoplication

b

Treatment A detailed account of the management of oesophageal perforation has been given in Chapter 4. If recognized intraoperatively, an oesophageal perforation should be repaired immediately
and the patient given broad-spectrum antibiotics. For a longitudinal split insert the sutures at right-angles to the long axis of
the oesophagus, taking care to narrow the oesophageal lumen as
little as possible. Close a circular defect transversely. The choice
of suture material for these repairs is a matter of personal choice.
Some surgeons prefer catgut, whereas others use non-absorbable
materials such as silk or Nuralon.

When an oesophageal perforation is suspected postoperatively
and confirmed radiologically the factors that determine treatment are as follows:

1 Extent of the perforation and leakage
2 Communication with the pleural cavity
3 Time interval since operation
4 Type of operation performed initially
5 Site of the perforation

If a hydropneumothorax is present, insert an underwater
sealed chest drain via the sixth intercostal space in the anterior
axillary line. Commence broad-spectrum antibiotics and intravenous feeding and withhold oral fluid and food. If the leak is
small and adjacent to the fundoplication, position a nasogastric

tube with multiple side holes above and below the perforation and connect it to gentle and continuous suction.

Benign oesophageal strictures should be dilated on a separate occasion prior to antireflux surgery. This avoids the risk of instrumental perforation of the oesophagus when the dilatation is performed immediately prior to the antireflux procedure. An alternative manoeuvre is to dilate the oesophageal stricture retrogradely, intraoperatively through a small gastrotomy. Dilatation from below is often safer and easier than from above. If instrumental perforation occurs following dilatation, the oesophageal defect is invariably large and communicates with the pleural cavity. Reoperation rather than medical management of the perforation is required. A full thoracotomy is necessary on the same side as the pneumothorax. The various methods that can be used to close the perforation are described in Chapter 4. The management of an intrathoracic oesophageal perforation discovered more than five days after operation is controversial. Sutures inserted into the friable oesophageal wall frequently cut out and rarely can a satisfactory closure be achieved. If the oesophageal leak is only small on contrast radiology, persevere with nonoperative treatment. However, if there is severe disruption, thoracotomy is required, and it may be necessary to completely excise the thoracic oesophagus if the patient is to survive. A cervical oesophagostomy is constructed and the gastro-oesophageal junction oversewn. A feeding jejunostomy is inserted for postoperative enteral nutrition. A gastrostomy should be avoided, for the stomach will later be used to anastomose to the oesophagus as a third procedure when all the intrathoracic sepsis has resolved.

Ensure by contrast radiology that the perforation has completely sealed before oral feeding is reintroduced. A benign stricture may develop at the site of the perforation and require dilatation. Wait at least three to four weeks after the perforation has closed before attempting the dilatation. Use Celestin's or Eder–Puestow's dilators passed over a guide-wire rather than blind dilatation using mercury-weighted bougies.

Bleeding

Bleeding may occur from the ascending branch of the left gastric, oesophageal, intercostal or internal mammary arteries or the spleen. Intraoperative damage to the inferior pulmonary vein during thoracotomy results in massive bleeding, which requires immediate treatment. Intrathoracic bleeding from either the inferior pulmonary ligament or from an intercostal vessel may be missed at the time of surgery and present as a postoperative haemothorax.

Splenic haemorrhage poses the greatest bleeding problem, particularly after transabdominal antireflux surgery. Traction on the spleen or omentum may tear an adhesion attached to the splenic capsule, producing bleeding from the splenic surface; traction on the gastrosplenic ligament may damage a branch of the splenic vein in the hilum.

Prevention　Divide adhesions between spleen, colon and omentum early in the procedure before traction-induced damage occurs. Insertion of a large moist abdominal pack behind the spleen displaces it anteromedially and reduces the risk of damage to hilar vessels. With a transthoracic approach be careful not to damage the ascending branch of the left gastric artery or the uppermost short gastric vessels. Check for evidence of bleeding, especially around the spleen, before the abdomen or chest is closed.

Recognition and　The management of bleeding depends on the time of recognition, *treatment*　mode of presentation and severity. Intraoperative bleeding is controlled initially by pressure, followed by identification and appropriate treatment of the bleeding point. If splenic damage occurs, splenic preservation is preferable to splenectomy whenever possible (Chapter 12). Splenectomy triples the complication rate of antireflux surgery (Rogers, Herrington & Morton, 1980).

Unrecognized and untreated bleeding leads to hypovolaemic shock. The signs of shock may improve with rapid transfusion but deteriorate again as the rate of transfusion is decreased. If there is no evidence of external blood loss perform an ECG to exclude cardiogenic shock due to myocardial infarction. If the diagnosis is still in doubt or if transfusion requirements are difficult to determine, monitor the central venous pressure. This will be low in a patient with hypovolaemic shock but high in cardiogenic shock. Do not be lulled into a sense of false security if no blood issues from an intraperitoneal drain. Both suction and tube drains can become blocked with clotted blood and conceal a major intraperitoneal haemorrhage. If hypotension occurs due to hypovolaemia the patient should be re-explored as soon as possible. Give plasma expanders to correct the hypotension until blood is available. This will reduce the risk of acute tubular necrosis of the kidney. At operation remove the intraperitoneal clot and locate the bleeding point. This may be difficult because of generalized oozing. A splenic capsular injury can usually be managed satisfactorily by a combination of local pressure, gentle diathermy coagulation and application of locally haemostatic substances such as oxidized regenerated cellulose (Surgicel gauze). If the bleeding is from the splenic hilum, a partial or total splenectomy may be necessary for complete control.

Intrathoracic bleeding is less of a problem. The inflated lungs cause a tamponade effect and the haemorrhage is rarely concealed, the blood draining readily through the chest drain. If hypotension occurs after thoracotomy, check that there is oscillation of fluid in the tube in the drainage bottle. The absence of oscillation could be due to a blood clot on the end of the chest drain, which should be flushed with sterile saline. Be careful not to cause a pneumothorax. If the patient has been hypotensive and there is a significant haemothorax on chest X-ray in the 24 hours after surgery, the chest should be reopened, the blood evacuated and the bleeding point controlled.

Gas Bloat Syndrome

Clinical features This syndrome is characterized by postcibal epigastric discomfort and distension associated with an inability to eructate or vomit. Air is swallowed during a meal, but because the fundoplication is 'super competent' the air becomes trapped in the stomach, causing the distension and discomfort. This syndrome occurs most frequently after total fundoplication, particularly when the wrap is more than 4 cm in length and when the operation is performed without an oesophageal dilator in position. The symptoms are worst in the immediate postoperative period and usually improve within the first few months of operation. Six months after a Nissen fundoplication only 2 or 3% of patients have troublesome gas bloat symptoms.

Management Explain the mechanism of the symptoms to the patient. Eating food dry and drinking between meals may reduce the amount of air entering the stomach in a short space of time. Repetitive dry swallows in an attempt to promote belching should be avoided as these will exacerbate rather than relieve the situation. If gas bloat symptoms persist for more than six months after operation, they are unlikely to resolve. A further laparotomy, with dismantling of the fundoplication and construction of either a 'floppy' repair or a partial fundoplication, may be necessary in a severely afflicted patient. Postprandial epigastric distension and fullness may be due to gastric stasis secondary to vagal damage. These patients usually have associated vomiting, thus differentiating them from patients with a true gas bloat syndrome. If there is any doubt, perform a radioisotope gastric emptying study. An insulin (Hollander) test may also be useful in determining whether gastric vagal denervation has occurred. A patient with gastric retention should be treated initially with metoclopramide or domperidone. If the symptoms fail to improve within a few weeks, then a gastric drainage procedure (pyloroplasty or gastroenterostomy) may be necessary. Try to avoid performing a drainage procedure whenever possible because of the duodenogastric bile reflux which will almost certainly follow.

Recurrent Gastro-oesophageal Reflux Symptoms

Clinical features Gastro-oesophageal reflux symptoms may be present following antireflux surgery. This may be *persistent reflux* due to an ineffective operation or *recurrent reflux* which develops some months or years after operation, following a period of effective reflux control. Brand et al (1979) have shown that in the long-term the effectiveness of an antireflux operation may diminish, although this is not necessarily associated with a return of reflux symptoms.

Reflux symptoms are present in 5–10% of patients following previous antireflux surgery. It is more likely after the Allison or Hill repairs or after anterior gastropexy than after partial or total fundoplication (Demeester, Johnson & Kent, 1974). Disruption of the wrap may be responsible for the recurrence of reflux symptoms. This may occur because of gastric distension in the immediate postoperative period and can be minimized by the insertion of a nasogastric tube for 48 hours after operation, until effective gastric contractions have returned. Disruption may also occur if the wrap is too tight.

Duodenal contents, particularly bile, may be responsible for reflux oesophagitis and persistent reflux symptoms in some patients may be due to uncontrolled bile reflux rather than acid reflux. If bile is seen in the stomach on endoscopy, consider the possibility of 'alkaline' oesophagitis. Twenty-four hour pH studies will probably be normal in these patients, but a ^{99m}Tc-HIDA scan may demonstrate oesophageal bile reflux.

Management Anatomical recurrence of a hiatus hernia will be seen in 50% of patients with recurrent reflux symptoms. Repeat the endoscopy to see if macroscopic oesophagitis is present. However, the absence of oesophagitis does not exclude the diagnosis of recurrent reflux and 24 hour ambulatory pH studies are of value in assessing this group of patients. Patients with demonstrable reflux should be treated medically initially and 50–70% will respond. Those patients whose recurrent symptoms are not controlled by medical treatment or in whom reflux complications such as a benign stricture or bleeding occur will need to have a further antireflux operation. Patients whose symptoms recur soon after the initial operation are more likely to require further surgery than those who develop symptoms some years after their first operation.

Operative technique A transabdominal approach is preferable irrespective of the type of operation that was performed initially, unless there is a large fixed intrathoracic hiatus hernia. A second thoracotomy is likely to involve difficult dissection of the lung from the pleura and it is unlikely that it would be more successful than the first in controlling the reflux symptoms.

Reopen the abdomen through an upper mid-line incision. Few adhesions will be encountered if a transthoracic operation was performed previously. If the first operation was transabdominal, carefully dissect the stomach from the undersurface of the left lobe of the liver. Patient, sharp dissection will eventually be rewarded by adequate exposure of the structures at the oesophageal hiatus. The stomach must be completely mobilized from the lower oesophagus before a further attempt at a fundoplication is made. Be careful to identify the vagus nerves, which are at greater risk of damage during a second procedure. The type of fundoplication performed is a matter of individual preference. Most surgeons would perform a Nissen fundoplication, acknowledging that this is most likely to give the best chance of control of reflux, but accepting the risk of dysphagia and the gas bloat syndrome.

An alternative surgical approach is to modify the nature of the refluxed material. Distal gastrectomy combined with a Roux-en-Y duodenal diversion will both reduce gastric acid secretion and prevent duodenal contents from reaching the oesophagus. This operation is especially applicable to patients with 'alkaline' oesophagitis. To prevent bile reflux it is important that the lower anastomosis of the Roux loop is made at least 50 cm from the gastrojejunal anastomosis. Good results have been claimed for this procedure, particularly in patients whose antireflux operation had been unsuccessful and for whom repeat fundoplication was considered hazardous (Washer et al, 1984). It has been claimed that an extensive gastrectomy is unnecessary, but the more limited the gastric resection the higher the occurrence of stomal ulceration as a late complication. If adhesions in the region of the oesophageal hiatus make repeat fundoplication difficult, then distal gastrectomy with Roux-en-Y diversion is an acceptable alternative operation.

Gastric Ulceration

A chronic gastric ulcer may develop following fundoplication and any patient who develops chronic epigastric pain following an antireflux procedure should have an endoscopy. I (CJS) have seen this complication twice. The ulcer is usually situated high on the lesser curve of the stomach, just below the fundoplication. It may develop in the early postoperative period and it has been suggested that it occurs more frequently when an antireflux procedure is combined with a highly selective vagotomy for duodenal ulceration. Alternatively, the gastric ulcer may develop months or years after the fundoplication. The exact aetiology of gastric ulceration after antireflux surgery is unknown. Vagal damage with gastric stasis has been implicated. Following highly selective vagotomy, the relative lesser curvature ischaemia secondary to devascularization may be more important. A patient may have gastro-oesophageal reflux and a duodenal ulcer, but there is no direct association between the two conditions.

Clinical features and management The patient may present with chronic epigastric pain suggestive of peptic ulceration or with a complication such as gastrointestinal bleeding or peritonitis due to perforation.

Any patient who develops epigastric pain following an antireflux procedure should be endoscoped. If a gastric ulcer is found, it must be biopsied to exclude malignancy. Having determined that the gastric ulcer is macroscopically and microscopically benign, treat the patient medically for eight weeks with an H2 receptor blocker, bismuth compound, carbenoxolone or other similar preparation and then repeat the endoscopy to assess ulcer healing. Complete healing can usually be achieved with medical treatment. If the patient presents with peritonitis and a gastrointestinal perforation, laparotomy is necessary. There are two treatment options for a perforated gastric ulcer:

1 Simple closure of the perforation
2 Definitive ulcer surgery by distal gastrectomy, including the ulcer, followed by Roux-en-Y anastomosis

Treatment by ulcer excision and some form of vagotomy is not technically feasible following an antireflux procedure. A Roux-en-Y anastomosis is the most acceptable form of gastric reconstruction, for it minimizes the risk of biliary gastritis and possible biliary oesophagitis. Simple closure of the ulcer is probably adequate treatment for an ulcer which develops after a combined highly selective vagotomy and antireflux procedure (Kennedy et al, 1979). In other circumstances we would opt for gastrectomy with Roux-en-Y anastomosis.

Pneumothorax

A postoperative pneumothorax may be due to a number of different factors related to the surgical approach.

Transabdominal operation	Transthoracic operation
Pleural damage	Lung damage
Complication of positive pressure ventilation	Failure of the lung to re-expand
	Disconnection of an underwater sealed chest drain

During a transabdominal operation inadvertent damage to the pleura may occur. The left pleura is affected more frequently than the right and this usually occurs just above the oesophageal hiatus during mobilization of the oesophagus and/or hiatus hernia. Air enters the left pleural cavity during operation, but the lung does not collapse because of the positive pressure ventilation. No adverse clinical sequelae result and the diagnosis is only made on a postoperative chest X-ray when a small apical pneumothorax is observed. Rarely does the pneumothorax exceed 20%. Check the patient at 15 minute intervals for an hour, then hourly, to ensure that a tension pneumothorax does not develop. Repeat the chest X-ray after four hours. If the pneumothorax has not increased in size, no active intervention is required and the air will be absorbed gradually over the next week. Chest X-rays should be performed daily. However, if the clinical signs and serial chest X-rays indicate that the pneumothorax is increasing, then it is more likely to be due to a ruptured emphysematous bulla on the lung surface. A chest drain should be inserted via the sixth intercostal space in the anterior axillary line and connected to an underwater seal. The air leak will often continue for as long as seven days, sometimes longer, but will generally stop. The chest drain can be removed when there has been no air leakage for over 24 hours.

Immediately following a transthoracic operation, a chest X-ray should be taken to ensure that the collapsed left lung has fully re-expanded. Failure to expand is often due to a bronchial mucus plug, which should be extracted with a bronchoscope and the lung then reinflated with positive pressure ventilation. Intra-operative damage to the lung may result in a persistent air leak from the intrathoracic drain postoperatively and there is frequently an associated small pneumothorax. The air leak is usually small and seals completely within 48 hours. A massive air leak with significant pneumothorax and collapse of the lung is extremely rare and indicates that there is a major tear in the lung or bronchial tree. Immediate facilities for assisted ventilation must be made available and further thoracotomy is required as soon as possible to identify, and repair, the damage.

If a patient who has been well postoperatively following a transthoracic operation suddenly develops cardiorespiratory embarrassment, check the connections on the chest drains to ensure that they have not become disconnected and the patient developed a pneumothorax. If so, clamp the chest drain with the clamps that are kept at the bedside, reconnect it to the underwater bottle, and release the clamps again. Deep breathing and coughing will hasten the re-expansion of the lung and evacuation of the pneumothorax.

Angelchik Prosthesis

A new concept in the control of gastro-oesophageal reflux, using a silicone prosthesis (Fig. 6.11a), was introduced by Angelchik in 1979. This device is positioned around the lower oesophagus, just above the gastro-oesophageal junction, after minimal mobilization of the lower oesophagus and fundus. The tapes attached to the prosthesis are securely tied, their ends cut 1 cm from the knot, and a haemostasis clip applied to prevent separation of the tapes (Fig. 6.11b). The prosthesis is not anchored to the oesophagus or the stomach in any way. A radio-opaque marking strip on the outer circumference of the prosthesis enables it to be easily located postoperatively by X-ray. It is intended that the device should be easy to insert, of a standard size for all patients, and that the operation should be quicker to perform than other

Figure 6.11
(a) Angelchik
antireflux prosthesis.
(b) Its final position
above the gastro-
oesophageal junction.

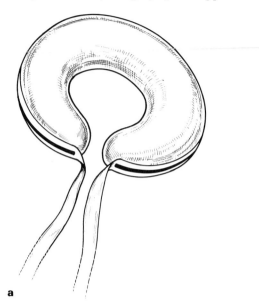

a

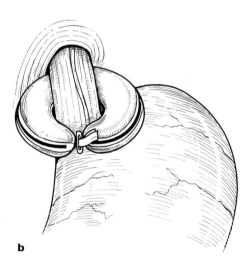

b

antireflux procedures. However, by virtue of the prosthesis, this particular technique has a number of unique complications that do not occur with other antireflux operations.

Migration of the prosthesis

Migration may be of two types:

1 Up the oesophagus into the mediastinum or down over the stomach

2 Into any other part of the abdominal cavity, owing to disruption of the tapes on the prosthesis.

Migration up the oesophagus is highly undesirable, for the prosthesis angulates in the mediastinum, compressing the oesophagus. This can only be relieved by operative removal of the device. The complication is preventable by careful repair of the margins of the right crus prior to insertion of the prosthesis. Migration downwards results in a significant narrowing of the body of the stomach. This is associated with early satiety and recurrence of reflux symptoms. This downward displacement can be avoided by minimal dissection of the gastro-oesophageal junction. If downward displacement does occur and the device is seen to be encircling the stomach on an abdominal X-ray, it must be removed by a further laparotomy. Insertion of a new prosthesis would only be complicated by a similar problem and an alternative antireflux operation, such as a Nissen or a Lind procedure, should be performed.

Disruption of the tapes, with migration of the prosthesis within the peritoneal cavity, usually down into the pelvis, was a problem associated with early batches of the prosthesis. The device has been modified so that the securing tapes pass around the entire circumference and tape disruption appears to have been overcome. However, if the tapes of an old device do give way, it may be removed at a second laparotomy and the surgeon has the option of inserting a new (modified) prosthesis or performing a 'standard' antireflux procedure.

Erosion

The Angelchik prosthesis is a foreign body and as such is hazardous to use in the presence of sepsis. The manufacturers state that insertion is contraindicated in the presence of infection anywhere in the body or where there is a possibility of contamination, particularly from the gastrointestinal tract, during the operation. Sepsis may result in abscess formation, with drainage of pus into the adjacent gastrointestinal tract. In a number of instances the prosthesis has actually entered the lumen of the bowel and been passed per rectum. The device should not be used if the gastrointestinal tract is opened.

If erosion into the stomach or oesophagus does occur, laparotomy is indicated. Operation will be difficult because of adhesions secondary to intra-abdominal sepsis. The prosthesis should be removed, any abscess encountered should be drained, but no attempt should be made to close a gastrointestinal perforation, for the sutures will merely cut out. Continuous nasogastric suction and total parenteral nutrition should be instituted. In the absence of distal obstruction the fistula should eventually close.

Dysphagia

Dysphagia is the commonest complication associated with this device. Severe dysphagia due to intrathoracic migration requires removal of the prosthesis, as indicated previously. Mild dysphagia occurs in 15–40% of patients postoperatively, which is similar to the prevalence after a Nissen procedure, but in the majority resolves within six months of surgery. If the dysphagia fails to resolve, perform a barium swallow to assess the degree of mechanical obstruction. The decision to remove a prosthesis will have to be based on the severity of the patient's symptoms, degree of weight loss and radiological appearances.

The long-term results with this device are as yet unknown, although some surgeons believe that the early results are promising.

Conclusions

Antireflux operations are generally straightforward and the incidence of complications can be reduced by careful selection of patients for surgery, choice of the appropriate operation and good operative technique. A good result should be achieved in over 90% of patients who undergo surgery. Poor results are more likely with an inexperienced surgeon, an obese patient and with the addition of a pyloroplasty or splenectomy. Many of the postoperative problems, such as dysphagia and the gas bloat syndrome, are both mild and transient. Persistent dysphagia is likely to require further surgery. Continued or recurrent reflux symptoms occur in up to 10% of patients, most of whom can be managed medically.

Persisting Controversies

- Best approach for an antireflux procedure—transabdominal or transthoracic
- Length of the fundoplication
- Role of the Angelchik prosthesis
- Aetiology of gastric ulcers after antireflux surgery
- Is the addition of a highly selective vagotomy to fundoplication dangerous?

Further reading
Angelchik, J.P., Cohen, R. & Kravetz, R.E. (1983) A ten-year appraisal of the anti-reflux prosthesis. *American Journal of Gastroenterology*, 78, 671–673.
Allison, P.R. (1951) Reflux oesophagitis, sliding hiatus hernia and the anatomy of repair. *Surgery, Gynecology and Obstetrics*, 92, 419–431.
Brand, D., Eastwood, I.R., Martin, D., Carter, W.B. & Pope, C.E., II. (1979) Oesophageal symptoms, manometry, and histology before and after antireflux surgery. *Gastroenterology*, 76, 1393–1401.

Bushkin, F.L., Neustein, C.L., Parker, T.H. & Woodward, E.R. (1977) Nissen fundoplication for reflux peptic oesophagitis. *Annals of Surgery*, *185*, 672–677.

Demeester, T., Johnson, L.F. & Kent, A.H. (1974) Evaluation of current operations for the prevention of gastro-oesophageal reflux. *Annals of Surgery*, *180*, 511–525.

Henderson, R.D. (1979) Nissen hiatal hernia repair: problems of recurrence and continued symptoms. *Annals of Thoracic Surgery*, *28*, 587–593.

Hill, L.D. (1967) An effective operation for hiatus hernia. An eight-year appraisal. *Annals of Surgery*, *166*, 681–692.

Kennedy, T., Magill, P., Johnston, G.W. & Parks, T.G. (1979) Proximal gastric vagotomy, fundoplication, and lesser-curve necrosis. *British Medical Journal*, *i*, 1455–1456.

Leonardi, H.K. & Ellis, F.H. (1983) Complications of the Nissen fundoplication. *Surgical Clinics of North America*, *632*, 1155–1165.

Lind, J.F., Burns, C.M. & MacDougall, J.T.A. (1965) 'Physiological' repair for hiatus hernia: manometric study. *Archives of Surgery*, *91*, 233–237.

Nissen, R. (1961) Gastropexy and 'fundoplication' in surgical treatment of hiatus hernia. *American Journal of Digestive Diseases*, *6*, 954–961.

Pearson, J.B. & Gray, J.G. (1967) Oesophageal hiatus hernia: long-term results of conventional thoracic operations. *British Journal of Surgery*, *54*, 530–533.

Polk, H.C. (1976) Fundoplication for reflux oesophagitis. Misadventures with the operation of choice. *Annals of Surgery*, *183*, 645–652.

Rogers, D.M., Herrington, J.L. & Morton, C. (1980) Incidental splenectomy associated with Nissen fundoplication. *Annals of Surgery*, *191*, 153–156.

Shackleford, R.T. (1978) *Surgery of the Alimentary Tract. Volume 1: Oesophagus*, 2nd edn. Philadelphia: W.B. Saunders.

Skinner, D.B. & Belsey, R.H.R. (1967) Surgical management of oesophageal reflux and hiatus hernia. *Journal of Thoracic and Cardiovascular Surgery*, *53*, 33–54.

Washer, G.F., Gear, M.W.L., Dowling, B.L., Gillison, E.W., Royston, C.M.S. & Spencer, J. (1984) Randomised prospective trial of Roux-en-Y duodenal diversion versus fundoplication for severe reflux oesophagitis. *British Journal of Surgery*, *71*, 181–184.

7 Complications of the Treatment of Achalasia

Achalasia is an oesophageal motor disorder characterized by a hypertensive lower oesophageal sphincter which fails to relax completely on swallowing. In the body of the oesophagus peristaltic waves are either absent or diminished in amplitude and are replaced by repetitive, non-propulsive, tertiary contractions. The aetiology of the condition is unknown. Histologically the ganglion cells in Auerbach's plexus degenerate or disappear, this degeneration being greater in the body of the oesophagus than in the region of the lower oesophageal sphincter. The mucosa often shows evidence of chronic oesophagitis. Electron microscopic examination of the vagus nerves reveals patchy Wallerian degeneration and autopsy studies suggest that there may be a reduction in the number of motor cells in the dorsal motor nucleus of the vagus in the brain stem (Cassella et al, 1964). Thus the pathophysiological changes in the oesophagus may be secondary to an abnormality in the vagal nucleus. There is some experimental evidence to support this hypothesis. A condition resembling achalasia can be produced by electrolytic destruction of the dorsal motor nucleus in cats and the nucleus ambiguus of dogs (Higgs, Kerr & Ellis, 1965). Genetic factors may be involved in the development of achalasia, for it can occur in siblings, in association with certain disorders which are known to be inherited as autosomal recessive conditions and also in certain in-bred communities, such as Apache Indians.

The symptoms and signs of achalasia are due to the failure of the lower oesophageal sphincter to relax. The patient develops dysphagia, sometimes associated with regurgitation of undigested food and this is later followed by weight loss. Recurrent chest infections are due to aspiration of pharyngeal contents. Powerful tertiary contractions in the body of the oesophagus can cause severe chest pain. The only abnormal signs on physical examination are due to weight loss and chest infection. A dilated oesophagus may be seen on an erect chest X-ray (Fig. 7.1), sometimes with an air/fluid level, and there may be evidence of aspiration pneumonia, usually affecting the posterior basal segment of the right lung. The lower end of the oesophagus has a characteristic bird's beak appearance on a barium swallow, with delayed passage of barium into the stomach. The oesophagus is

Figure 7.1
Erect chest X-ray of a
patient with achalasia
showing an
enormously dilated
oesophagus
containing food
debris and an air/fluid
level.

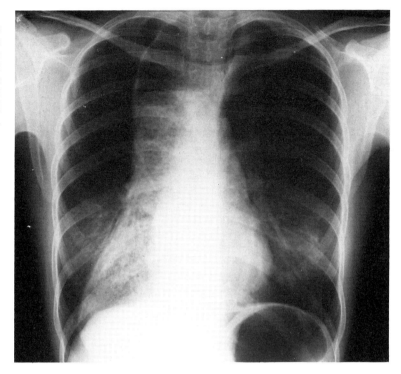

frequently dilated and may contain a column of barium. Incomplete oesophageal emptying leads to chronic retention oesophagitis which may predispose to the development of an oesophageal carcinoma.

Treatment of Achalasia

The pathophysiological changes are irreversible and the aim of treatment is to give symptomatic relief by decreasing the resistance at the lower end of the oesophagus. There are three alternative forms of treatment:

Drugs
Anticholinergic agents, glyceryl trinitrate and α-adrenergic blocking drugs have all been used, but with little success. Calcium-blocking agents such as nifedipine 10–20 mg sublingually before meals reduce the lower oesophageal sphincter pressure for over an hour and may give improvement in up to 70% of patients with mild or moderate symptoms. The patients need to take a tablet before each meal and have to continue to do so for life.

Forceful dilatation of the cardia

Oesophageal dilatation with mercury-weighted bougies is of no lasting value. However, forceful dilatation, which probably achieves its effect by disruption of oesophageal muscle fibres, can produce a permanent symptomatic cure. The dilators which can be used are shown in Table 7.1.

Oesophagomyotomy

This operation can be performed via an abdominal or thoracic approach. The longitudinal and circular muscle fibres of the lower oesophagus are incised and dissected back to expose at least 50% of the circumference of the oesophageal mucosa beneath (Fig. 7.2). The incision should extend for 0.5 cm below the gastro-oesophageal junction and for a minimum of 6 cm up the oesophagus and thus well above the narrow segment. The narrow segment on barium swallow and the high pressure zone on manometry is never more than 4 cm in length and an extended myotomy as far as the aortic arch is unnecessary. Since it is easy to perform a 6 cm oesophageal myotomy from the abdomen, this approach is preferable. The operation time is shorter and the postoperative complications of thoracotomy are avoided.

The choice of treatment is determined by personal preference and available facilities. Drug treatment may be successful in the early stages but as symptoms worsen the therapy becomes less effective. Good long-term results are achieved in up to 75% of patients who undergo forceful dilatation. Operation is avoided but multiple dilatations may be necessary. After oesophagomyotomy good results have been reported in 70–85% of patients. There has been only one prospective randomized study reported comparing forceful dilatation with oesophagomyotomy (Csendes et al, 1981), which concluded that surgical treatment gives better long-term results but has a higher prevalence of postoperative gastro-oesophageal reflux. A similar conclusion was reached in the large retrospective study from the Mayo Clinic (Okike et al, 1979) in which the results of treatment of 899 patients were compared. Excellent or good results were commoner after myotomy (85% versus 77%), with a similar early morbidity and mortality. The choice of myotomy or forceful dilatation for the initial treatment of achalasia remains controversial. One widely accepted view is that dilatation should be the initial treatment

Table 7.1 Dilators used for forceful dilatation of the cardia		
Starck dilator	Mechanical device with expanding metal arms	
Pneumatic dilators	Browne–McHardy or Rider–Moeller	
Hydrostatic dilator	Plummer bag	
Progressive pneumatic dilator	Series of bags with increasing diameter up to 4.5 cm	

Figure 7.2
The extent of the
myotomy.

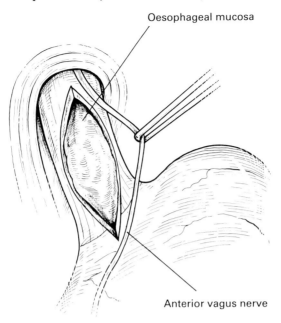

Oesophageal mucosa

Anterior vagus nerve

for all patients and cardiomyotomy reserved for those who remain symptomatic after several dilatations. Young patients with achalasia and those with symptoms of less than 5 years duration are more likely to require eventual oesophagomyotomy.

Complications of Forceful Dilatation

The commonest technique currently used is pneumatic dilatation with a Browne–McHardy or Rider–Moeller dilator. This can be done under general anaesthesia or local anaesthetic and sedation. The former, although more inconvenient, is applicable to almost all patients including children and the mentally handicapped and additionally affords protection for the airway. Oesophageal pain during dilatation may be a problem when a general anaesthetic is not used. The position of the cardia must be accurately determined and the dilator positioned across it before inflation. This can be done by prior endoscopy or preferably by radiological screening during the dilatation procedure.

The oesophagus must not contain food residue at the time of dilatation because of the risk of mediastinal contamination if a perforation occurs. Do not give food or fluid for twelve hours before dilatation, and if the oesophagus is distended, thorough lavage should be performed using a wide-bore naso-oesophageal tube. When the Rider–Moeller dilator is used the patient should first be endoscoped so that a guide-wire can be passed through the biopsy channel into the stomach. The dilator is then slid over the guide-wire. Once correctly positioned it is inflated to 200 mmHg for 1 minute, 300 mmHg for a further minute and then deflated and withdrawn. Endoscopy can be repeated to exclude oeso-phageal perforation. After treatment examine the patient regularly for clinical evidence of perforation and perform an erect chest X-ray after four hours to exclude mediastinal emphysema. If there is no perforation, oral feeding can be recommenced and the patient discharged the following day. If a progressive pneumatic dilatation technique is used, begin with a bag of 3 cm diameter and gradually increase to 4.2 or even 4.5 cm.

The results of treatment can be assessed simply by symptomatic review or by barium swallow or manometry. Repeat the dilatation if dysphagia remains or recurs. Between 50 and 60% of patients only require one dilatation, but repeated dilatation will be necessary in the others. Failure to achieve lasting symptomatic improvement after three or four dilatations is an indication for oesophagomyotomy.

Oesophageal perforation
The reported incidence of oesophageal perforation after forceful dilatation is between 1 and 4%. It is usually longitudinal, 2 to 3 cm in length and situated just proximal to the gastro-oesophageal junction, on the left lateral wall of the oesophagus. It may communicate with the pleural cavity. Perforations following forceful dilatation are rarely fatal. Mediastinal contamination is less severe and communication with the pleural cavity less frequent than in patients with a spontaneous oesophageal perforation (Boerhaave syndrome).

An oesophageal perforation may occur at the site of dilatation, just above the gastro-oesophageal junction (most commonly), or in the cervical oesophagus, owing to instrumentation (rarely). A lower oesophageal perforation may be recognized endoscopically, but if the perforation only becomes obvious during the next few hours by clinical examination or chest X-ray, then a radiological study of the oesophagus should be performed using a water-soluble contrast medium, e.g. Gastrografin, to determine the site of perforation. A cervical oesophageal perforation should be treated as described in Chapter 4. If the perforation is in the lower oesophagus, then the two treatment options are:

- Conservative treatment
- Immediate thoracotomy, with repair of the perforation ± oeso-phagomyotomy

The majority of perforations can be treated conservatively. Position a nasogastric tube with multiple side holes across the perforation and attach it to continuous low suction. Withhold oral fluids and food, give broad-spectrum antibiotics and total parenteral nutrition and perform a Gastrografin swallow seven days later to see if the perforation has sealed. This treatment is unsuitable for children and mentally handicapped patients or when there is communication with the left pleural cavity. In these patients the perforation should be repaired in two layers via a left thoracotomy. This should be combined with a definitive oesophagomyotomy if mediastinal contamination is not excessive. After closing the perforation rotate the oesophagus through 180° and make the myotomy incision opposite the tear. This incision must extend across the gastro-oesophageal junction and the oesophageal muscle be dissected back to expose at least 50% of the circumference of the underlying mucosa.

Gastro-oesophageal reflux
Heartburn due to gastro-oesophageal reflux is less of a problem after pneumatic dilatation than after oesophagomyotomy. It is often transient and is rarely severe. Postural control of reflux is important because of the poor oesophageal peristalsis. Antacids, H2-receptor blocking agents or alginate preparations may be used, but dopamine antagonists should be avoided.

Recurrent dysphagia
Recurrent dysphagia occurs in 40–50% of patients treated by pneumatic dilatation. The risk is highest in patients under the age of 45 years and in those whose symptoms were present for less than five years prior to the first dilatation. It can be treated by a repeat dilatation or oesophagomyotomy. Unless the patient refuses dilatation, this should be advised, for a further 10–15% will achieve satisfactory long-term relief from their dysphagia. However, young patients and those in whom more than four dilatations are necessary, particularly if the interval between the dilatations is short, are unlikely to achieve long-term symptomatic control if the dilatation is simply repeated. This group should be advised to have surgery.

Complications of Oesophagomyotomy

Operative technique is important in reducing the incidence of postoperative complications.

Operative technique Heller first performed an anterior and posterior extramucosal myotomy for the treatment of achalasia in 1914 and this operation was modified in 1923 by Zaaijer, who used just a single anterior incision. Oesophagomyotomy can be performed via the transthoracic or transabdominal routes and opinions differ as to which is the best approach. Whilst thoracotomy permits the myotomy incision to be extended up to the aortic arch if necessary, the narrow segment at the lower end of the oesophagus is never more than 4 cm in length and can be incised quite easily from beneath the diaphragm. Patients with vigorous achalasia and frequent tertiary contractions *are* probably best treated by extended myotomy, but they form only a small proportion of the total number of patients with achalasia. The majority can be treated adequately by the transabdominal route.

The myotomy incision should be adequate in length and depth. From the level of the gastro-oesophageal junction it should extend at least 6 cm up the oesophagus, but no more than 0.5–1.0 cm down onto the stomach. Extending the incision further onto the stomach substantially increases the risk of gastro-oeso-phageal reflux. All circular muscle must be divided throughout the length of the incision and the underlying mucosa and submucosa exposed. Begin the myotomy with a 1 cm longitudinal incision using a knife and starting just above the cardia. Be careful not to breach the mucosa. Separate the longitudinal muscle fibres by gently inserting and opening a pair of Nelson's scissors. By opening the scissors again between the circular muscle fibres, the plane between the mucosa and circular muscle will become apparent. Pass the scissors into this plane and then elevate and divide the circular muscle. Pott's angled scissors are ideal for this manoeuvre. Use a knife to continue the myotomy across the gastro-oesophageal junction, for the plane between the mucosa and muscle is less readily apparent at this level. Diathermy of small vessels in the submucosa may be necessary. Throughout the procedure the anterior vagus nerve should be gently retracted to avoid inadvertent damage. The margins of the myotomy incision should be dissected back to expose at least half of the oesophageal circumference. This will ensure that all muscle fibres are divided and will prevent linear healing of the muscle edges with recurrence of dysphagia. Carefully inspect the exposed mucosa for evidence of a small mucosal tear. If present, this should be repaired with interrupted chromic catgut sutures. A nasogastric tube should be left in situ for 48 hours postoperatively until postoperative motor activity returns to the stomach.

Gastro-oesophageal reflux

Although oesophagomyotomy relieves the cardiospasm, complete division of the lower oesophageal sphincter predisposes to gastro-oesophageal reflux, and some authors have advocated that an antireflux procedure should always be performed after oesophagomyotomy. Patients with achalasia have poor oeso-phageal peristalsis, thus an individual reflux episode may result in a prolonged low intraoesophageal pH, which can lead to oesophagitis and possibly a benign oesophageal stricture. There is a great variation in the reported incidence of postoperative reflux symptoms, figures varying from 3 to 48% having been published. The figure tends to be greater the longer the period of postoperative follow-up. There is a positive correlation between the occurrence of reflux and the length of myotomy incision onto the stomach. When the distance exceeds 2 cm the incidence of significant reflux approaches 100%, but when the myotomy incision crosses the gastro-oesophageal junction by only a few millimetres, the incidence of troublesome reflux is low. A routine antireflux procedure is unnecessary if the operative technique described earlier is followed carefully. A fundoplication in a patient with achalasia and an adynamic oesophagus is not without its risks for it may cause dysphagia due to obstruction. If an antireflux procedure *is* performed after oesophagomyotomy, then a partial, as opposed to a total, fundoplication is preferable. In the surgical treatment of achalasia the authors' preference is for oesophagomyotomy without an antireflux procedure, ensuring that the incision only crosses the gastro-oesophageal junction by a few millimetres.

Treatment Reflux symptoms should be treated in the usual manner. Emphasis must be placed on postural methods of reflux control because of the impaired oesophageal peristalsis. Antacids and H2-receptor blocking agents are useful. Development of a benign peptic stricture indicates a significant reflux problem. The stricture should be dilated, preferably using Celestin dilators passed over a guide-wire. Mercury-weighted dilators are best avoided for they may curl in the oesophagus, rather than traverse the stricture, and an oesophageal perforation can occur. Following dilatation, intensive medical treatment to combat further reflux is necessary. If reflux symptoms cannot be controlled medically, or if the stricture recurs after dilatation, an antireflux operation should be considered. The decision to reoperate should be based on careful symptomatic assessment, endoscopic findings, 24 hour ambulatory oesophageal pH studies and the patient's suitability for further surgery.

A transabdominal partial fundoplication is the operation of choice for patients with troublesome reflux. Careful dissection around the hiatus is necessary to avoid opening the oesophageal mucosa anteriorly or damaging the anterior vagus nerve. Thorough oesophageal mobilization is required before the fundoplication is performed. The point at which the gastric fundus can be anchored to the oesophagus is dependent on the available musculo-fibrotic tissue at the lower end of the oesophagus following the previous oesophagomyotomy.

Oesophageal perforation
An oesophageal perforation is recognized intraoperatively in up to 5% of patients. A quantity of gastric juice appears on the submucosa, usually through a hole of less than 3 mm in diameter. The perforation is at the level of the gastro-oesophageal junction where the mucosa and circular muscle are most difficult to separate. The hole should be closed with interrupted catgut sutures and the patient given a single intravenous dose of a prophylactic broad-spectrum antibiotic.

Postoperative perforation occurs in approximately 1% of patients, which is less than after forceful dilatation. It arises following unrecognized intraoperative damage to the oesophageal mucosa. If the defect is large, the patient develops increasing abdominal pain in the immediate postoperative period, with pyrexia, tachycardia and signs of peritonitis. These symptoms and signs may be masked by administration of narcotic analgesics or confused with other postoperative infective problems, particularly chest infection. If the diagnosis is in doubt, a radiological examination of the oesophagus should be performed using a water-soluble contrast medium, rather than barium. A large perforation, which is recognized within 48 hours of laparotomy, should be treated by repeat laparotomy, peritoneal lavage and closure of the defect.

A small perforation with only limited peritoneal contamination usually results in a left subphrenic abscess. The patient develops a tachycardia and swinging pyrexia 4 or 5 days postoperatively. Chest examination and X-ray may reveal a pleural effusion, and ultrasound scan may confirm the diagnosis. Perform a Gastrografin swallow and look for evidence of an oesophageal leak. If the diagnosis of a subphrenic abscess due to oesophageal perforation is confirmed, stop oral intake, give total parenteral nutrition and antibiotics and wait for the abscess to 'mature' before draining it on or around the tenth postoperative day, via a left subcostal incision. Once the abscess has been drained repeat the Gastrografin swallow weekly until the perforation is seen to have closed radiologically. Oral feeding can be recommenced a few days later.

Recurrent dysphagia

It is worth re-emphasizing that the aim of oesophagomyotomy is to relieve the 'obstruction' at the lower end of the oesophagus. It will not reverse the pathophysiological abnormalities that occur in achalasia, and peristalsis in the body of the oesophagus will always be abnormal. Although an oesophagomyotomy may successfully relieve dysphagia, a grossly dilated oesophagus will never return to normal size.

Recurrent dysphagia may be due to a variety of causes (Table 7.2). In the early postoperative period it is generally secondary to either an incomplete myotomy or a fundoplication combined with myotomy. Incomplete myotomy occurs most often after a transthoracic operation in which the incision is not carried far enough downwards, across the gastro-oesophageal junction (Fig. 7.3). Late recurrence is usually due to an oesophageal stricture,

Table 7.2	
Causes of postoperative dysphagia following oesophagomyotomy	1 Inadequate myotomy
	2 Linear healing of myotomy scar
	3 Peptic stricture secondary to reflux
	4 Stricture due to chronic oesophagitis
	5 Benign stricture following healing of a perforation
	6 Motility disorder in body of oesophagus
	7 Fundoplication
	8 Oesophageal carcinoma

Figure 7.3
Barium swallow of a
patient with recurrent
dysphagia six years
after transthoracic
oesophagomyotomy.
At a second operation
the previous myotomy
incision was found to
end 2 cm above the
gastro-oesophageal
junction.

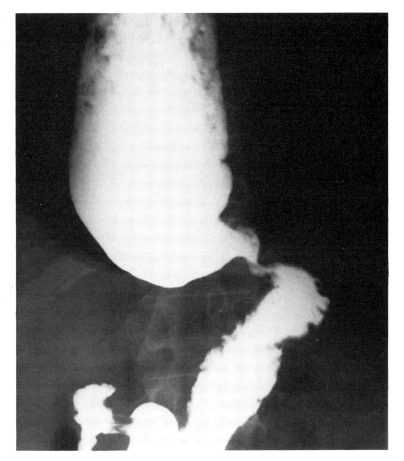

carcinoma or motility disorder. Endoscopy should be performed and all strictures biopsied. When there is no stricture or carcinoma the lower oesophageal sphincter pressure should be measured manometrically. If the pressure is high, then the available options are:

- forceful dilatation
- repeat myotomy

The treatment selected is again dependent on personal preference and local facilities. There is no increase in the incidence of oesophageal perforation with forceful dilatation after previous oesophagomyotomy. If surgery is performed, an abdominal approach is preferable so that the gastro-oesophageal junction can be adequately seen. Be careful not to damage the anterior vagus nerve. If the myotomy was incomplete, it should be completed, taking care to follow the instructions for operative technique given earlier in this section. Oesophageal strictures should be treated by dilatation, combined with antireflux measures when the stricture is due to reflux. Treatment of a patient with a grossly dilated oesophagus but adequate myotomy is less straightforward. Oesophagectomy without thoracotomy has been advocated on the grounds that the oesophagus will never function again as an effective conduit with good peristalsis and there is an increased risk of carcinoma. It has a significant mortality rate, however, and thus needs further careful evaluation.

Carcinoma

Patients with achalasia are at a slightly greater risk than normals of developing an oesophageal carcinoma. The carcinoma is usually of the squamous cell variety. Primary oesophageal adenocarcinomas develop in patients with severe reflux and a columnar-lined oesophagus. The site of the tumour in achalasia differs from that in oesophageal carcinoma in general, occurring most frequently in the middle third rather than the lower third. However, the sex incidence is similar to that of oesophageal carcinoma in general, with a marked preponderance of males. These patients tend to develop their carcinoma on average 10 years younger than those who do not suffer from achalasia.

Oesophageal carcinomas in achalasia are generally attributed to chronic retention oesophagitis. The tumour may be advanced at the time of presentation because the symptoms are thought by the patient (and sometimes by the attending physician) to be due to a recurrence of the original condition. All achalasia patients with worsening or recurrent dysphagia should have an endoscopy to exclude carcinoma.

Whether an effective myotomy reduces the risk of carcinoma is controversial. Many cases of carcinoma have been reported following oesophagomyotomy, often many years after operation. In some instances the operation had been symptomatically successful, but in others the patients still had stasis in a dilated oesophagus. It has been suggested that oesophagomyotomy early in the course of achalasia may reduce the risk of carcinoma, but as yet this is unproven. Because the role of myotomy in reducing the risk of carcinoma is still unclear and because these patients tend to have a lower age of presentation and poorer prognosis, it is reasonable to advise that all patients with achalasia should have regular endoscopy and biopsy at 1–2 yearly intervals looking for either dysplasia or invasive carcinoma. Carcinoma should be treated by either radiotherapy or oesophagectomy. Patients with dysplasia should have endoscopy and biopsy at more frequent intervals, such as six monthly, looking for evidence of carcinoma in situ.

Conclusions

Achalasia is an irreversible condition. Treatment is aimed at relieving the spasm at the lower end of the oesophagus. Oesophagomyotomy has a lower incidence of oesophageal perforation but a higher incidence of gastro-oesophageal reflux than forceful dilatation. Recurrent dysphagia may be due to a variety of causes, including carcinoma. Regular postoperative endoscopic assessment of patients with achalasia is desirable.

Persisting Controversies

- Should forceful dilatation or oesophagomyotomy be the initial treatment for achalasia?
- Does successful treatment reduce the risk of development of an oesophageal carcinoma?
- Does a long extension of the myotomy onto the stomach increase the risk of postoperative gastro-oesophageal reflux?
- What is the place of oesophagectomy in treatment of achalasia?

Further reading

Cassella, R.R., Brown, A.L. Jr., Sayre, G.P. & Ellis, F.H., Jr (1964) Achalasia of the oesophagus. Pathologic and etiologic considerations. *Annals of Surgery, 160,* 474–487.

Csendes, A., Velasco, N., Braghetto, I. & Hewiquez, A. (1981) A prospective randomised study comparing forceful dilatation and oesophagomyotomy in patients with achalasia of the oesophagus. *Gastroenterology, 80,* 789–795.

Ellis, F.H., Gibb, S.P. & Cozier. P.E. (1980) Esophagomyotomy for achalasia of the esophagus. *Annals of Surgery, 192,* 157–161.

Harley, H.R.S. (1978) *Achalasia of the Cardia.* Bristol: John Wright.

Higgs, B., Kerr, F.W.L. & Ellis, F.H., Jr (1965) The experimental production of oesophageal achalasia by electrolytic lesions in the medulla. *Journal of Thoracic and Cardiovascular Surgery, 50,* 613–618.

Okike, N., Payne, W.S., Neufeld, D.M., Bernatz, P.E., Pairolero, P.C. & Sanderson, D.R. (1979) Oesophagomyotomy versus forceful dilatation for achalasia of the oesophagus: results in 899 patients. *Annals of Thoracic Surgery, 28,* 119–125.

Stoddard, C.J. & Johnson, A.G. (1982) Achalasia in siblings. *British Journal of Surgery, 69,* 84–85.

Vantrappen, G. & Janssens, J. (1983) To dilate or to operate? That is the question. *Gut, 24,* 1013–1019.

8 Complications of Variceal Surgery

There are two strategies for the treatment of variceal haemorrhage: one for stopping the acute bleed and the other for the prevention of recurrent bleeding. Both of these strategies require a judicious selection from the available treatments, namely vasoactive drugs, balloon tamponade, endoscopic sclerotherapy, oesophageal transection and portal–systemic shunting. Considerable experience is necessary and in many situations the choice of treatment may be dictated by local factors, such as special interest, experience, proximity of a referral centre and, of course, the clinician's own prejudices. Whatever the method of treatment used, complications are frequent, since the patient population with bleeding oesophageal varices is usually debilitated from underlying liver disease. Before discussing the complications of the various treatments, it is necessary to review the systemic effects of the portal hypertension.

Effects of Portal Hypertension on the Patient

Most patients in the UK, presenting with bleeding oesophageal varices suffer from cirrhosis, often of alcoholic origin, and thus have some degree of liver failure. Moreover, many of these patients have encephalopathy, disorders of coagulation and possibly renal failure. In addition, alcoholic patients may have additional problems such as gastritis, chronic pancreatitis, malabsorption, and vitamin deficiencies. However, other patients with extrahepatic blocks have near normal liver function and consequently are at less risk from some of the complications of treatment.

Ideally the deleterious effects of portal hypertension should be treated prior to embarking on treatment of the varices so that the risk of complications is reduced. This is often difficult in an emergency situation, but is more easily accomplished in the elective management of these patients.

Liver failure
Liver failure leads to a reduction in serum albumin and causes various amino-acid imbalances. Furthermore, the coagulation factors produced by the liver, factors II, V, IX, X and fibrinogen, are usually reduced. These abnormalities, especially when coupled with malnutrition, often prejudice healing. As yet there is no

convincing evidence that total parenteral nutrition improves healing in cirrhotic patients. Empirically, vitamin supplements should be given to patients with malnutrition. Continuation of alcohol abuse accelerates liver failure and thus stringent efforts must be made to promote alcohol abstinence. Joint management by surgeon and hepatologist is valuable, the latter advising specifically on the medical management of the liver disease.

Encephalopathy

The causes of hepatic encephalopathy are multifactorial and extremely complex. Encephalopathy is usually either acute or chronic. Acute hepatic encephalopathy is usually related to some precipitating event such as a recent haemorrhage, diuretic administration, infected ascites or a dietary indiscretion. Chronic hepatic encephalopathy results from deterioration of liver function or the creation of a portal–systemic shunt. The management of acute hepatic encephalopathy is usually successful after the causative factor has been identified and removed. Most commonly acute encephalopathy is precipitated or aggravated by a recent bleed. This is best treated with lactulose by mouth (or nasogastric tube) 30 ml t.d.s. and a daily laxative (magnesium sulphate enema).

Haemopoietic disturbance

The secondary hypersplenism that invariably accompanies portal hypertension leads to a pancytopenia in approximately 30% of patients. The anaemia is often compounded by other causes such as chronic gastrointestinal oozing from varices, gastritis or a peptic ulcer. Correction of the anaemia by blood transfusion should be undertaken when the haemoglobin is less than 10 g/dl. The reduced platelet count coupled with the depletion of coagulation factors may lead to clotting anomalies. When acute variceal haemorrhage occurs or elective surgical treatment is contemplated, it is desirable to correct the clotting anomaly. A good rule of thumb is that when the prothrombin ratio is greater than 1.5, fresh frozen plasma should be given, and if the platelet count is $< 35 \times 10^9/l$, a platelet transfusion should be administered. Also, give vitamin K 15 mg i.m. daily.

If the acute haemorrhage is promptly controlled, then total blood loss should seldom be more than 6 units. If difficulties are encountered in controlling the acute haemorrhage, then larger quantities of blood may be needed. If there is any suggestion of a significant clotting disorder, perform a platelet count and measure the serum fibrin degradation products and fibrinogen level in order to exclude intravascular coagulation. It is usually wise if there is a serious clotting disorder to consult a haematologist for further advice about treatment.

Ascites

Ascites is common in advanced liver failure and adds to morbidity and mortality if it should become infected. When the patient has had a recent onset of abdominal pain or acute encephalopathy for no apparent reason, 20 ml of ascitic fluid must be obtained by aseptic needle aspiration for microbiological examination. In view of the high mortality of infected ascites (> 50%), treatment must be commenced before the results of cultures are available if the ascitic fluid (i) is cloudy; (ii) has a high white cell count (> 300 WBC/mm^3); or (iii) contains organisms on Gram staining. Ninety per cent of the isolated organisms are sensitive to a combination of a cephalosporin, an aminoglycoside and metronidazole. Therefore parenteral antibiotic treatment must be vigorously pursued if infection is suspected or proven.

Uninfected ascites should be treated, particularly if a laparotomy is contemplated. This is best achieved by a low-salt diet, fluid restriction to around 750 ml per day and spironolactone 100 mg daily, increasing by 100 mg daily on alternate days to a maximum of 600 mg per day, aiming for a weight loss of approximately 0.5 kg daily. There is no place for abdominal paracentesis.

Other remedial factors
Many of the patients presenting with bleeding oesophageal varices suffer from chest diseases requiring pre- and postoperative physiotherapy to avoid respiratory complications. If the patient is already on steroids, they may need to be increased depending on the treatment planned.

Child's classification
Child's classification (Table 8.1) is the traditional grading system that is used to measure the overall effects of liver dysfunction. It does correlate with operative mortality and survival, especially after shunt surgery. In particular, Child's C patients have a much worse prognosis than Child's A or B patients.

Methods of Treatment

Most clinicians use treatments with which they are familiar and which have an acceptable morbidity and mortality. There is

Table 8.1 Criteria for Child's classification	*Group A*	*Group B*	*Group C*
Serum bilirubin (μmol/l)	34.0	34.0–51.0	51.0
Plasma albumin (g/l)	35.0	30.0–35.0	30·0
Ascites	None controlled	Easily controlled	Poorly
Encephalopathy	None	Minimal 'coma'	Advanced
Nutrition	Excellent	Moderate	Poor
Risk of operation	Good	Moderate	Poor

much controversy concerning the ideal treatment for patients with bleeding oesophageal varices. Indeed, there is no ideal treatment but rather selection of the most appropriate treatment for a particular patient.

Acute variceal haemorrhage

Generally, most clinicians who have an interest in variceal bleeding control the acute haemorrhage with a combination of vasoactive drugs and balloon tamponade, reserving oesophageal transection for those patients who fail to respond to the initial treatment. However, in my own practice I (J. N. Baxter) prefer to perform endoscopic sclerotherapy (often followed by balloon tamponade) as soon as possible after the diagnosis of variceal haemorrhage has been made, even if the patient is actively bleeding (see p. 166). Thus, endoscopic sclerotherapy is performed within six hours of referral and repeated five days later. If no further bleeding has occurred, then the acute haemorrhage is considered controlled.

There is no place for portal–systemic shunting as an emergency treatment for acute variceal haemorrhage, since the operative mortality is in excess of 50%. Once the acute haemorrhage has been controlled, it is necessary to carry out further treatment to prevent recurrent variceal haemorrhage.

Prevention of recurrent variceal haemorrhage

Endoscopic sclerotherapy is currently the best treatment for the prevention of recurrent variceal bleeding. However, some surgeons prefer oesophageal transection, whilst others, particularly in the USA, prefer portal–systemic shunting.

Endoscopic sclerotherapy should be performed at three-weekly intervals until the varices have been obliterated. Patients must then have an endoscopy every six months to detect any recurrence of the varices. Any such recurrences must be further injected.

Complications of Treatment

Vasoactive drugs

Vasoactive drugs, such as vasopressin or somatostatin can be used intravenously to control acute bleeding, though they are only used as a first-line treatment if balloon tamponade is not possible (e.g. no experience, excessive length of previous tamponade, presence of a hiatus hernia, etc.). Oral beta-blockers can be used to prevent recurrent variceal bleeding.

Vasopressin

The most widely used vasoactive drug for the control of acute variceal haemorrhage, despite little convincing evidence of its efficacy, is vasopressin. Vasopressin is given as a continuous i.v.

infusion starting at 0.4 unit/min, increasing to 0.6–0.8 unit/min until control is achieved. The rate of administration should then be reduced to 0.4 unit/min. Unfortunately, vasopressin administration is often associated with severe abdominal colic, which may necessitate discontinuing the infusion. Reducing the rate of administration can be tried in order to reduce the severity of abdominal colic, but it is usually necessary to stop the infusion completely.

More importantly, vasopressin may cause systemic hypertension with left ventricular failure, requiring immediate cessation of the infusion and initiation of specific cardiac therapy (digoxin and diuretics). An infusion of nitroprusside (1–5 μg/kg body weight/min) concurrently with vasopressin will reduce cardiovascular toxicity, but this is rather arduous to administer and requires constant monitoring in an intensive care unit. Consequently, it is easier to administer vasopressin alone and to resort to balloon tamponade if cardiovascular side-effects should occur.

Somatostatin
Somatostatin is a better vasoactive drug than vasopressin in the control of acute variceal haemorrhage (Jenkins et al, 1984). Somatostatin is administered as a 250 μg/hour infusion following a 250 μg bolus (over 2 min) and can be safely infused for as long as five days if necessary. This drug is associated with significantly less side-effects and is more effective than vasopressin in controlling variceal haemorrhage (Jenkins et al, 1984). It is very important that a loading bolus (250 μg) is administered and that the continuous infusion is uninterrupted. If there is ever any doubt about the continuity of the somatostatin infusion, a further bolus (250 μg) should be administered.

Beta-blockers
Beta-blockers have no place in the emergency control of variceal bleeding. Indeed, their place in the prevention of recurrent variceal bleeding is uncertain. It is certainly worth remembering that if a patient is taking a beta-blocker to prevent recurrent variceal haemorrhage and then presents with another variceal bleed, resuscitation may be difficult because of the depressive effect of the drug on the myocardium (beta-1 effect). It may be necessary under these circumstances to administer inotropic agents (such as digoxin) to antagonize the cardiac effect of the beta-blocker.

Balloon tamponade
It has been recognized for many years that the use of balloon tamponade for the control of acute variceal haemorrhage has potentially dangerous complications, but with improvements in the design of balloon tubes and, more particularly, experience in their use, the risk of complications has been reduced. Thus balloon tamponade is still the most widely used technique for

controlling acute variceal haemorrhage. However, the passage of a balloon tube by an inexperienced clinician is accompanied by the risk of significantly more complications. Thus, anyone who is prepared to treat these patients should be thoroughly familiar with the technique of insertion and subsequent management. The initial haemorrhage is controlled in over 90% of cases. However, rebleeding often occurs following removal of the tube, resulting in an overall control rate of approximately 75%. All patients must be managed in an intensive care or high-dependency unit.

Important technical points

1 Use a Minnesota or four-lumen Sengstaken–Blakemore tube.
2 Test the gastric and oesophageal balloons before insertion.
3 Pass the well-lubricated tube into the stomach up to at least 50 cm. The position of the gastric balloon can be checked by listening over the stomach with a stethoscope whilst rapidly introducing air into the gastric channel. After the insertion of 250 ml of air into the gastric balloon, the tube is pulled up until the gastric balloon impacts at the gastro-oesophageal junction.
4 Inflate the oesophageal balloon with saline mixed with Conray until a pressure of 35–40 mmHg is obtained; then tape the tube to the patient's face without traction. Perform a chest radiograph immediately after insertion to check the tube position.
5 It is important to maintain continuous low-pressure suction on the oesophageal channel and to aspirate the stomach hourly. The pressure in the oesophageal balloon must be checked every four hours.
6 Never apply more than 12 hours continuous oesophageal compression without an interval of decompression. If necessary, a second 12 hour period of compression can be applied, provided that there has been at least 30 min of decompression. No more than 24 hours total oesophageal compression must be applied over a 48 hour period.

The complications of balloon tamponade are shown in Table 8.2.

Difficulty of insertion
Rarely, some difficulty may be encountered in inserting the balloon tube. This is particularly so if the patient is not very co-

Table 8.2
Complications of
balloon tamponade

Difficulty of insertion
Failure to control bleeding
Oesophageal rupture
Pulmonary aspiration
Respiratory obstruction
Discomfort

operative and the tube is too pliable. The tube can be stiffened by placing it in a refrigerator, but the urgency of the situation usually does not allow time for this. The best solution is to use a stiff guide-wire from a large ureteric or Fogarty catheter, threaded through the lumen of the tube.

Failure to control bleeding
Overt signs of continued haemorrhage after balloon tamponade of the oesophagus has been undertaken, usually implies that bleeding is occurring from a source other than the oesophageal varices, often a bleeding gastric varix. However, before a diagnosis of bleeding of an extravariceal origin can be confirmed, it is necessary to check the position of and pressure in the oesophageal balloon, in order to eliminate incomplete compression of the oesophageal varices. If bleeding is still not controlled after checking the balloon tube, then repeat the gastroscopy to make a precise diagnosis of the source of bleeding. The use of a gastroscope with a wide-bore suction channel (e.g. Olympus GIF-1T) is very useful in this situation. If a gastric varix or peptic ulcer is demonstrated to be the origin of the bleeding, then an immediate laparotomy should be undertaken to deal with it. A bleeding gastric varix should be underrun with prolene, and if circumstances permit, all visible gastric varices should also be underrun (see p. 176). It is not necessary to perform an oesophageal transection, as this would only add unnecessarily to the risk of morbidity and mortality.

Occasionally repeat gastroscopy reveals erosive gastritis as the source of haemorrhage. This is a very sinister cause of bleeding in patients with concomitant varices and usually only responds to an emergency portal–systemic shunt. However, before embarking on a shunt it is worth trying intensive conservative measures with intragastric administration of low-sodium antacids (e.g. aluminium hydroxide 4%, 400 ml over 24 h by nasogastric tube) and cimetidine 75 mg/hour i.v. If this fails to rapidly control the haemorrhage (e.g. within 4–6 hours), then an emergency end-to-side portacaval shunt must be performed. Do not perform a total gastrectomy, as this is much less satisfactory in controlling the bleeding.

Oesophageal rupture
Oesophageal rupture usually occurs *early* (within 24 hours), from accidental over-distension of the oesophageal balloon, but may occur *later*, following oesophageal necrosis secondary to prolonged balloon compression. Neither problem should occur if there is scrupulous attention to detail in inserting and inflating the balloon tube, as described above. When this complication is recognized the patient is usually moribund and salvage is impossible. Thus if any patient develops respiratory distress with pain, fever and possibly surgical emphysema, order an immediate chest radiograph to detect air in the mediastinum. If an *early*

rupture has occurred, carry out an immediate exploration through a left thoracoabdominal incision. It may be possible to perform a local repair of the ruptured oesophagus along with an oesophageal transection. An oesophagogastrectomy may be the only option open if the oesophagus is extensively damaged, although this procedure is associated with a very high operative mortality. Methods of oesophageal repair following perforation are considered later in this chapter (p. 177) and also in Chapter 4 (p. 68).

Pulmonary aspiration
Pulmonary aspiration is usually the result of aspiration of saliva from inadequate oesophageal suction or from aspiration of blood following a difficult tube insertion. Chest symptoms and signs (fever, tachypnoea, tachycardia, pleuritic pain) rapidly develop and require intensive chest physiotherapy and parenteral broad-spectrum antibiotic administration. Since physiotherapy is impossible until the balloon tube is removed, this should be expedited once the haemorrhage has been arrested. In spite of aggressive measures the patient's condition may deteriorate and blood gas measurements often reveal that respiratory failure has supervened. This requires positive pressure ventilation in an intensive care unit.

Respiratory obstruction
Respiratory obstruction may occur from one of two causes. First, a faulty gastric balloon may deflate and be regurgitated. Second, a large sliding hiatus hernia with a high gastro-oesophageal junction may allow the oesophageal balloon to rise into the pharnyx. This latter problem requires considerable ingenuity to overcome. The best solution is to use a Linton tube if one is available. This tube has a gastric balloon of relatively small size which can be drawn up into the hiatus hernia and impacted at the gastro-oesophageal junction (Fig. 8.1a). Some traction is necessary to compress the varices. Another solution is to wind strong adhesive tape around the proximal oesophageal balloon of a Minnesota tube to reduce its length by one-half. The tube is inserted, the gastric balloon inflated with 100 ml of air and then impacted at the gastro-oesophageal junction. This position can be maintained with 1 kg of traction (Fig. 8.1b). If this fails to control the bleeding, then the oesophageal balloon can be inflated. Instruct the nurses to maintain a careful watch on the patient and be prepared to deflate the oesophageal balloon at the first sign of respiratory distress.

Discomfort
No patient tolerates a balloon tube without some discomfort. Occasionally it is necessary to sedate a severely distressed patient. Diazepam 5–10 mg i.v., repeated every 4–6 hours, is usually sufficient.

Figure 8.1
Methods of balloon
tamponade of
oesophageal varices
associated with a
large hiatus hernia.
(a) Using a Linton
tube. (b) Using a
modified Minnesota
or Sengstaken–
Blakemore tube (see
text).

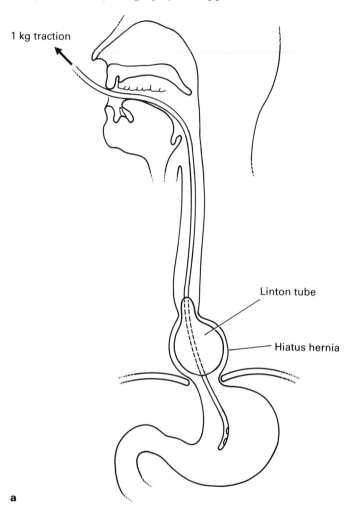

Figure 8.1
Methods of balloon tamponade of oesophageal varices associated with a large hiatus hernia. (a) Using a Linton tube. (b) Using a modified Minnesota or Sengstaken–Blakemore tube (see text).

1 kg traction

Linton tube

Hiatus hernia

a

Endoscopic sclerotherapy

Most clinicians perform sclerotherapy with a flexible endoscope, such as an Olympus GIF-K, fitted with an injection needle passed down the suction channel, with or without a Williams' overtube. The use of the aspiration channel for the injection needle makes aspiration of blood difficult if active variceal bleeding is encountered. Some clinicians claim that a rigid endoscope allows better suction under these conditions, although with persistence and ingenuity actively bleeding varices can be injected using the flexible endoscope. There is considerable debate about: (i) whether injection should be performed when varices are actively bleeding or after a period of conservative treatment; (ii) the necessity of a Williams' overtube; (iii) what substance to use as a sclerosant; (iv) where to inject the sclerosant; (v) how much of the

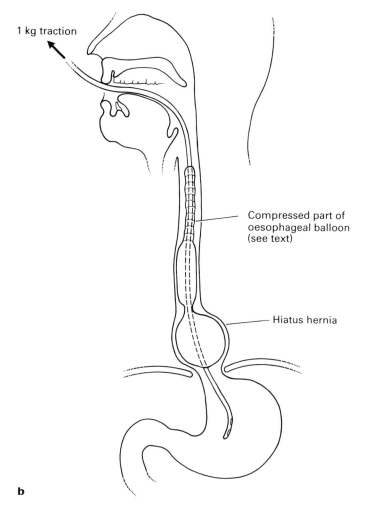

1 kg traction

Compressed part of
oesophageal balloon
(see text)

Hiatus hernia

b

sclerosant should be injected and how frequently it should be injected; and (vi) whether adjuvant treatment, e.g. balloon tamponade, may be useful after injection. Most of these questions cannot be answered until adequately performed clinical trials have been reported.

There is general agreement at present that 5 ml of ethanol-amine oleate per varix, injected intravariceally using a flexible endoscope and a Williams' overtube, provides good results. I (JNB) prefer to use general anaesthesia and inject the varices within six hours of admission to hospital, whether actively bleeding or not. Sedated patients are reported to tolerate injection sclerotherapy using a Williams' overtube. However, if treatment is performed during active bleeding or soon after, general anaesthesia and endotracheal intubation are necessary in order to prevent aspiration of blood.

Other technical points

1 The Williams' overtube must be well lubricated, especially at its end, to facilitate atraumatic insertion through the upper oesophageal sphincter.

2 All injections should be intravariceal, the needle being repositioned if a submucosal bleb is being raised.

3 The point of injection should be as near the cardia as possible and only varices in the last 5 cm of the oesophagus need be obliterated.

4 Tamponade with the Williams' tube should be performed for at least ten minutes after completion of injection. Careful inspection of the oesophagus should then be carried out to confirm adequate haemostasis. If the varices are still bleeding, perform a second ten-minute tamponade, and only if bleeding does not stop, carry out a balloon tamponade.

5 Always order a chest radiograph immediately after injection sclerotherapy to check for inadvertent oesophageal perforation.

The complications that may occur with endoscopic sclerotherapy are shown in Table 8.3.

Early bleeding

Recommencement of active haemorrhage often results from the attempt to perform sclerotherapy. This often occurs prior to actual injection if a lengthy endoscopy is performed, with removal of clot overlying the ruptured varix. Furthermore, placement of the Williams' tube sometimes disturbs a clot and causes renewed haemorrhage. In either event, patience and persistence will be rewarded by successful injection into the bleeding varix. Rotate the Williams' tube through 90° to compress the bleeding varix, then wait for five minutes before attempting to inspect the area. Perform copious washing with saline solution down the Williams' tube, coupled with aspiration through a long sucker to remove clots, then slowly rotate the Williams' tube back to its original position. This usually allows adequate visualization of the offending varix for injection. It is

Table 8.3
Complications of
endoscopic
sclerotherapy

Early	Late
Bleeding	Interval bleeding
Oesophageal perforation	Bleeding secondary to oesophageal ulceration
Pain	Perforation secondary to oesophageal necrosis
Pyrexia	Stricture
Adult respiratory distress? syndrome	Motility disorders (reflux or dysphagia)

important to inject the actual varix which is bleeding if this can be identified. An aid to sclerotherapy under these difficult circumstances is to use a simultaneous infusion of somatostatin (see p. 164) to reduce bleeding. In practice I have never had to do this. Following a difficult sclerotherapy for active bleeding, it is wise to employ balloon tamponade of the oesophagus for 12 hours.

If great difficulty is encountered in performing sclerotherapy in the face of active bleeding, consider aborting sclerotherapy and inserting a Minnesota tube, with a view to repeating the sclerotherapy 24 hours later. In practice I have never had to do this.

In a few patients bleeding recurs within hours after an apparently successful sclerotherapy. These patients can be tamponaded for 12 hours, and if necessary, a further 12 hours, provided an interval of at least 30 minutes is allowed without compression between the two episodes of balloon tamponade. The second period of compression can be combined with an infusion of somatostatin (see p. 164), if this drug is available. The somatostatin infusion can be continued for 2–5 days after the cessation of tamponade. If bleeding recurs again shortly after the second period of oesophageal tamponade, then emergency oesophageal transection should be carried out. It is unwise to delay the decision to operate if bleeding is not controlled by two 12 hour periods of balloon tamponade.

Perforation
Oesophageal perforation may be recognized *early* after sclerotherapy (within 24 hours), or *late*. Early perforation is nearly always from a small rupture of the cervical oesophagus, which is often related to some difficulty in inserting the endoscope with the Williams' tube through the upper oesophageal sphincter. On other occasions it occurs after effortless passage of the endoscope and Williams' tube and thus presumably results from perforation of the oesophagus by cervical osteophytes. In either case the first suspicion of an oesophageal rupture is that the patient develops surgical emphysema or a routine post-sclerotherapy chest radiograph shows air in the upper mediastinum and soft tissues of the neck. On examination the patient may have surgical emphysema in the neck but is well and oblivious of the complication. Treatment is conservative with i.v. fluids, i.v. broad-spectrum antibiotics and nil by mouth for at least 72 hours, after which oral fluids can be cautiously restarted. If at any time fever supervenes and there is evidence of increasing spread of extravasated material, then operative intervention must be considered. This should take the form of drainage and total parenteral nutrition with i.v. antibiotics. Fortunately this is very rarely necessary after instrumental perforation of the cervical oesophagus.

A thoracic perforation usually presents late (after 10–14 days), in some cases being heralded by sudden deterioration of the patient's condition, with respiratory distress, fever and chest pain. Septicaemic shock may rapidly supervene. However, in other cases there may only be pyrexia of unknown origin. The cause is usually a full-thickness oesophageal wall necrosis. If any doubt exists about the diagnosis, a Gastrografin swallow must be immediately performed.

Technical aspects of the injection sclerotherapy are probably causative, e.g. too large a volume of sclerosant (which should not exceed 25 ml in total), paravariceal rather than intravariceal injection, inexperience, etc. Use of balloon tamponade following sclerotherapy has sometimes been quoted as undesirable and possibly adding to morbidity from oesophageal necrosis. This has never been my experience. Any persistent post-sclerotherapy bleeding should be treated with immediate balloon tamponade for at least six hours, although a better alternative would be to use a somatostatin infusion.

Treatment of late thoracic perforation should be relatively conservative, with resuscitation, antibiotics, cardiovascular support, nasogastric suction drainage of the oesophagus above the perforation, mediastinal toilet and intercostal drainage through a small thoracotomy (on the side on which the Gastrografin extravasates), gastrostomy, and feeding jejunostomy (Fig. 8.2). Gunning and Kingsnorth (1979) recommend local applications of 20% sodium hydroxide via an endoscope at weekly intervals until the perforation closes. Mortality is very high following late thoracic oesophageal perforation in patients with oesophageal varices.

Early thoracic perforation (within 24 hours) if recognized should be treated along traditional lines by immediate local repair. Oesophageal transection should be performed at the same time if the oesophageal tear is large enough and positioned such that the stapler can be readily inserted through it to the correct position for such a procedure.

Pain

Some retrosternal discomfort is usually present for 24–48 hours following sclerotherapy, especially if a Williams' overtube is used. This may be associated with dysphagia. Local factors such as oesophagitis, perioesophagitis and temporary motility dysfunction are probably causative. They require no treatment apart from simple analgesics and reassurance.

Pyrexia

A transient post-injection pyrexia is seen in up to 25% of patients following sclerotherapy. The pyrexia may be due to chest complications. However, many of these patients have no obvious cause for their fever and it is speculated that it arises from injection phlebitis or perioesophagitis. Some clinicians report dramatic resolution of the fever with steroids, dexamethasone phosphate, 4 mg i.m., 12 hourly for 3–5 days. However, if chest

Figure 8.2
Management of late
perforation of the
thoracic oesophagus.

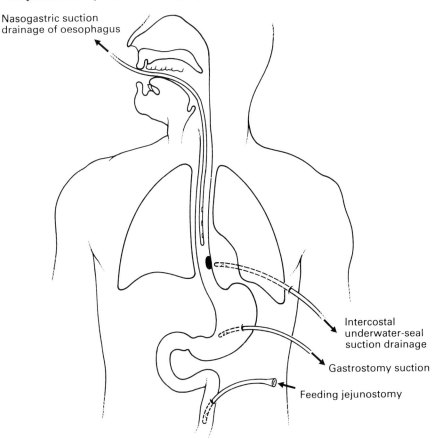

Nasogastric suction
drainage of oesophagus

Intercostal
underwater-seal
suction drainage

Gastrostomy suction

Feeding jejunostomy

infection is excluded, specific therapy is not recommended as the fever always resolves in a few days without any sequelae.

Adult Respiratory Distress Syndrome (ARDS)
Patients may develop ARDS following sclerotherapy, although this complication is very rare in its fulminant form (Monroe et al, 1983). The development within 8–36 hours following sclerotherapy of dyspnoea and hypoxaemia, and a chest radiograph showing bilateral alveolar/interstitial infiltrates should alert one to this possibility. A respiratory physician should be urgently consulted, as the diagnosis and management of this condition is complex. Clearly, avoidance of intravariceal injections of large volumes of sclerosant (> 25 ml) lessens the likelihood of this complication.

Interval bleeding
Interval bleeding is defined as recurrent variceal bleeding while the patient is receiving maintenance sclerotherapy, before obliteration has been achieved. This can be expected in up to 50% of

patients. Fortunately, the recurrent bleeding episodes are often mild in nature when compared with the first variceal haemorrhage and are often not life-threatening. These patients, however, should be treated according to the clinician's protocol for a patient presenting with a first bleed, i.e. emergency sclerotherapy or balloon tamponade followed by sclerotherapy. Following control of the rebleeding episode, the patient should be put back into the maintenance sclerotherapy programme. There is some controversy about the optimum interval between injection treatments. Too-frequent injections may lead to an increased incidence of local complications, e.g. stricture, mucosal ulceration, etc., while infrequent injections may increase the frequency of interval bleeds. Most clinicians compromise with a three-week interval between injections until obliteration is achieved. Furthermore, after obliteration there is a propensity for varices to return and bleed although the exact frequency of this complication is uncertain. This means that all patients will need life-long follow-up to monitor and treat rebleeding.

In some patients interval bleeding is frequent and massive. Moreover, inspection of the varices in these patients reveals little progress towards obliteration. Although no precise guidelines can be given, there is a place for either oesophageal transection or a portal–systemic shunt, especially if the patient has had three or four life-threatening bleeds. Surgery should only be performed electively, if possible. If the patient is Child's C grade (see p. 178), then oesophageal transection only should be performed. If the patient is young and Child's A or B grade, then a portal–systemic shunt can be considered (preferably an end-to-side portacaval), although at present most surgeons in the UK would prefer to perform an oesophageal transection. Considerable judgement is necessary. Where there is any doubt, do not delay referring the patient to an experienced surgeon.

Bleeding secondary to ulceration
Not uncommonly a secondary bleed may occur 7–10 days following sclerotherapy and repeat oesophagoscopy shows this to be from an oesophageal ulcer at the site of previous injection sclerotherapy. This usually results from paravariceal injection, although even after intravariceal injection there is always some paravariceal leakage and occasional ulceration. Treatment can be expectant with somatostatin infusion if active bleeding is occurring. Alternatively, balloon tamponade can be used to control the bleeding, though it should be ensured that the pressure in the oesophageal balloon does not exceed 40 mmHg. Repeat sclerotherapy at this stage is pointless and dangerous.

Stricture
Following sclerotherapy there is a 5–10% incidence of late stricture development with associated dysphagia. This is probably related to excessive fibrosis and is suspected of being more

common after paravariceal than intravariceal injection. These strictures are always soft and pliable and easily dilated with Celestin, Eder–Puestow or, perhaps better, Maloney's dilators (Fig. 6.9). Sometimes the stricture develops after only a few injection treatments, before variceal obliteration has been achieved. In this situation oesophageal dilatation can be performed and sclerotherapy continued until the varices are obliterated.

Motility disorders
There is some evidence to suggest that lower oesophageal sphincter function and motility may be disturbed following sclerotherapy. However, there are no convincing data to support an increased incidence of motility symptoms. In particular, there is no evidence that the incidence of gastro-oesophageal reflux is increased following sclerotherapy; therefore, the practice of prescribing antireflux therapy has no basis.

Oesophageal transection
If oesophageal transection is necessary, most surgeons favour a transabdominal approach and perform the transection with an EEA stapler. This is usually combined with some degree of local oesophageal devascularization.

Oesophageal transection is often reserved for the patient who presents with an acute variceal bleed which has failed to be controlled with vasoactive drugs, balloon tamponade, sclerotherapy or a combination of these. Clearly if conservative treatments fail, there should be no delay in proceeding with oesophageal transection. The mortality is high in Child's grade C patients but there is no viable alternative. Emergency portal–systemic shunting has a prohibitive mortality, especially in Child's C patients.

Important technical points
Technical points that may reduce the incidence of complications following oesophageal transection include the following:

1 Use a midline incision, though occasionally it is necessary to convert this into a thoracoabdominal incision if the left lobe of the liver is excessively large and impeding progress.
2 Ligate all perioesophageal veins and bare the oesophagus for at least 5 cm, taking care to preserve the anterior vagus nerve. This can be very difficult when there has been previous sclerotherapy, since the perioesophageal tissues are very fibrotic; patience and care are necessary.
3 If possible, use the American EEA pattern stapler with a 28 mm head and perform the transection within 1 cm of the gastro-oesophageal junction.
4 Ligate the left gastric pedicle (including the left gastric vein).
5 Through a generous gastrotomy inspect the fundus of the stomach and underrun with prolene or polyglycolic acid any

obvious gastric varices (Fig. 8.3). It is important to start the suturing of the gastric varices as high as possible, into the oesophagus if necessary. A long, curved thin blade retractor inserted into the oesophagus will make these apex sutures easier to insert.

6 Insert a nasogastric tube intraoperatively.
7 Do not insert an intraperitoneal drain.
8 Administer prophylactic antibiotics, e.g. a cephalosporin and metronidazole.

Avoid the temptation to do a splenectomy, since postoperative splenic vein thrombosis may aggravate the portal hypertension. It is exceedingly rare to have to perform a splenectomy for secondary hypersplenism. After oesophageal transection, follow-up all patients with endoscopy at yearly intervals to detect return of the varices.

The complications that occur following oesophageal transection are shown in Table 8.4.

Early bleeding
Early bleeding generally implies that the transection was performed too high or that bleeding was originally from a gastric varix which was missed at operation. In either case perform

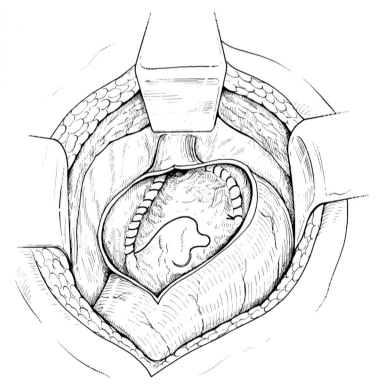

Figure 8.3
Method of underrunning gastric varices. Use a prolene or polyglycolic acid suture, starting the underrunning as high as possible.

Table 8.4
Complications
following
oesophageal
transection

Early	Late
Bleeding	Stricture and dysphagia
Oesophageal perforation	Recurrent bleeding
Ascitic fluid leak	
Chest complications	
Liver and other organ failure	

endoscopy to exclude a haemorrhagic gastritis and then undertake reoperation as soon as possible. Underrun a bleeding gastric varix with prolene and also any other gastric varices if the situation permits. Bleeding from the oesophagus can be controlled by directly underrunning the varices at the gastro-oesophageal junction with the aid of a wide gastrotomy and good retraction. A reanastomosis with the stapler must not be attempted, as this would result in an isolated avascular segment, which invariably undergoes necrosis.

Perforation
Perforation is the result of unrecognized accidental damage to the oesophagus during transection or an anastomosis which has leaked. This is usually discovered late after at least 24 hours, although, if diagnosed radiologically within 24 hours (using a thin barium swallow), immediate reoperation and direct repair should be performed. In addition to local repair, pass a nasogastric tube to 30 cm and insert a gastrostomy tube. Both tubes should be maintained on continuous low-pressure suction and the patient commenced on total parenteral nutrition. A late perforation requires immediate re-exploration, with sump drains inserted around the anastomosis, and nasogastric and gastrostomy tubes inserted as above.

Ascitic fluid leak
Any laparotomy in a patient with portal hypertension is often followed by the development of ascites, even if ascites was not present preoperatively. Thus an intraperitoneal drain should not be inserted to avoid protein and fluid loss through an artificially created fistula. Moreover, drains are likely to increase the incidence of infection of the ascitic fluid. Even if no drain is inserted, there is often a transient leak of ascitic fluid from the laparotomy wound. This should not be treated as a significant wound dehiscence. A skin stitch should be inserted at the site of the leak and the wound fitted with a colostomy bag to collect the drainage. Spironolactone therapy and salt and fluid restriction should then be commenced (see p. 161). The wound usually dries up in 1–2 weeks.

Chest and other organ complications

Postoperative chest complications such as atelectasis and pneumonia are more common in these patients. Thus, pre- and postoperative chest physiotherapy should be prescribed and specific antibiotics administered according to the sensitivities of the cultured organisms.

Some degree of exacerbation of pre-existing liver failure is inevitable following laparotomy, especially in emergency situations. This may be accompanied by an exacerbation of encephalopathy. Acute renal failure may develop in circumstances where there has been prolonged hypotension, the aetiology of which may be complex. The help of a renal physician is desirable, as the management is often not straightforward.

Stricture and dysphagia

Some minor dysphagia is common following oesophageal transection, but this usually settles in a few months. However, in approximately 15% of patients it is more persistent and requires oesophageal dilatation. This is easily accomplished with Maloney's, Eder–Puestow or Celestin dilators. There is some evidence that this problem may be more common if the transection is performed too high and less common if it is performed as near the gastro-oesophageal junction as possible.

Late recurrent bleeding

Many episodes of late recurrent bleeding following oesophageal transection are the result of lesions other than oesophageal varices, e.g. gastritis, peptic ulcer, etc.; however, recurrent bleeding from varices can be expected in 6–10% of patients following oesophageal transection. The cause in some cases may be from reformation of variceal channels, whilst in others the transection may have been placed too high in the oesophagus. In either case sclerotherapy should be carried out until the varices have been obliterated. Rarely, if sclerotherapy is proving ineffective, a portal–systemic shunt should be electively performed.

Portal–systemic shunts

Regardless of the type of shunt performed, emergency shunting has a prohibitive operative mortality of 45%, rising to 70% for Child's C patients. Clearly, therefore, shunts should only be performed electively, although exceedingly rarely it may be necessary to perform an emergency shunt if all else has failed. It has become clear that (i) the operative mortality of the various types of shunts in experienced hands is similar; (ii) the reduced incidence of encephalopathy following a distal splenorenal shunt is short lived and certainly by the end of a year the incidence is the same as that of a total (e.g. end-to-side portacaval) shunt; (iii) a Child's grade C patient should never be shunted because of the high operative mortality; (iv) a mesocaval shunt with synthetic graft material should be avoided, as the thrombosis rate is almost

50%, with return of the bleeding risk; and (v) no procedure is more effective at preventing recurrent variceal haemorrhage than a portacaval shunt. Thus in the very rare, emergency situation, an end-to-side portacaval shunt is the only shunt that should be performed, since it is faster and easier to perform than most other shunts and is more certain of decompressing the portal circulation.

Portal–systemic encephalopathy is the major factor preventing more widespread use of shunts. However, although it cannot be denied that some 5% of patients may experience severe chronic encephalopathy, many clinicians, especially those in the USA, feel that this is easier to manage than continuing admissions to hospital with recurrent bleeding. The minor degree of encephalopathy that other patients may experience is easily controlled with medical treatment and often of little inconvenience to these patients. However, considerable judgement is necessary to choose which patients may be suitable for a shunt. Moreover, at present, the methods used for selecting patients for shunting are wanting. However, there is general agreement that patients with good liver function, especially Child's grade A patients, are likely to do best. An end-to-side portacaval shunt is the best procedure, as it is relatively simple and can be readily performed by a well-trained general surgeon.

Apart from the general complications, mentioned above, that result from performing a laparotomy on any patient with portal hypertension, the specific complications that ensue from portal–systemic shunts are shown in Table 8.5.

Portal–systemic encephalopathy

Subclinical and mild encephalopathy can be easily controlled with restriction of dietary protein to approximately 50 g/day and the use of lactulose, initially at 30 ml t.d.s. with meals. The lactulose dosage should be altered to produce at least two semi-solid bowel actions, but not frank diarrhoea, per day. If this does not work, neomycin 3 g/day can be tried in place of lactulose. Although neomycin alone is almost as effective as lactulose, it can be complicated by nephrotoxicity, ototoxicity, staphylococcal or *Clostridium difficile* colitis and malabsorption.

It is most important to exclude any cause of acute encephalo-

Table 8.5 Complications following portal–systemic shunts	
	Portal–systemic encephalopathy
	Deterioration in liver function
	Rebleeding
	Liver and other organ failure
	Ascites
	Haemosiderosis
	Pancreatitis

pathy, e.g. recent haemorrhage, infection (especially of ascitic fluid), constipation, increased intake of dietary protein, uraemia, electrolyte imbalance (especially hypokalaemia due to diuretic administration), and analgesic and sedative overuse. If bleeding, constipation or increased dietary protein are causative, prescribe cathartic agents such as magnesium sulphate enemas.

In the very few patients who have the refractory severe form of encephalopathy it is worth trying bromocriptine (a dopamine agonist) 15 mg/day and oral metronidazole 400 mg t.d.s. (to reduce bacterial ammonium production), although success with these agents is poor. There are only two alternatives remaining: (i) dismantling the shunt; and (ii) colon exclusion or excision. If possible, the shunt should be taken down. (This is impossible for an end-to-side portacaval shunt but possible for most others.) The shunt is best exposed and a ligature applied to the actual shunt. This can be readily performed in mesocaval, distal and central splenorenal shunts. A side-to-side portacaval shunt requires surgical division of the shunt, with repair of the portal vein and inferior vena cava. There have been some reports of the application of a rubber sling around the shunt (including side-to-side portacaval shunts), with gradual occlusion over a period of six weeks by external application of tension to the sling (Bismuth, Houssin and Grange, 1983). The proponents of this technique claim that gradual occlusion of the shunt makes early rebleeding less likely, although they also perform an oesophageal transection during the operation. In spite of encouraging results with this technique, it is clearly hazardous, as the sling has to cut through the shunt over the six weeks, with a risk of internal haemorrhage.

Whichever method is used, dismantling the shunt invariably cures the problem, though the risk of rebleeding returns. Thus injection sclerotherapy should be carried out to obliterate the varices prior to dismantling a shunt. However, oesophageal transection may be a viable alternative if there is not enough time to perform sclerotherapy.

Subtotal colectomy with an ileorectal anastomosis or colon exclusion are the only options open in patients with an end-to-side portacaval shunt. These operations have a high postoperative mortality of approximately 25%. However, they are usually performed in moribund patients who have end-stage liver disease. The results in the survivors are by and large very good. However, it must be stressed that this operation should never be carried out in a patient with untreated portal hypertension (e.g. a thrombosed shunt), as the risk of postoperative haemorrhage is too high. Furthermore, the patient should have good liver function and no end-stage liver disease.

If intensive medical therapy has failed, colon excision or exclusion should be carried out sooner rather than later. Colon excision with an ileosigmoid or, better, ileorectal anastomosis gives the best results. Colon exclusion (i.e. ileorectal anastomosis with ileal and sigmoid mucous fistulas leaving the colon in situ) may result in bacterial overgrowth in the remaining colon, with worse results.

Deterioration of liver function

After an end-to-side portacaval shunt has been performed there is a temporary disturbance of standard liver function tests (bilirubin, liver enzymes), owing to complete absence of portal blood flow. However, the liver function tests return to preoperative values gradually, after 3–6 months. It is generally thought that global liver function is only marginally impaired in the long term as a result of a total shunt. Thus, no specific therapy is necessary for this complication, although it is necessary to exclude other causes of disturbed liver function, e.g. continued alcohol abuse. The promise of maintenance of portal flow by a selective shunt, e.g. a distal splenorenal shunt, is now uncertain and in all probability most selective shunts are near total shunts.

Rebleeding

This complication generally implies that the shunt has thrombosed, although other causes of bleeding have to be excluded. Shunt thrombosis can be confirmed by performing coeliac axis or superior mesenteric arteriography. The shunt that has thrombosed is invariably a mesocaval type. In this situation it is possible to perform another shunt, e.g. a portacaval shunt, although most surgeons would opt for sclerotherapy or oesophageal transection in the first instance.

Rarely, the angiogram demonstrates that the portal–systemic anastomosis is stenotic rather than occluded. Moreover, measurement of wedged hepatic venous pressure demonstrates that portal hypertension persists. There are recent reports of successful transvenous dilatation of these strictures with balloon catheters, resulting in a reduction of portal pressure and bleeding risk.

Ascites

Ascites is very common following a distal splenorenal shunt but it is usually satisfactorily controlled with medical treatment. If ascites persists in spite of aggressive medical measures, then a Le Veen peritoneovenous shunt should be performed. A Le Veen shunt will block in 19% of patients and a further 50% will develop disseminated intravascular coagulation; only in a few percent does it become clinically significant. Septicaemia resulting in death may occur following peritoneovenous shunt insertion if the ascites becomes infected.

Hepatic haemosiderosis

This complication occurs in the long term, following certain shunt procedures. It is of no clinical significance and thus requires no treatment.

Pancreatitis

Pancreatitis rarely occurs following construction of any shunt requiring dissection of the pancreas, especially the distal splenorenal shunt. There is often a history of prior pancreatitis and technical difficulty with the dissection. A pseudocyst may develop and should be drained by ultrasound or CAT scan guided percutaneous needle aspiration.

Conclusion

The management of these difficult patients is best undertaken by a clinician who is interested and experienced in the various treatment options. A clear treatment strategy, scrupulous attention to technical detail, high dependency unit monitoring and the availability of a hepatologist, haematologist, renal and chest physician will all help to reduce the complication rate in these patients.

Persisting Controversies

- What is the place of endoscopic sclerotherapy and oesophageal transection in preventing recurrent variceal haemorrhage?
- What is the long-term efficacy of endoscopic sclerotherapy?
- Which patients are suitable for a shunt?
- Which type of shunt should be performed?

Further reading

Bismuth, H., Houssin, D. & Grange, D. (1983) Suppression of the shunt and esophageal transection: a new technique for the treatment of disabling postshunt encephalopathy. *American Journal of Surgery*, *146*, 392–396.

Bredfeldt, J.E., Pingoud, E.G., Groszmann, R.J., Tilson, M.D. & Conn, H.O. (1981) Balloon dilatation of stenotic portacaval anastomosis. *Hepatology*, *5*, 448–451.

Crossley, I.R. & Williams, R. (1984) Progress in the treatment of chronic portasystemic encephalopathy. *Gut*, *25*, 85–98.

Gunning, A.J. & Kingsnorth, A. (1979) Treatment of chronic oesophageal perforations with special reference to an endoscopic method. *British Journal of Surgery*, *66*, 226–229.

Henderson, J.M., El Khishen, M., Millikan, W.J., Sones, P.J. & Warren, W.D. (1983) Management of stenosis of distal splenorenal shunt by balloon dilation. *Surgery, Gynecology and Obstetrics*, *157*, 43–48.

Jenkins, S.A., Baxter, J.N., Corbett, W., Devitt, P., Ware, J. & Shields, R. (1985) A prospective randomised clinical trial comparing somatostatin and vasopressin in controlling acute variceal haemorrhage. *British Medical Journal*, *290*, 275–278.

Monore, P., Morrow, C.F., Millen, J.E., Fairman, R.P. & Glauser,

F.L. (1983) Acute respiratory failure after sodium morrhuate esophageal sclerotherapy. *Gastroenterology*, *85*, 693–699.

Picone, S.B., Donovan, A.J. & Yellin, A.E. (1983) Abdominal colectomy for chronic encephalopathy due to portal–systemic shunt. *Archives of Surgery*, *118*, 33–37.

Sarfeh, I.J., Juler, G.L., Stemmer, E.A. & Mason, G.R. (1982) Results of surgical management of haemorrhagic gastritis in patients with gastroesophageal varices. *Surgery, Gynecology & Obstetrics*, *155*, 167–170.

Soderlund, C. & Wiechel, K. (1983) Oesophageal perforation after sclerotherapy for variceal haemorrhage. *Acta Chirurgica Scandinavica*, *149*, 491–495.

Weber, F.L. (1983) Therapy of portal–systemic encephalopathy; the practical and the promising. *Gastroenterology*, *81*, 174–181.

Westaby, D., MacDougall, B.R.D. & Williams, R. (1982) *Variceal Bleeding*. London: Pitman.

9 Complications Common to Gastrectomy and Vagotomy With Drainage

The indications for gastric resection have changed dramatically over the past 40 years. Previously most gastrectomies were performed for the cure of duodenal ulcer. Today vagotomy has removed primary duodenal ulcers from the list of indications for gastrectomy. The most frequent indication is now gastric carcinoma, followed by resection for chronic gastric ulcer, with a relatively small number being performed for recurrent peptic ulcer following vagotomy. This change has influenced the frequency, especially of burst duodenal stump and postgastrectomy symptoms.

Early Complications

Bleeding

Causes The stomach is extremely vascular and intraluminal bleeding may follow any incision and closure with inversion, as follows gastrectomy, gastroenterostomy with anastomosis or pyloroplasty. The duodenal stump may bleed following a Polya partial or total gastrectomy. A missed ulcer may bleed. After operation an acute ulcer or erosion can develop rapidly and bleed. Haemorrhage sometimes occurs from diagnosed or unsuspected lesions, such as oesophageal or gastric varices. At operations performed to control gastric bleeding, the source, such as a peptic ulcer, may not be recognized, may not be controlled, or if controlled, may recur.

Extraluminal bleeding follows gastrectomy if a gastric vessel is damaged but not invaginated sufficiently to bleed into the lumen. External gastric vessels that are divided during a resection may not be properly controlled or may stop and produce postoperative reactionary bleeding. Arterial bleeding may develop as the pressure rises or venous bleeding may occur as the result of straining that increases the venous pressure, causing a clot to be dislodged. Secondary bleeding is rare. During major resections bleeding may be caused from damage to the spleen, diaphragmatic crus, omentum, pancreas, liver lobe, or small or large bowel. During the fashioning of a jejunal conduit, mesenteric vessels may be damaged and subsequently bleed. Within the chest, mobilization of the lung may result in damage to the vessels at the lung root: especially at risk is the lower left pulmonary vein, as the lower lobe is elevated. On the right the azygos venous system may be damaged.

A vessel may retract within a bulky ligature (see p. 12) and form a haematoma that only later bursts into the abdomen or chest. The raw edges of cut viscera may continue to bleed. Inadvertent damage to the spleen and liver may be missed during operation. An occasional cause of major bleeding is damage to the left hepatic vein, when the left lobe of the liver is mobilized to improve the view of the diaphragmatic hiatus when carrying out radical gastrectomy and vagotomy (Fig. 9.1).

A generalized bleeding tendency is seen in patients treated with anticoagulant drugs, jaundiced patients, and those with clotting and vascular defects which are sometimes induced by drugs, including cytotoxics.

Prevention Recognize and treat before operation those patients with an increased tendency to bleed, and correct anaemia, if necessary delaying an elective operation.

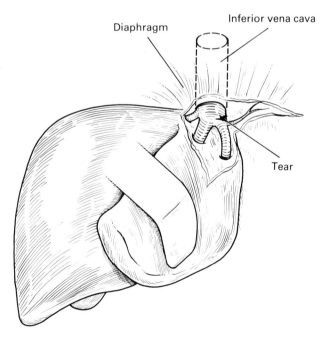

Figure 9.1
Injury to left hepatic vein or inferior vena cava behind mobilized left lobe of liver.

At operation carefully control major blood vessels before dividing them. Check all raw surfaces, including cut viscera. When suturing oesophagus, stomach, duodenum and jejunum, use the over-and-over continuous haemostatic stitch (see p. 14) or release clamps, identify and individually ligate blood vessels in the edge of the cut bowel, if a non-haemostatic Connell type of stitch is to be used. Stapled anastomoses are not immune from bleeding.

On completion of the operation carefully check all the major blood vessels, the viscera such as liver, spleen and pancreas, and in particular the divided mesenteries and omenta. A notorious source of bleeding is from the splenic ends of divided left gastroepiploic or short gastric vessels, which drop deeply into the abdomen, bleed into the gastrosplenic omentum, sometimes forming a haematoma that may be mistaken on a casual glance for a portion of the spleen. If a left hepatic vein has been nicked while mobilizing the liver, place a pack in the angle between the diaphragm and the left lobe of the liver for five minutes by the clock. This nearly always controls the bleeding. It may now be possible to suture it. If not, try placing a strip of haemostatic gauze in the angle and replacing the left lobe, gently compressing it with a retractor placed over a pack. These manoeuvres will virtually always control the bleeding in this low-pressure system. Be patient and do not rush into medial sternotomy to display the inferior vena cava, or caval clamping. If necessary insert a gauze roll pack, leave it for 48 hours and then gently remove it.

At an operation to control bleeding, as from peptic ulceration, make sure that the bleeding is fully controlled at the first operation. Failure to do so now is a potent cause of postoperative bleeding. The majority of bleeding posterior chronic duodenal ulcers can be controlled through a gastroduodenotomy. Severe bleeding in the base of the ulcer is from the gastroduodenal artery or one of its branches. Place deep sutures of non-absorbable material on an eyeless needle through the base of the ulcer above and below the site of bleeding (Fig. 9.2). When the bleeding is confidently controlled the gastroduodenotomy can be closed as a pyloroplasty. Truncal vagotomy is carried out to reduce gastric acid secretion and prevent progression of the ulcer.

Bleeding from very large ulcers cannot always be controlled in this manner and demand Polya partial gastrectomy. It is sometimes possible to transect the duodenum proximal to the ulcer, evert the edges, insert haemostatic stitches, and then safely close the duodenum in two layers (Fig. 9.3). With a very proximal ulcer it is sometimes better to transect the duodenum distal to it for safe closure, leaving the ulcer base exposed for the insertion of haemostatic stitches (Fig. 9.4).

Do not lightly dissect distally in the duodenum beyond an extensive or post-bulbar ulcer. Be prepared to perform Nissen's manoeuvre (Fig. 9.5). Transect the duodenum through the

Figure 9.2
Insert stitches to
control duodenal
ulcer bleeding.

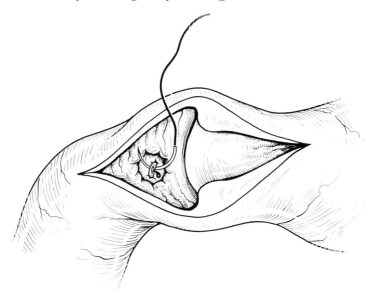

anterior wall as far proximal as possible. Insert non-absorbable sutures to control the bleeding. Suture the anterior duodenal wall to the distal edge of the ulcer, thus closing the duodenum. If possible now fold the duodenal wall proximally to cover the ulcer base, suturing it to the proximal ulcer edge.

If you cannot safely close the duodenum by any method after controlling the bleeding, do not hesitate to place a purse-string suture around the cut end, place in a large latex tube, tighten the purse-string suture, and then bring the tube to the surface through a separate stab wound (Fig. 9.6). Perform Polya hemigastrectomy. Connect the tube to a collecting bag and remove it after 10 to 14 days. Provided there is no distal obstruction, the fistula invariably closes.

For bleeding gastric ulcer the most effective operation is Billroth I partial gastrectomy, including the ulcer. If the ulcer base is in the pancreas or liver, make sure that bleeding is controlled here with carefully placed non-absorbable sutures. On occasion in a frail patient, with a high bleeding ulcer, it is satisfactory to perform anterior gastrotomy, underrun the ulcer base from within the stomach to control the bleeding, and then close the stomach, and perform truncal vagotomy and pyloroplasty (Fig. 9.7). In my (RMK's) view there is no logic in attempting proximal gastric vagotomy in these emergency circumstances, and, anyway, the nerves of Latarjet may well be caught within the non-absorbable stitches used to control the bleeding. An alternative, if the part of the stomach containing the ulcer is accessible, is to excise the ulcer, control the bleeding from the edges, close the stomach, and then perform vagotomy and

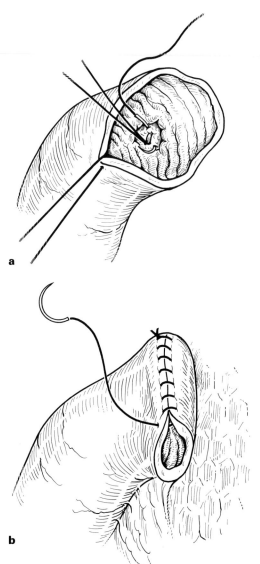

pyloroplasty (Fig. 9.8). For control of variceal bleeding, see p. 160.

Features   Intraluminal bleeding becomes evident if a nasogastric tube is in place, since the aspirate is bloodstained, being 'coffee-ground' if it has been in contact with acid. The patient may vomit blood even with a tube in place. Blood has a laxative effect, so it is passed rectally or is apparent on the glove after rectal examination. Blood that has been in contact with gastric acid is black and tarry.

Figure 9.4
Transection of the
duodenum for closure
distal to an ulcer.

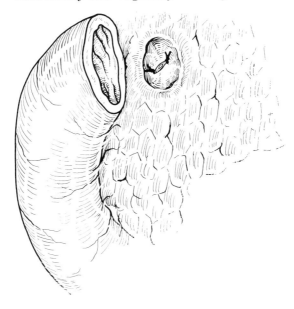

Bleeding within the duodenal and afferent jejunal loop from a duodenal ulcer or cut duodenal edge sometimes presents atypically. The blood often distends the loop but does not pass on into the stomach or jejunum. In a thin patient, the distended loop may produce a visible and palpable abdominal swelling.

Extraluminal bleeding into the abdomen or into the chest following thoracoabdominal gastrectomy initially produces the general signs of hypovolaemia, with restlessness, pallor, peripheral vascular shutdown, rising pulse rate, falling blood pressure and rapid shallow respiration. It may be heralded by a discharge of blood through drains or through the wound. However, absence of a dischage does not exclude intra-abdominal or intrathoracic bleeding.

Intra-abdominal bleeding results in distension, measured by increasing girth if the level at which it is taken is carefully marked. Intrathoracic bleeding is evident because the pleural cavity becomes filled with blood, causing respiratory distress, dullness to percussion and absent breath sounds.

Investigations   Plain posteroanterior chest X-ray demonstrates intrathoracic bleeding as mediastinal widening, or intrapleural opacity and pulmonary collapse. In the lower chest, mediastinal widening is obscured by the cardiac shadow. Intra-abdominal bleeding produces a raised diaphragm. Plain abdominal films may suggest intra-abdominal bleeding by producing a diffuse opacity. However, if there is doubt, ultrasound examination is valuable and can be carried out at the bedside. It is especially useful to demonstrate a collection of clotted blood, for example around an

Figure 9.5
Nissen's closure.
(a) The duodenum is
closed by suturing the
anterior wall to the
distal edge of the
ulcer. (b) If possible
suture the anterior
duodenal wall to the
proximal edge of the
ulcer.

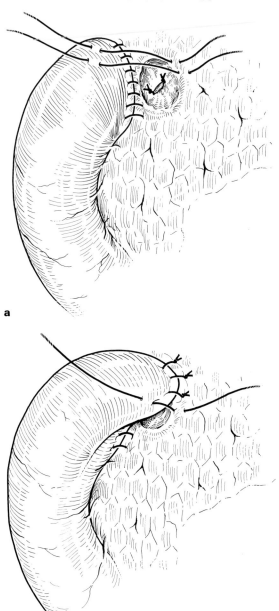

a

b

injured spleen or liver. The scan is obscured beneath the wound, however. Blood can be aspirated from the chest if it does not emerge through the drains and the drains can be resited. If there is doubt about intra-abdominal bleeding, it is reasonable to run in 500 ml of sterile saline through a needle, leave it for 30 minutes and aspirate it to see how heavily bloodstained it is.

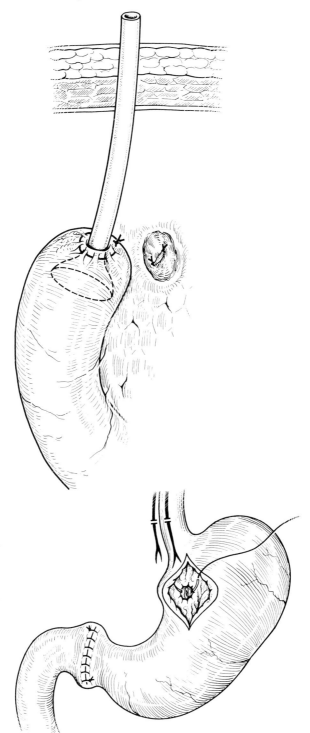

Figure 9.6
If the duodenum cannot be safely closed, insert a large tube (here a Winsbury White catheter). Hold it in place with a purse-string suture.

Figure 9.7
Control of bleeding high gastric ulcer in poor-risk patient. Perform anterior gastrotomy, underrun the ulcer and close the gastrotomy. Carry out truncal vagotomy and pyloroplasty.

Figure 9.8
Ulcer excision to
control bleeding
gastric ulcer. The
defect is closed
transversely. Truncal
vagotomy and
pyloroplasty are
carried out.

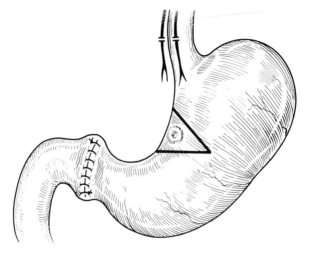

Figure 9.8
Ulcer excision to control bleeding gastric ulcer. The defect is closed transversely. Truncal vagotomy and pyloroplasty are carried out.

If there is doubt about intraluminal bleeding, it is wise to carry out endoscopy. Instill the minimum of air, and aspirate it after inspecting each suspect area.

Management   If blood emerges from the wound or around a drain, remove a skin stitch and gently explore to see if it is merely a superficial vessel that can be compressed or clipped with a haemostat.

Intraluminal bleeding occurring early after operation is almost certainly suture line bleeding or arises from failure to control a source, such as bleeding peptic ulcer or varices. For the management of varices see p. 160. Bleeding from the suture line requiring transfusion, or causing features of shock, demands return of the patient to the operating theatre as soon as possible, after arranging for at least four units of blood to be crossmatched. Re-explore the patient after removing the sutures, and take down the anterior suture line.

Do not, as is frequently advised, create a fresh incision. Suture line bleeding is almost invariably from the anterior line, since the over-and-over posture suture line is haemostatic and I have only once seen bleeding from this. Therefore cut a stitch in the middle of the anterior suture line of the seromuscular stitch and unpick it in each direction. Cut and unpick the all-coats stitch in a similar manner (Fig. 9.9). A suture line bleed will be revealed. Carefully control the bleeding edge, if necessary compressing it gently with a swab-holding forceps, wiping the edge and then gently releasing the swab-holding forceps, while a haemostatic forceps is accurately applied to the vessel. Apply a second forceps with projecting tips below this, so that a satisfactory ligature can be tied. Alternatively but not so certainly, insert an 'X' stitch to obliterate the vessel (Fig. 9.10). When haemostasis is complete, aspirate blood from within the bowel lumen and close the

Figure 9.9
Postoperative
intraluminal bleeding.
Open the anterior
suture line.

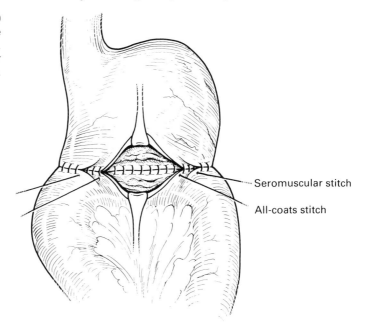

Seromuscular stitch

All-coats stitch

Figure 9.10
Control of bleeding
from posterior suture
line with 'X' stitch.

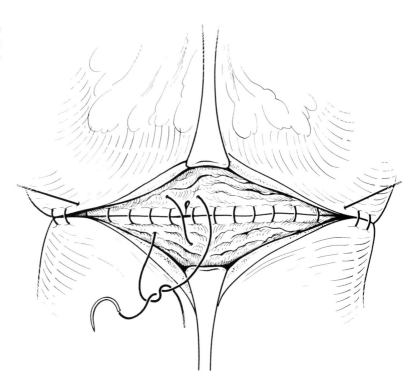

anterior suture line using an over-and-over all-coats stitch, tying the unpicked ends to the new suture line ends. Similarly place a seromuscular stitch and tie the unpicked ends to the new suture line ends.

When bleeding occurs following operation to control bleeding from an ulcer that has been left, the rebleeding is nearly always from the ulcer base. It is wise to attempt endoscopy in the anaesthetic room before reopening the abdomen. If necessary wash out all the blood before passing the endoscope and use an instrument with a wide suction channel. If the ulcer is indeed still bleeding, reopen the abdomen and the bowel to explore the ulcer. Determine not to close the abdomen until the bleeding is controlled. First identify exactly where the bleeding is coming from. Place a finger in the crater and gradually move it aside while holding a fine sucker in the other hand to aspirate blood (Fig. 9.11). Once the bleeding point is identified, insert 2/0 silk sutures on eyeless needles to control the bleeding. If this is a duodenal ulcer, the gastroduodenal artery or one of its branches has not been controlled at the previous operation. If the duodenal ulcer was previously treated by duodenotomy, and underrunning of the ulcer, followed by pyloroplasty and truncal vagotomy, do not lightly convert this to a gastrectomy, since this of itself will

Figure 9.11
The index finger controls the bleeding ulcer crater while deep stitches are inserted to control it.

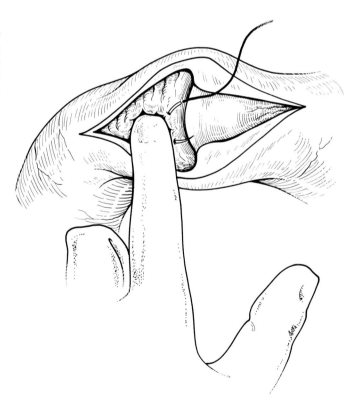

not control the bleeding. If a bleeding gastric ulcer was initially treated by gastrotomy, and underrunning of the ulcer, carrying out a gastrectomy will not of itself control bleeding from the ulcer base if this is eroding another structure. However, if the bleeding is from a vessel in the gastric wall, ulcer excision, usually by performing a Billroth I gastrectomy, allows the surgeon to control the supplying vessels and at the same time to carry out a definitive operation. Do not, however, carry out the gastrectomy as a demonstration. Remember that you are operating for the primary purpose of controlling bleeding by the simplest method. You are not operating for the primary purpose of curing the ulcer—that may be achieved without surgery, and if surgery proves necessary, elective surgery is safer than emergency surgery.

Ulcer re-bleeding
Insert non-absorbable stitches
Resect only if this increases control
Do not close up until bleeding completely controlled

When the bleeding is controlled, reclose the bowel and the abdomen.

Preliminary endoscopy may have demonstrated that bleeding is from another source. Erosive bleeding is treated more conservatively than ulcer bleeding. If this fails, however, then Billroth gastrectomy is indicated. Fortunately most erosions occur in the distal stomach.

Carcinoma is an infrequent cause of bleeding requiring emergency surgery. Ideally, in a fit patient radical surgery is preferred, but if you are tempted to carry out an incomplete resection in a potentially curable patient, you would be better to control the bleeding by underrunning the bleeding point and to plan to carry out adequate elective radical surgery after an interval. There are times, however, when inadequate resection is forced upon the operator in an unfit patient with a combination of bleeding and perforation. Quite severe bleeding very occasionally develops from ulceration at the cardia, when a nasogastric tube has been in place for an extended period. A patient who has retched or vomited during the postoperative period sometimes develops a Mallory–Weiss tear. Both of these stop bleeding spontaneously.

Leakage

Causes   Anastomoses may leak and the union most at risk is the one to the oesophagus following total or upper partial gastrectomy (see p. 93). The long gaps to be bridged attenuate the blood supply and occasionally thrombosis or external compression blocks the supply. If the patient becomes hypotensive or hypoxic, the bowel healing and viability are threatened. Organisms flourish in the lumen and as the mucosa and then the rest of the wall becomes gangrenous and eventually gives way, surrounding tissues are flooded with infected toxic contents. The powerful longitudinal muscle of the oesophagus distracts the ends and unless all the sutures grasp all the coats, poorly placed stitches cut out. The great distensibility of the oesophagus allows large gaps to develop between stitches unless they are placed close together.

Gastrojejunostomy, following gastrectomy or as a drainage procedure to bypass a peptic or malignant irremovable stricture, and as a 'drainage' procedure following truncal vagotomy, rarely leaks. It is technically easy to perform and both stomach and jejunum heal well. Pyloroplasty suture lines occasionally leak but as a rule not calamitously.

A most feared leak following Polya partial gastrectomy is burst duodenal stump. This rarely follows gastrectomy for cancer but nearly always occurs after operations for duodenal ulcer. It follows technically imperfect closure, usually of a scarred duodenal stump, ischaemia resulting from excessive mobilization, and, most potently, mechanical obstruction of the afferent jejunal loop, usually from excessive invagination at the gastroenterostomy. Obstruction of the afferent loop results in distension, with duodenal secretions, pancreatic juice and bile, which catastrophically disrupt the sutured closure or occasionally cause gangrene and disruption of the lateral wall (Fig. 9.12).

Figure 9.12
Burst duodenal stump caused by technical failure of closure, combined with tension caused by afferent loop obstruction.

Site of obstruction

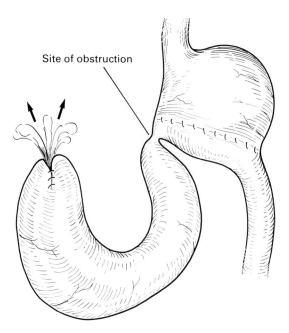

A notorious source of leaks following Billroth partial gastrectomy used to be at the junction of the gastroduodenal and gastric lesser curve suture lines. Technical advances have now made this a rarity. Very occasionally the upper end of the lesser curve suture line leaks from imperfect closure, especially when the lesser curve excision is taken high to include a high gastric ulcer or to ensure wide excision of a distal carcinoma (Fig. 9.13).

Vagotomy alone infrequently results in leakage, although during truncal vagotomy the lower oesophagus may be damaged and complete transection has been reported, usually because the anatomy at the hiatus has not been elucidated by the surgeon. Following proximal gastric vagotomy a rare complication is ischaemic necrosis of the gastric lesser curve, which then breaks down causing leakage (see Fig. 11.2). There is no known technical failure to account for this, since it does not occur following extensive gastric mobilization. It is now infrequently reported.

Prevention Leakage is almost entirely preventable by taking care to determine the anatomy, to avoid ischaemia and to employ accurately placed all-coats sutures.

The anastomosis most at risk is one made to the oesophagus. The gap to be bridged is large and the conduit, whether stomach, jejunum or colon depends on an extended blood supply. Take special precautions in mobilizing bowel to create anastomoses with the oesophagus (see p. 95).

Burst duodenal stump is preventable by ensuring that the

Figure 9.13
On the left, the line of resection of a high gastric lesion is indicated. On the right, the first stitch is being inserted.

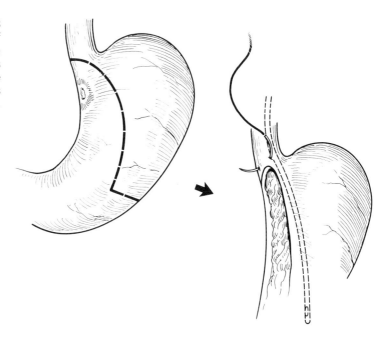

closure is sound. In the absence of duodenal ulcer, the first part of the duodenum can be mobilized for 1.5–2.0 cm beyond the point of transection by keeping close to the duodenal wall. A loose over-and-over all-coats 2/0 catgut stitch on an eyeless needle includes the thin, e.g. Lang–Stevenson, occluding clamp, which is then withdrawn as the stitches are tightened seriatim (Fig. 9.14). A purse-string seromuscular stitch is now inserted 1 cm distally. The closed stump is invaginated and the purse-string suture is tied (Fig. 9.15). A stitch now picks up the right gastric vascular pedicle, the anterior duodenal wall, the right gastroepiploic stump and the peritoneum over the head of the pancreas and draws them together over the purse-string suture (Fig. 9.16).

The method can be used proximal to a distal ulcer (pre-ulcer closure) or distal to a proximal ulcer (post-ulcer closure). Occasionally neither of these is possible. It is nowadays rarely necessary to carry out gastrectomy in the face of severe duodenal ulcer except for occasional bleeding ulcers; the Nissen procedure is described on p. 186. For severe stenosing duodenal ulcers, vagotomy and gastroenterostomy is an excellent combination that avoids the need to dissect the duodenum.

Very rarely, perhaps when operating upon a recurrent ulcer and carrying out vagotomy and gastrectomy, the Plenck manoeuvre of prepyloric closure is necessary, but the decision must be taken before tying the right gastric and gastroepiploic vessels so that the blood supply to the distal antrum can be preserved. Transect the antrum 3–4 cm proximal to the pylorus. Now elevate the mucosa distally from the cut edge. I (RMK) find this most easily achieved by first injecting sterile 1:300 000 adrenaline in physiological saline into the submucosa. Strip the mucosa as a cuff to the pylorus, sealing submucosal vessels with point diathermy (Fig. 9.17). Close the duodenal mucosa with a transfixion stitch and excise the antral mucosa. Now insert a purse-string suture within the muscular wall just proximal to the duodenal closure, tighten and tie it. Insert and tie two further purse-string sutures to securely close the antrum. I employ mucosal gastric resection (Kirk, 1984) to avoid the need to close the duodenum. This is in essence a Billroth I gastrectomy, removing only the mucosa.

If a safe closure is impossible, do not hesitate to abandon attempts. Instead create a controlled fistula. Insert a purse-string suture around the transected duodenum. Insert the end of a latex catheter of 20–24 F gauge, tighten and tie the purse-string around it (Fig. 9.6). Lead the tube to the exterior through a stab wound and allow it to drain for 10–14 days before removing it. Unless there is distal obstruction it will reliably heal.

Prevention of afferent loop obstruction demands care in fashioning the gastroenterostomy. It is important not to invaginate jejunal wall too generously. On completing the anastomosis carefully check that the lumen is not obstructed by ensuring that the jejunal wall can be invaginated into the stomach (Fig. 9.18)

Figure 9.14
Safe closure of the duodenal stump. Above, loose, over-and-over, sutures are inserted to enclose the cut duodenal stump and Lang–Stevenson forceps. The Lang–Stevenson forceps are then withdrawn, and the sutures are tightened seriatim. Guard against twisting by inserting the forceps tips through the loose loop as it is tightened.

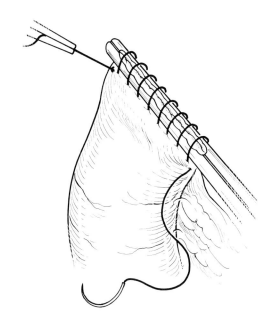

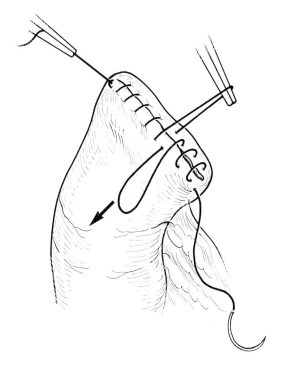

Figure 9.15
Purse-string suture.

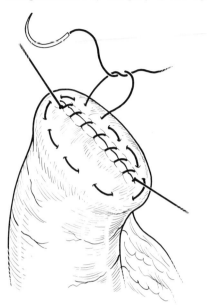

Figure 9.16
The purse-string
suture has been tied.
A third stitch picks up
the peritoneum over
the pancreas, the
right gastroepiploic
and right gastric
vessels, and the
anterior duodenal
seromuscularis.

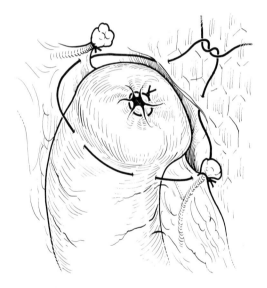

with the index finger. If it cannot, take down the anastomosis and refashion it.

Lesser curve necrosis following proximal gastric or highly selective vagotomy should theoretically occur more frequently when the spleen is injured and has to be removed, since this deprives the proximal stomach of its remaining blood supply. However, this has not been associated with any of the reported cases. It is doubtful whether reperitonealization of the lesser curve is a real protection. The rarity of gastric necrosis following

Figure 9.17
Plenck manoeuvre.
The antral mucosa is
excised above the
ligature and the antral
seromuscularis is
closed with sutures.

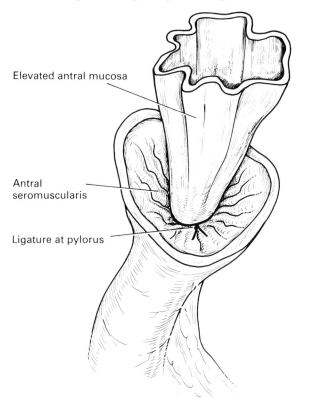

Elevated antral mucosa

Antral
seromuscularis

Ligature at pylorus

Figure 9.18
Invaginate the jejunal
wall through the
anastomosis with an
index finger.

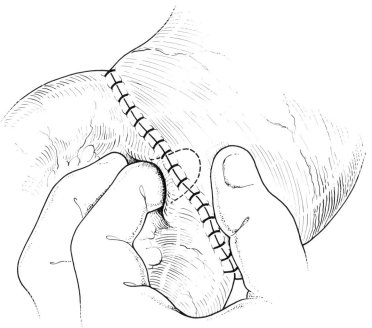

mobilization for oesophagogastric anastomosis suggests that we do not yet know the true explanation for this infrequent and capricious complication, and therefore cannot take effective steps to avoid it.

Billroth I gastrectomy is rarely complicated by leakage. Make sure that there is no tension by performing Kocher's mobilization of the duodenum. Securely invaginate the walls at the meeting of the lesser curve closure and the gastroduodenostomy. Make sure the upper end of the new lesser curve is securely closed and carefully invaginate it. Do not fear that this will obstruct the cardia, provided a nasogastric tube is in place.

Pyloroplasty rarely leaks, provided it is carried out only when the distal and proximal ends of the incision in the stomach and duodenum can be easily brought together without tension (Fig. 9.19). It does not matter whether the sutures are inserted as a single edge-to-edge layer or as a two-layer inverting suture. If the duodenum is stiffly scarred and fixed deeply in an obese abdomen, so that Kocher's duodenal mobilization cannot be performed, it is safer to carry out gastroenterostomy.

Features   Many small leaks are undetected and resolve spontaneously. Clinically evident leaks present in a variety of ways. Postoperative cessation of function usually prevents much leakage, especially if nasogastric or nasoenteric aspiration is used to keep the bowel empty until function returns after three to four days. Recovery ceases, the patient feels less well, may or may not suffer pain and tenderness, and continues to deteriorate. The bowel which was recovering ceases to function, but clinically remains paralysed and becomes distended (see p. 27). Following duodenal and small bowel leakage, absorption of bile from the peritoneal cavity may cause jaundice. Sometimes the leak produces sudden and catastrophic collapse, which may be mistaken for a cardiorespiratory disaster. The presentation is often related to the extent of the leak but differs from patient to patient, so that someone with a small leak may be very shocked, while another patient with a major leak shows minimal features. Sometimes a fistulous track rapidly forms to the surface, with bowel content emerging from the wound or through a drain track. If the patient swallows a little methylene blue dye, the emerging fluid is rapidly stained by it. The efflux may erode the surrounding skin.

Leak into the mediastinum often presents no physical signs apart from general, and sometimes catastrophic deterioration. As a rule the mediastinal pleura is not intact, so fluid drains into one or other pleural cavity, producing dullness to percussion and collapse of the lower lung lobe. Aspiration of the fluid allows inspection, and, if necessary, chemical analysis to confirm that this is bowel content.

It is probable that some of the silent leaks progress to abscesses that become clinically evident after a prolonged period. Patients occasionally present with pain, rigors and swinging pyrexia

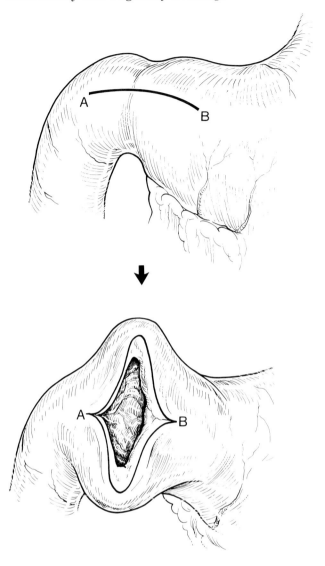

Figure 9.19
A safe pyloroplasty can be formed only if the two ends of the gastroduodenotomy (marked A, B) can be brought together without tension.

weeks or months after an operation from which recovery appeared to have been uneventful. An abscess is discovered that is likely to have developed as a result of a silent leak following the operation.

Investigation A dramatic abdominal or chest catastrophe self-evidently demands early exploration. Less dramatic and insidious leaks may be difficult to detect. Radiology is valuable. A plain chest X-ray may reveal mediastinal widening, air emphysema, and if a leak has drained into the pleural cavity, a pleural effusion or hydropneumothorax with collapse of the lung. In the abdomen a plain X-ray shows a sudden increase in free gas, fluid levels outside the bowel and usually dilated bowel loops also with fluid levels (see p. 27). Radiological studies using swallowed water-soluble contrast medium usually reveal the site and extent of leakage. A HIDA scan is useful to confirm a suspected duodenal stump leak following a Polya partial gastrectomy (Fig. 9.20). Ultrasound and CT scanning help detect the site of a collection (see p. 36). If lesser curve necrosis following proximal gastrectomy or highly selective vagotomy is suspected, carry out endoscopy using the minimum of air insufflation to confirm or exclude the diagnosis.

Management

Following a major leak restore the shocked patient's condition as much as possible by intravenous fluid and electrolyte replacement. Cross match blood and administer a versatile antibiotic combination active against aerobic and anaerobic organisms, such as a third-generation cephalosporin with metronidazole. As soon as possible return the patient to the operating theatre to explore the operation site.

If the operation involved an oesophageal anastomosis that has leaked, repair is almost always impossible. The leak usually results from ischaemic breakdown or tension disruption, thus precluding repair. The safest course of action is to drain the leak, defunction the oesophagus, possibly by a cervical oesophagostomy, and to create a distal feeding stoma such as a jejunostomy (see p. 4). Occasionally, however, when the fundus of the stomach has been brought into the chest, there is sufficient mobility to bring it up over the repair to give an 'ink-well' effect (Fig. 9.21).

Figure 9.20
HIDA scan showing pooled radioactivity around a leaked duodenal stump, just below the liver.

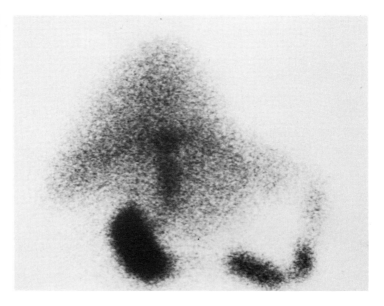

Damage to the oesophagus following vagotomy can usually be repaired because ischaemia is not involved. To carry out a full assessment and achieve a satisfactory repair may require extension of the upper abdominal incision into a left thoraco-abdominal exposure. Repair the damage carefully. This is an ideal circumstance to reinforce the repair. In the presence of hiatal hernia there is excessive, stretched peritoneum and phreno-oesophageal ligament that can be wrapped and sutured over the repair. Alternatively, the fundus of the stomach can be mobilized and used to reinforce it, or even can be used to patch a defect as described by Thal (see p. 81). Beware, however, if a proximal gastric or highly selective vagotomy was carried out because excessive division of the short gastric vessels could theoretically impair the blood supply to the upper stomach, since the left gastric vessels have already been disconnected.

Leakage from a ruptured duodenal stump demands two actions. The first is to create a controlled fistula. Place an all-coats purse-string suture around the edges of the rupture, if necessary mobilizing the duodenal stump minimally. Insert a large catheter such as 24 F into the duodenum and tie the purse-string suture around it. Sometimes the emerging catheter can be wrapped with omentum. Bring the end of the catheter out through the abdominal wall through a stab wound. Secondly, exclude obstruction of the afferent loop, looking in particular at the point where it reaches the stomach (Fig. 9.22). If necessary, take down the anastomosis and refashion it. This may be inappropriate if the patient is very ill, so note the obstruction and

Figure 9.21
'Ink-well' inversion of oesophagogastrostomy.

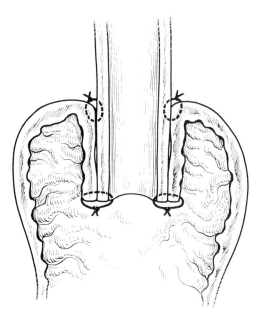

Figure 9.22
Revision of afferent loop obstruction. (a) The incision produces a longitudinal defect, as shown in (b) and (c). The defect is sutured as a transverse line.

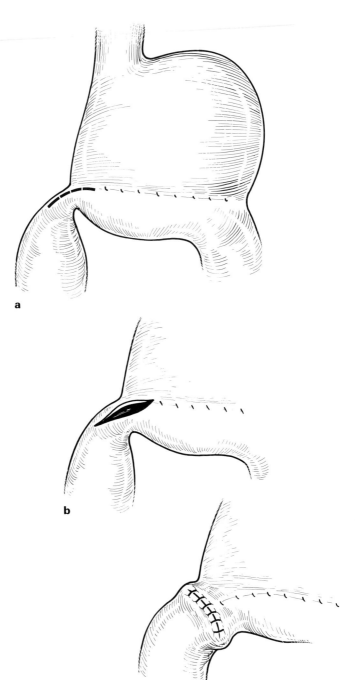

determine to reoperate on the patient as soon as he has recovered. Plan to remove the tube after 10 to 14 days, provided the obstruction at the gastroenterostomy is overcome. The fistula will then rapidly heal.

Lesser curve necrosis following proximal gastric or highly selective vagotomy appears to be an infrequent 'all or none' ischaemic phenomenon. It demands immediate resuscitation and operation. Approach the stomach through the original incision. Confirm the diagnosis and aspirate the leaked contents, particularly from the depths of the lesser sac. The reason for the leak was lack of blood supply and it is therefore useless merely to sew up the necrotic area. The wall must be cut back until healthy bleeding stomach is reached and this can usually be achieved only by gastrectomy, transecting the stomach well above the area of necrosis.

Leakage following Billroth I gastrectomy and pyloroplasty is infrequent. Very occasionally a small leak can be treated in the same way as an anterior duodenal ulcer perforation. Sutures are inserted to close the defect and tied over a fold of omentum. Larger defects require defunctioning of the stomach. In the case of Billroth I gastrectomy it is possible to separate the duodenum and carefully close it, trimming the ends and mobilizing a further part of the wall. The gastric stump is then resected further back and converted to a gastrojejunostomy. If a pyloroplasty is seriously disrupted, the same conversion may be performed. In both cases, however, it is often unsafe to close the duodenal stump. A controlled fistula should be created by inserting a wide-bore latex tube held in place with a purse-string suture, led to the surface and removed after 10 to 14 days. The patient is fed parenterally meanwhile.

After operations for leakage insert drains down to the leaked area. Closed drainage systems have largely replaced corrugated drains. Ensure, however, that there is no pressure from the drain on any repaired or doubtful viscus. As a rule feed the patient parenterally, although it may be possible to initiate jejunostomy feeding in some cases.

Infection

Causes   Apart from leakage, severe infection is relatively uncommon following gastrectomy and vagotomy, when compared with colonic and complex biliary tract operations. Contamination occurs principally from spillage of upper gastrointestinal contents which, although normally almost sterile, allow organisms to flourish in the presence of ulceration, obstruction or neoplasm. Organisms from the patients' nasopharynx, skin or large bowel may result in infection, apart from those introduced from the exterior. Infection may develop in the wound. It may develop within the peritoneal cavity, presenting immediately, or after a delay, especially if it is hidden by antibiotic treatment.

Prevention   The surgical principles of adequate preparation, relief of obstruction and careful technique to avoid spillage, haemorrhage, ischaemia or leakage (see p. 22) apply.

Features   The patient may fail to improve, with no definite features apart from intermittent pyrexia, raised white cell count, and, if the infection is within the peritoneal cavity, delayed recovery of gut function because of adynamic ileus. There may be a palpable tender swelling, but this cannot be relied on. Often rectal examination is most helpful in demonstrating a tender, boggy swelling in the prerectal pouch.

A wound infection presents with redness, swelling and discharge of pus spontaneously after probing or the removal of sutures. Leakage with inevitable infection usually but not always produces severe and often sudden deterioration (see p. 27). Smouldering infection perhaps from a small leak or infected haematoma may remain undetected. The patient develops toxic symptoms, rigors and pyrexia after days, weeks or even months. Clinically, radiologically or using scanning techniques, a collection is discovered.

Investigation   The best guide to the presence of infection, apart from the clinical findings, is the temperature chart, which has an exaggerated diurnal swing. The white cell count is raised and there is a granulocytosis, with a shift to the left. The nitrogen balance demonstrates catabolism. Plain X-ray of the chest and abdomen may indicate an opacity or intraperitoneal air with a fluid level, especially well seen below the diaphragm. Ultrasound scan is valuable and can be performed at the bedside. CT scan is very useful, especially in obese patients. Gallium scanning or indium-111-labelled white cells often localize obscure infection (see p. 36), and in the future NMR will be valuable.

Management   Wound infection is treated by removing sutures, and separating the edges. A swab is sent for culture. Antibiotics should be avoided at this stage, unless there is cellulitis or toxaemia.

The management of leakage is dealt with on p. 204. Other intra-abdominal infections require surgical or other types of drainage. The indications for each method are not fully established (see p. 41). I (RMK) employ surgical drainage whenever infection is certain but cannot be localized or defined and the cause is uncertain. I also employ it if there are multiple sources, or if multiple abscesses are discovered. Finally, surgery is necessary if the patient is toxic, catabolic, jaundiced with swinging pyrexia and has a high white cell count.

On the other hand, percutaneous direct or scan-guided insertion of drainage tubes is suitable if the cause appears to no longer act, the abscess is single, static and well defined, and responds to drainage. Of course take blood for culture and administer effective versatile antibiotics, such as a third-generation cephalosporin.

When operating for intra-abdominal sepsis, attempt first to localize it by radiology, ultrasound or a CT scan or by a radioactive gallium or indium scan. If it is localized, it may then be approached directly and drained, but if it cannot be localized, or is diffuse, reopen the original wound. As a rule it is possible only to arrange drainage. If there is a continuing cause, such as a leak, either bring the affected bowel to the surface, which is usually not possible, or drain the leak to the surface. If infection is associated with ischaemic tissue or bowel, do not close the wound without first correcting it. Remove any foreign material. Send swabs for aerobic and anaerobic culture and to determine sensitivity.

The catabolic effect of intrathoracic or intra-abdominal sepsis can be dramatic. Total parenteral nutrition is usually necessary if bowel function is impaired. If this is not already implemented, insert a central venous feeding catheter under the strictest sterile precautions before dealing with the infection.

In spite of the most thorough operation to drain sepsis and remove the cause, it may continue, especially if the organisms are virulent and insensitive to antibiotics. Do not ignore the need to carry out further surgery if necessary, or to leave the abdominal wound completely open if the sepsis is extensive (see p. 40).

Dysphagia

Occasionally patients develop dysphagia following gastrectomy or vagotomy. This may be caused by irritation from the nasogastric tube or reflux of acid and bile into the lower oesophagus. It may occur as a result of injury or leakage, with local abscess formation, or when performing a high sub-total gastrectomy for gastric ulcer or carcinoma, when the lower oesophagus may be constricted as the lesser curve is closed. Some temporary hold-up is frequent following total gastrectomy and replacement with jejunum or colon. This is partly from oedema at the anastomosis and partly from a delay in peristaltic adaptation of the conduit. Rarely the surgeon obstructs the loop with stitches: when suturing the anterior wall he picks up the posterior wall.

Prevention When performing high gastrectomy make sure a medium sized, e.g. 14–18 F, nasogastric tube is in place and close the lesser curve securely around it, without excessive turn-in. Any narrowing is only temporary. Take great care not to injure the oesophagus. As soon as possible raise the head of the bed or sit the patient upright. Do not leave the nasogastric tube in place a moment longer than necessary, but remember that stagnant bile is just as irritant to the lower oesophagus and cardia as is acid.

Management Ensure that the patient can be fed by an alternative route, either parenterally or by jejunostomy or gastrostomy. If the exact cause of dysphagia is in doubt, order a radiological examination of the patient while he swallows a water-soluble contrast medium to determine if there is mechanical blockage, leakage, failure of peristalsis, or obstruction beyond. If this does not clarify the cause, perform endoscopy to inspect the anastomosis or site of hold-up, to relieve or push through a food bolus, or, rarely, to cut a constricting stitch.

The type of leak that causes a local hold-up alone may be amenable to conservative management, but if dysphagia is but one feature, then exploration may be indicated not for the dysphagia itself but for correction of the leak. A moderate stricture at the anastomosis, or following closure of the high lesser curve during partial gastrectomy, will almost certainly improve spontaneously. A bolus of soft food swallowed by the patient is a safer dilator than surgical bouginage. A narrow stricture may require surgical dilatation, although some respond to autobouginage, using a Hurst's mercury-filled bougie (see p. 114). The patient sits in a chair. His throat is sprayed with lignocaine and he swallows a well-lubricated bougie, which is allowed to fall through by its own weight. If necessary the site of the lower end is checked with an X-ray. Alternatively, a swallowed balloon may be distended under X-ray control to dilate the stricture. These methods are valuable especially when an Eder–Puestow guide-wire cannot be advanced beyond a stricture to perform endoscopically controlled dilatation.

Reflux

Causes   Following any operation on the oesophagus or stomach, reflux may develop. Following gastrectomy with gastroenterostomy, bile may flood from the afferent loop into the stomach and reflux up the oesophagus. Any dissection around the cardia during vagotomy, clearance of glands, or mobilization for resection or anastomosis may interfere with continence. Even the presence of a nasogastric tube may prejudice competence and result in reflux. The mechanism of competence is complex and the cause of reflux in some cases and the reason for its absence in others is not clear.

Prevention   As a general rule surgeons try to retain, repair and restore the anatomical features around the cardia. There is no evidence that repair of the hiatus following vagotomy reduces the incidence of postoperative reflux. Gastric resections for carcinoma must as a primary necessity extend well clear of growth. Replacing the stomach with a jejunal loop is likely to favour bile, pancreatic and duodenal juice reflux. Side-to-side anastomosis of afferent to efferent loops is an uncertain method of diverting irritant fluid from the anastomosis. A Roux-en-Y anastomosis (see p. 224) is the most effective method, though even this is not totally reliable. A second layer of sutures is sometimes inserted to draw the conduit over the oesophagus to form a non-spill 'ink-well' effect (see Fig. 9.21), in the hope of preventing reflux.

Management The best safeguard against reflux is a competent cardiac sphincter mechanism. If this must be damaged, resected or bypassed, then reflux may still not occur (but see p. 114).

Obstruction and retention

Causes Following gastric operations involving anastomoses or suture lines, especially with two-layer closure, the inevitable oedema produces some obstruction after operation. This resolves after a few days. Rarely the surgeon may inadvertently pick up the posterior wall while completing the anterior closure. This resolves after two to three weeks if the suture material is absorbable, although cross-union of the mucosa can occur in part or whole.

Proximal gastric vagotomy without drainage may result in retention from duodenal stenosis and this may be avoided with duodenoplasty (Fig. 9.23). Truncal vagotomy and drainage are indicated for pyloric stenosis. Vagotomy, either truncal or selective, may produce atony and this can last for days or even weeks. Truncal vagotomy is carried out whenever the stomach is mobilized for anastomosis to the oesophagus following resection. Atony may, for no apparent reason, follow gastrectomy, gastro-enterostomy, or indeed any gastric operation.

Following partial or total gastrectomy with continuity restored using jejunum, the afferent loop may be obstructed, usually by excessive inturning at the anastomosis. If the obstruction does not provoke rupture of the closed duodenal stump, it gradually resolves with gushes of duodenal juice, bile and pancreatic juice flooding into the stomach or oesophagus.

The efferent loop may become obstructed, especially as it passes through the diaphragm or mesocolon or if it becomes adherent to the parietes or other viscera. Rarely the surgeon may obstruct the bowel by inserting stitches into it while closing the abdomen, and a knuckle of bowel may protrude into the wound and obstruct.

Occasionally the efferent loop undergoes spastic contraction which causes obstruction. It may resolve spontaneously and is perhaps ischaemic in origin.

Adynamic ileus can complicate leakage, infection, pancreatitis and ischaemia and occur in general conditions, may suggest uraemia and electrolyte disturbances or may follow unrelieved mechanical obstruction.

Features Initially the volume of aspirate from the nasoenteric tube is high, remains high, or having been small, increases. If the patient has no nasoenteric tube in place, he may vomit. Abdominal pain is often difficult to interpret in the postoperative period, but the patient may get typical colic. If there is ischaemia or strangula-

Figure 9.23
Duodenoplasty
overcomes
postpyloric bulbar
stenosis.

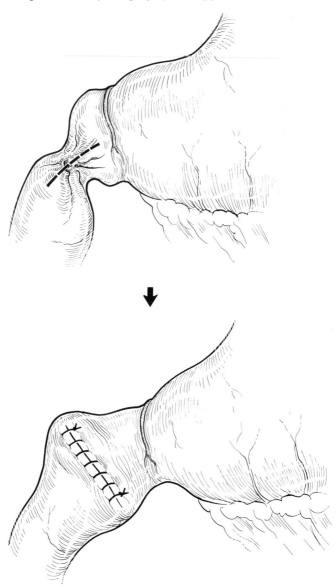

tion, the pain is classically continuous, but in the presence of adynamic ileus it may be absent. Bowel sounds are absent if the patient has a nasoenteric tube in place because the air is removed from the gut. The passage of flatus and faeces may stop or never start. Sometimes in partial obstruction, however, there is spurious diarrhoea.

Tenderness is sometimes localized to the site of the obstruction, but distension often obscures it by tensing the abdominal wall. The abdominal circumference increases unless nasoenteric aspiration is effectively continued. Rectal examination often reveals distended bowel loops or bogginess if fluid collects in the pelvis. Leak of infection producing paralytic ileus causes toxicity, pyrexia, and sometimes collapse with hypotension.

Investigations Chest X-ray and erect and supine films of the abdomen are valuable in localizing the site and severity of the obstruction or hold-up. Water-soluble contrast medium can be used to study progress of the medium and to determine the site of the leakage. Endoscopy is helpful, especially if the gastric outlet is obstructed. Afferent loop distension is sometimes best demonstrated using ultrasound or CT scanning techniques.

Treatment Gastric retention from obstruction caused by oedema of invaginated suture lines can be seen at endoscopy, and no action need be taken, since the oedema will gradually subside. If stitches are seen to cross and obstruct the anastomosis, it should be possible, after waiting for healing to take place, to cut them with scissors passed down a fibreoptic endoscope biopsy channel.

The gastric atony that occasionally follows any gastric operation does not usually respond to active measures. Aspiration of the stomach, restoration of electrolyte and fluid balance and nutritional support parenterally are all that can usually be achieved. However, make sure that there is no mechanical, vascular, or intra-abdominal infective cause.

Afferent loop obstruction requires surgical relief. It may not be necessary to unpick the whole anastomosis. Instead, cut the stitch and unpick it in both directions. Refashion the anastomosis to avoid excessive inturning and obstruction of the afferent loop and tie the unpicked threads to the ends of the newly inserted stitches (see Fig. 9.22).

Small intestinal obstruction may follow any operation, resulting from adhesions, kinks, and obstruction as it passes through the diaphragm or mesenteric defects. Simple obstruction may become strangulation, which is even more difficult to distinguish than in an operated abdomen. Since it is difficult to distinguish adynamic ileus from obstruction with subsequent paralysis, or a secondary phenomenon of peritonitis, explore such patients after excluding general causes such as uraemia and electrolyte disturbances.

Reopen the original wound. If the cause is obvious, deal with it but determine to explore the whole area of the previous operation. Release obstructed bowel and decompress it if it is grossly distended, either by getting the anaesthetist to pass through the mouth or nostril a long suction tube, which can then be manoeuvred onwards by the operator, or insert a suction tube through a purse-string suture placed on the antimesenteric border of the middle of the distended segment. Have an assistant hold up the loop while you pass the tube in each direction, feeding the bowel over the tube to resemble a concertina. When the bowel is empty remove the sucker, tighten and tie the purse-string suture, and reinforce it with a second seromuscular invaginating stitch.

Drain an abscess or leak, and resect gangrenous bowel.

Many senior surgeons misjudge the features of gangrene resulting from severe mechanical obstruction. Bowel that has been trapped and sustains venous congestion turns plum coloured and blood exudes from the vessels in the subserous coat. This does not represent gangrene, but will not disappear after a few minutes. Truly gangrenous bowel is often not tensely distended by slack, with patchy greenish areas of total necrosis, loss of sheen and sometimes the exuding of faeculent smelling fluid. The sites of entrapment are rarely dark but are initially white and well-localized rings (see p. 48). Make sure that these recover their pink colour—they are more potentially dangerous than the shiny plum coloured bowel between the constriction wings. Occasionally, in time of doubt, with a desperately ill patient, close the abdomen, spend 24 to 48 hours resuscitating the patient, then reopen the abdomen and reinspect the bowel. If a resection is necessary, try to avoid anastomosis. Prefer to bring the cut bowel ends to the surface, suturing mucosa to skin.

The bowel will not function for some time following such an operation, so ensure there is an adequate central venous feeding line for total parenteral nutritional requirements.

Late Complications

Grading of chronic late sequelae

A number of sequelae, including the dumping syndrome, recurrent ulcer and miscellaneous digestive disturbances, may follow gastric operations. It is usual to classify the severity of the postgastrectomy or postvagotomy symptoms following operation for peptic ulcer by some modification of the Visick ratings. Visick grade 1 is an excellent result, in which the patient has no postprandial symptoms. In grade 2 are placed those patients who have mild symptoms that do not seriously interfere with lifestyle and which can be avoided by simple measures. When both the patient and surgeon are satisfied with the result, the patient is placed into one of these categories. Into grade 3 are placed those patients with moderate symptoms that cannot be avoided or relieved entirely by simple measures, but which are not incapacitating. Either the patient, the surgeon, or both feel disappointed with the result. Visick grade 4 implies a completely unsatisfactory result and includes patients with recurrent ulceration, incapacitating dumping or diarrhoea or other severe symptoms. The assessment is preferably made by an independent questioner who does not know what procedure has been carried out. It is best made after at least one year following operation, since, except for recurrent ulceration, most symptoms improve with time.

Grading of the result of operation has played an important part, especially in peptic ulcer surgery. Together with mortality rates, it has allowed a comparison of the results of various operations that have been claimed to be effective in curing the ulcers. Thus one operation may be safer but less effective than another, while an effective operation may carry an unacceptable risk of postprandial disturbances. Secondly, it offers some guidelines when contemplating revisionary surgery. Grade 4 patients should normally only be considered for a further operation if no other relief can be offered and an improvement is a reasonable probability.

Dumping syndrome

Causes   This is named for the supposed cause of the features. Food and fluid are dumped into the small bowel when the normal antral and pyloric metering is destroyed, denervated or bypassed. The syndrome was originally described following gastrectomy. When truncal vagotomy came into use it was not associated with dumping, but when the drainage operations of gastroenterostomy, pyloroplasty and distal gastrectomy were added, symptoms similar to those following gastrectomy were noted. Dumping after proximal gastric vagotomy is infrequent and rarely severe, since the pylorus remains intact and innervated.

When it occurs during or soon after eating, dumping is termed 'early'. The small bowel may be overfilled, causing colic and intestinal hurry. If the contents are hypertonic, fluid is attracted into the gut, acting by its bulk as a laxative. The fluid leached from the vascular compartment depletes it, causing cardiovascular features of faintness and dizziness.

'Late' dumping occurs after an interval following a meal. If the dumped contents contain sugars, these are rapidly absorbed, causing hyperglycaemia, triggering a sudden release of insulin, which produces an overswing of hypoglycaemia.

Some features of dumping are possibly mediated by gut peptides.

Incidence   Dumping syndrome is reported to follow gastrectomy for ulcer in 20–30%, and truncal vagotomy and drainage operations in 10–20% of cases. The severity varies from mild to severe and incapacitating. It is rare but not unknown following proximal gastric vagotomy without drainage. Remarkably few patients complain of dumping of any severity following partial or total gastric resection for cancer. Of course it must be understood that the incidence of dumping depends on what questions are asked and who asks them.

Features   Depending on the mechanisms involved, dumping features are usually divided into 'early' and 'late'. Early dumping, resulting mainly from mechanical and osmotic effects, produces distension, colic and watery diarrhoea. The cardiovascular effects may produce weakness, dizziness and fainting. The late symptoms of hypoglycaemia give the patient a feeling of shakiness, hunger, weakness, tachycardia and sweating, especially after taking sugars.

Investigations   Dumping can be provoked by giving the patient 150 ml of 50% hypertonic glucose solution. Thereafter the symptoms are carefully noted and haematocrit readings are taken at regular intervals. The patient may develop urgent diarrhoea. The rate of gastric emptying can be measured by radiology or scans of radioisotope-labelled food. It is worth screening peptide hormones. Diarrhoea is investigated by sigmoidoscopy, stool examination, faecal fat estimation, and with radiology, small bowel mucosal biopsy and pancreatic function tests in selected cases. It is important to exclude incidental conditions and not to assume that all diarrhoea is the result of postoperative dumping. Rarely a gastroileostomy is discovered.

Prevention   The most important single step is to make certain that the operation is necessary, that the diagnosis is certain, and that the symptoms are caused by the discovered pathology. Many of the postgastrectomy and postvagotomy syndromes of the past were but modifications of undiagnosed dyspepsia, lightly attributed to peptic ulcers.

Dumping is best avoided by eschewing, whenever possible, the operations that cause it. Polya gastrectomy is no longer indicated for the primary elective treatment of uncomplicated duodenal ulcer, and the most generally popular operation at present is proximal gastric vagotomy without drainage. If a drainage operation is necessary, for example in a patient with pyloric stenosis, select truncal vagotomy and gastroenterostomy in preference to truncal vagotomy with pyloroplasty, since pyloroplasty is usually irrevocable, at least from a functional standpoint, whereas gastroenterostomy is not. Proximal gastric vagotomy with duodenoplasty allows an innervated pylorus to remain intact while widening of a duodenal bulbar stenosis is overcome (see p. 211). In the past innumerable papers were written extolling the virtues of Polya gastrectomy and gastroenterostomy with antecolic or postcolic anastomosis, gastrectomy with afferent loop to the greater or lesser curve, and closure of part of the gastroenterostomy stoma during gastrectomy to act as a restricting 'valve'. There is no evidence that any of these refinements were important. Polya gastrectomy is usually employed now in reconstructions following gastrectomy for cancer in preference to Billroth I gastrectomy, precisely because a full-width stoma offers protection against recurrent tumour-causing stomal obstruction.

Billroth I gastrectomy retains its popularity as a surgical treatment for gastric ulcer and infrequently results in severe sequelae. The selection of procedures for cancer depends on the need to eradicate or control the disease; the possibility of postprandial sequelae is a secondary consideration.

Treatment   Dumping symptoms tend to improve, especially during the first year after operation. Simple rules help and the avoidance of sweet food and drinks, the taking of meals dry, with drinks taken between meals, are often helpful. It is usually beneficial for the patient to rest for a few minutes after eating. Some patients are at least temporarily intolerant of eggs, milk, cheese, butter and fried foods. Each patient should watch to see if individual foods cause upset and avoid them completely at first, cautiously reintroducing them after an interval.

A variety of drugs have been tried, including antispasmodics, cyproheptadine and pectin. I (RMK) have personally found the (presumed) placebo effect of a simple antacid tablet placed in the vestibule between the lower molar teeth and the cheek to be as effective as any other method of treatment.

Many surgical procedures have been described for the correction of dumping syndrome following gastrectomy and vagotomy accompanied by a drainage operation. Never embark upon a conversion operation without confidently excluding other possibilities and being certain of the diagnosis. Always estimate gastric acid output. Vagotomy may need to be added if it is high. The decision must be a joint one with the patient after frankly discussing the possibilities. It is wise to have someone else present, since the patient's memory of what took place may be distorted if he does not obtain the hoped-for result. Indeed, it is often valuable to obtain a second opinion from a physician, surgeon or psychiatrist.

Conversion operations have one feature in common—they all produce excellent results in the hands of their originators. The placebo effect of an abdominal operation is powerful (Kirk, 1976) and in the short-term most patients are improved. The operations are sometimes difficult to perform and are best left in the hands of those who regularly perform revisionary gastric surgery and are therefore able to acquire a reasonably balanced view of the likely benefit. Unfortunately many of these patients are passed from one surgeon to the next until someone agrees to reoperate. Revision may follow revision and the only virtue of some procedures is to demonstrate what bizarre mechanical distortions of the gut the body will tolerate.

At operation carry out a thorough exploration to exclude the possibility that the symptoms stem from an unexpected alternative cause.

Dumping following Polya partial gastrectomy for duodenal ulcer is often treated by conversion to Billroth I gastrectomy, based on the doubtful logic that since Billroth I gastrectomy is associated with a lower incidence of dumping than Polya gastrectomy, conversion will reduce the symptoms. Carefully dissect out the closed duodenal stump. Identify the gastroenterostomy suture line, open it anteriorly to avoid spillage, and totally disconnect it. Trim the edges of stomach and jejunum. Close the longitudinal defect in the jejunum as a transverse suture line in two layers (Fig. 9.24). Close the lesser curve half of the stomach in two layers, leaving the greater curve half open. Mobilize the duodenal stump by Kocher's manoeuvre and open the end of the stump to match the gastric defect. Create a gastroduodenostomy using a two-layer anastomosis. Sometimes a longitudinal incision in the anterior wall of the duodenal stump better matches the cut end of the stomach.

Figure 9.24
Conversion of a Polya gastrectomy to a Billroth I gastrectomy. The defect in the jejunum is closed transversely.

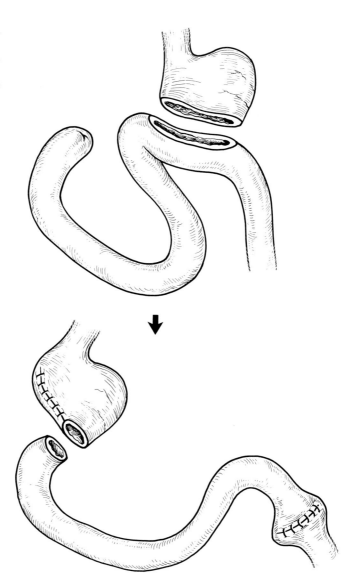

Another technique that has a vogue is to slow the rate of gastric emptying by interposing a reversed 10–12 cm segment of efferent jejunal loop at the gastric outlet. The duodenal stump is first identified, and then carefully mobilized using Kocher's manoeuvre. The anastomosis is disconnected, the cut gastric and jejunal edges are trimmed, and the jejunal stoma is closed as a transverse suture line. The lesser curve half of the stomach is then closed, provided that a valved gastrectomy has not been performed. The proximal jejunal blood supply is carefully examined in the segment just distal to the closed stoma. A segment is chosen and measured. The blood vessels are divided towards the base of the mesentery, preserving a good arterial and venous flow. The bowel is transected at each end and rotated 180°. Its distal end is united to the stoma left on the greater curve of the stomach, using a two-layer suture. The proximal end is united to a matched stoma created at the tip or anterior wall of the duodenal stump. The cut ends of jejunum remaining after the exclusion of the reversed segment are united to restore continuity (Fig. 9.25). The length of reversed jejunum is critical and is difficult to estimate since there is individual variation. If it is too long, it produces gastric retention; if it is too short, it is ineffective. If the original operation was for duodenal ulcer, it is wise to carry out a vagotomy, since the conversion increases the risk of recurrent ulcer.

Fortunately dumping infrequently follows Billroth I gastrectomy, but the interposition of a reversed 10–12 cm jejunal loop between the gastric remnant and the duodenum has been used in the few patients with severe symptoms following Billroth gastrectomy.

Following vagotomy and a drainage operation, dumping is attributable to the drainage operation. If the original operation was truncal vagotomy and gastroenterostomy, then simply disconnecting the gastroenterostomy and closing the defects in the stomach and jejunum usually cures the symptoms, provided that the gastric outlet is not stenosed (Fig. 9.26).

Pyloroplasty can be reversed by incising along the suture line, restoring the pyloric ring and resuturing the gastroduodenostomy (Fig. 9.27). The anatomical effect is excellent, but in my experience the long-term results have been disappointing. An alternative procedure is to disconnect the stomach and duodenum in the line of the pyloroplasty and interpose a reversed 10 cm segment of jejunum. I have never used this method.

Diarrhoea
This may be part of the dumping syndrome or may occur separately. Following any gastric operation the patient may develop a degree of steatorrhoea, and will be found to excrete more than 6 g of fat in a three-day stool collection. Sometimes a gastric operation may uncover a supposedly latent milk intolerance or similar condition. Of course the patient may develop any

Figure 9.25
Interposition of an
antiperistaltic jejunal
segment to slow
gastric emptying.

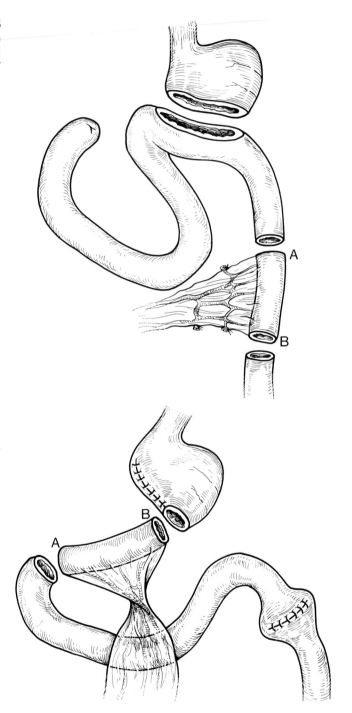

Figure 9.26
Provided that the
normal gastric outlet
is not stenosed,
dumping following
truncal vagotomy and
gastroenterostomy
can be improved by
disconnecting the
gastroenterostomy.

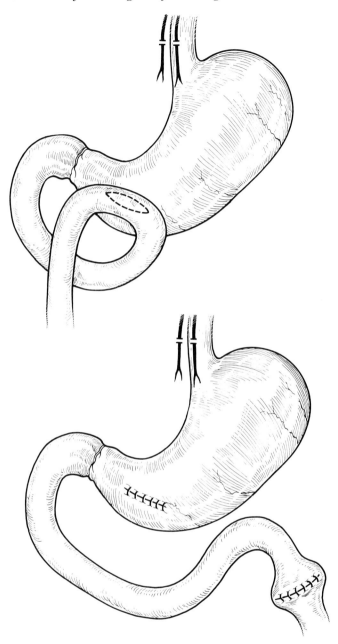

of the other causes of diarrhoea, including inflammatory bowel disease, so always exclude them, especially if there are no associated dumping symptoms.

Many patients can be satisfactorily controlled by taking codeine phosphate tablets 15–30 mg four-hourly as necessary, or

Figure 9.27
Reversal of
pyloroplasty. The scar
is excised and the
defect is closed as a
longitudinal suture
line.

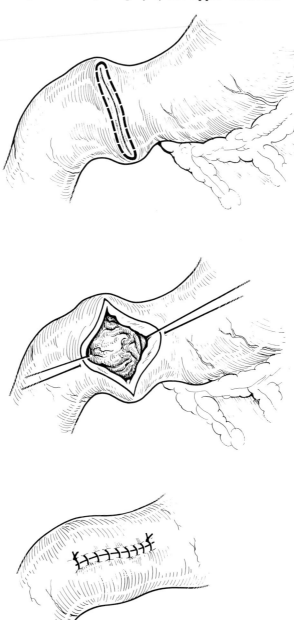

diphenoxylate hydrochloride (Lomotil) 5 mg six-hourly, or phtha-
lylsulphathiazole 1 g four times a day. Only a few are incapaci-
tated, and these patients are rarely seen now, with the replacement of truncal vagotomy and a drainage operation by proximal
gastric vagotomy without drainage.

A very rare technical mistake is gastroileostomy. This is discovered when a barium follow-through X-ray is ordered. The patient is totally relieved by an operation to take down the anastomosis, close the defect in the ileum as a transverse suture line and create a gastrojejunostomy.

In the absence of a mechanical cause for the urgent diarrhoea, reversal of an ileal segment has been introduced. A 10–12 cm segment is isolated with its blood supply intact, 40 cm proximal to the ileocaecal valve. It is reversed and re-anastomosed to restore continuity (Fig. 9.28). The length of bowel is critical: too short

Figure 9.28
Reversal of a
10–12 cm ileal loop
40 cm proximal to the
ileocaecal valve to
control intractable
diarrhoea.

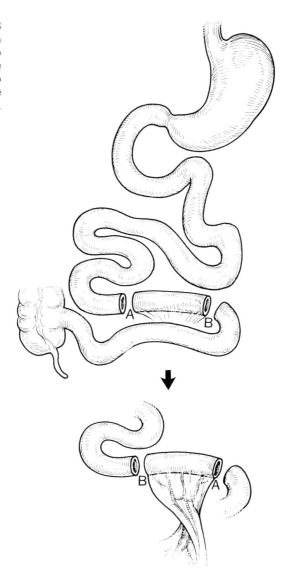

and it is ineffective; too long and it produces obstruction. This procedure must be rarely called for now.

Bile reflux
This deserves separate consideration from the dumping syndrome, although it may occur with it. Whenever the pylorus is damaged, resected or bypassed, bile may reflux into the stomach and regurgitate up the oesophagus. The patient's mouth suddenly fills with bitter yellow fluid. As a rule there is no food or other fluid.

This distressing symptom is occasionally the only sequel of gastrectomy, usually of Polya type. It may occur following total gastrectomy with oesophagojejunostomy, when an intact loop of jejunum is employed instead of the more usual Roux-en-Y segment. Enteroenterostomy between the afferent and efferent loops is an uncertain safeguard.

Management   If the symptoms are incapacitating, and occur alone, this is one of the few conditions that merits surgical revision. When Polya partial gastrectomy was the initial operation, two procedures are valuable. The first is to convert the gastrectomy to a Roux loop. The afferent loop is transected where it joins the stomach and the gastric end is closed. The proximal end is united end-to-side into the efferent loop at least 40 cm distal to the stomach (Fig. 9.29). The Tanner 'Roux-19' is an easier operation. The free part of the afferent loop is transected at its middle and the upper cut end is joined end-to-side into the efferent loop at a convenient site near the stomach. The lower cut end is joined end-to-side into the efferent loop 40 cm distally (Fig. 9.30). It is wise to perform truncal vagotomy if this has not already been carried out, to protect the patient from recurrence if the original operation was for duodenal ulcer.

Following total gastrectomy using an intact loop of jejunum enteroanastomosis is often recommended (Fig. 9.31), but in my (RMK's) experience it neither gives absolute protection against bile reflux nor reliably cures it. Since the anastomosis is high in the abdomen or in the chest, a Tanner Roux-19 operation performed through the abdomen is the operation of choice (Fig. 9.32).

Following Billroth I gastrectomy or pyloroplasty, severe bile reflux is unusual, though it is occasionally encountered. This is most suitably controlled by transecting the gastroduodenostomy or separating the stomach from the duodenum at the level of the pyloroplasty. Now isolate a 12–15 cm segment of proximal jejunum with its blood supply intact, rejoining the cut ends to restore continuity. Insert the isolated segment in an isoperistaltic manner between the distal stomach and the proximal jejunum (Fig. 9.33). This acts as a one-way 'valve', preventing bile reflux into the stomach. I have not found anatomical reconstruction of

Figure 9.29
Roux-en-Y
conversion for bile
diversion.

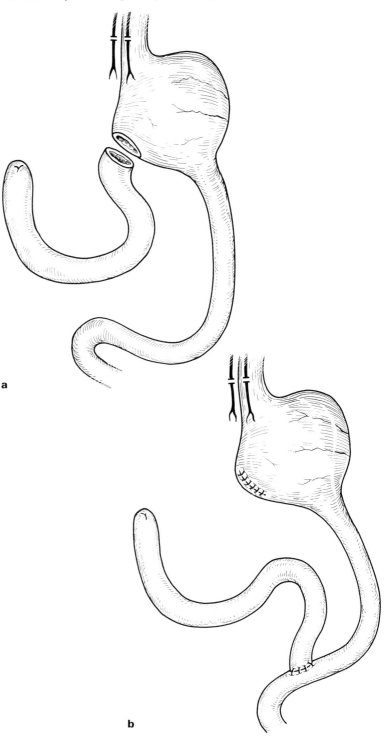

a

b

Figure 9.30
Tanner 'Roux-19'
operation for bile
diversion.

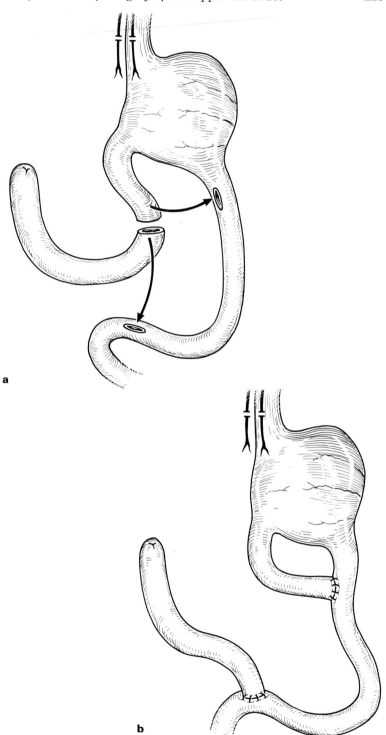

a

b

Figure 9.31
Side-to-side
enteroanastomosis
does not reliably
prevent or cure
bile reflux following
end-to-side
oesophagojejunostomy.

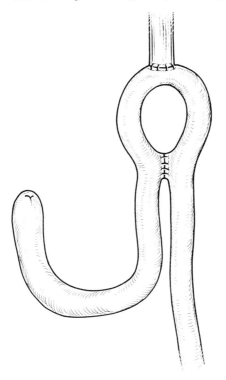

Figure 9.31
Side-to-side
enteroanastomosis
does not reliably
prevent or cure
bile reflux following
end-to-side
oesophagojejunostomy.

the pylorus to be effective in giving a return of function following pyloroplasty.

Recurrent peptic ulcer

Incidence   Duodenal ulcer recurrence rates vary between different reports. Recurrence follows Polya partial gastrectomy in about 2–5% of cases, truncal vagotomy and drainage in 5–10%, and proximal gastric vagotomy in more than 10% in early series but well below this in many later reports. Recurrence following distal gastrectomy and vagotomy has the lowest rate of below 2%, but this operation is rarely performed in Britain.

Gastric ulcer recurrence follows Billroth I gastrectomy in about 1% of cases. Proximal gastric vagotomy and ulcer excision is as effective as Billroth I gastrectomy. Gastric ulcer occasionally develops following truncal vagotomy without drainage for duodenal ulcer.

Causes   Duodenal ulcer usually heals when gastric acid secretion is reduced below 50% of the level at which ulceration developed. This entails a two-thirds gastrectomy, truncal vagotomy, or proximal gastric vagotomy that completely denervates the gastric parietal cell mucosa. Inadequate gastrectomy or incomplete vagotomy risks further ulceration. Roux conversion following

Figure 9.32
When an oesophageal anastomosis has been made in the chest to an intact jejunal loop, bile reflux is prevented by transabdominal Tanner Roux-19 conversion

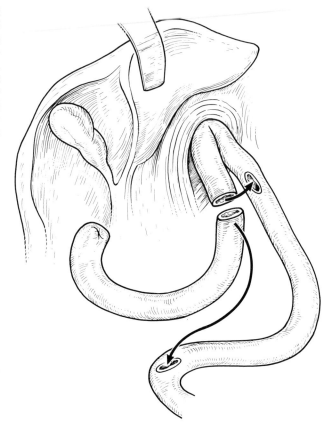

Polya gastrectomy increases the susceptibility to ulceration. If gastric antrum is left in the duodenal stump closure following Polya partial gastrectomy, the risk of ulceration is also increased because G-cells hypersecrete gastrin if they are in an alkaline medium.

In spite of adequate surgery, ulcers may recur in the presence of the Zollinger–Ellison syndrome in which a tumour or hyperplasia of non-beta cells of the pancreas secretes high levels of gastrin. G-cell hyperplasia may also develop in the gastric antrum. Parathyroid adenoma may be associated with recurrent ulcer. Recurrent ulcer occurs in the multiple endocrine adenopathy syndrome type 1 (MEA 1), which may be familial.

The reason for the occasional gastric ulcer recurrence is often obscure. Gastric retention is often indicted, but it is uncommon for patients with pyloric stenosis to develop gastric ulceration.

Prevention The standard elective operation for uncomplicated duodenal ulcer is at present proximal gastric vagotomy (highly selective vagotomy). Of course the results obtained by experts cannot be

Figure 9.33
Interposing an
isoperistaltic jejunal
loop to prevent bile
reflux following
Billroth I gastrectomy.

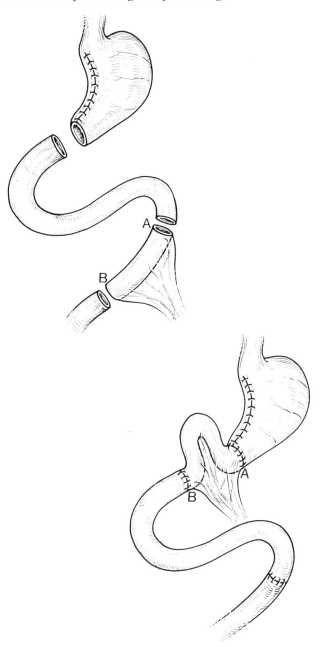

extrapolated to the whole body of surgeons, many of whom are
inexperienced. At least 7 cm of lower oesophagus must be
demonstrably denervated: many surgeons complete this anteriorly but fail to rotate the oesophagus to ensure that the
posterior—and especially the left posterior—surface is denuded

of fibres. This must be achieved without damaging the highest short gastric vessels, which are stretched and brought into view if the oesophagus is violently rotated (Fig. 9.34). Remember that the antrum is not extensive in duodenal ulcer patients and the distal extent of vagal separation must not leave acid-secreting mucosa innervated. It may be necessary to divide one or two proximal branches of the crow's foot, where the nerves of Latarjet break up, to leave only 5–6 cm of antrum supplied (Fig. 9.35).

When carrying out truncal vagotomy with a drainage procedure, identify the abdominal oesophagus by feeling the nasogastric tube. Make an incision over it, through both the peritoneum and phreno-oesophageal ligament, picking up each of these with forceps to avoid inadvertently cutting the anterior vagus nerve (Fig. 9.36). Identify the trunk, and ensure that it gives off gastric and hepatic branches before continuing as the anterior nerve of Latarjet. Elevate the trunk and gently strip the oesophagus from it as high as possible, before excising all that can be safely exposed. Attempt to encircle the oesophagus with finger and thumb. They are separated by a dorsal 'mesentery' in

Figure 9.34
The upper stomach is pushed to the right behind the oesophagus to ensure there are no intact posterior fibres.

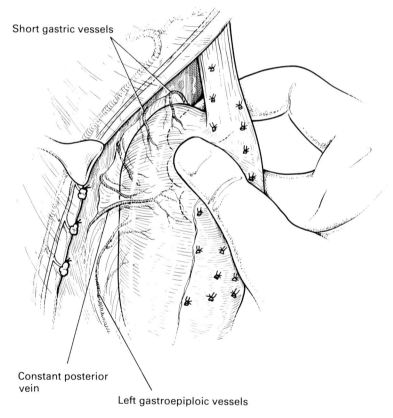

Short gastric vessels

Constant posterior vein

Left gastroepiploic vessels

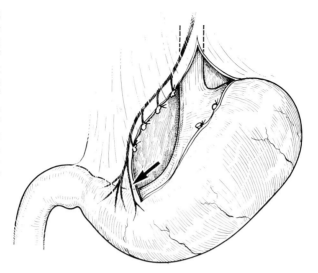

Figure 9.35
Carefully decide how extensive the distal innervation will be if the crow's foot is left intact. Should some of the proximal part of the crow's foot be divided [see arrow]? Remember the antrum is rarely more than 5–6 cm long in duodenal ulcer patients.

which lies the posterior trunk. Break through the connective tissue anterior and posterior to the nerve, and push it to the right to grasp it. Ensure that the main nerve passes distally towards the coeliac axis, that a branch continues as the posterior nerve of Latarjet and other branches pass to the lower oesophagus and stomach (Fig. 9.37). Gently strip oesophagus from the nerve above, and excise as long a segment as can be safely achieved. By performing vagectomy there is less chance of leaving intact branches than after performing mere vagotomy. Inspect the whole circumference of the lower 5 cm of oesophagus to detect and divide separate vagal branches.

Polya partial gastrectomy is no longer electively performed alone for duodenal ulcer. A three-quarters gastrectomy produced few recurrences, but hemigastrectomy resulted in up to 5% recurrent ulcers. When carrying out Polya gastrectomy for duodenal ulcer ensure that there is no antral mucosa in the duodenal stump.

Billroth I partial gastrectomy is almost always effective for gastric ulcer, provided that the ulcer is completely excised.

Recurrent peptic ulcers are likely in the presence of Zollinger–Ellison syndrome. Many surgeons do not carry out acid-secretion studies before operation. However, the ulcers have already demonstrated themselves to be resistant to adequate medical treatment, so it is wise to study acid secretion in the few patients who now present for surgery. If both maximal acid output and basal secretion are high, establish whether the serum gastrin is raised (see p. 240). Always at operation, carefully explore the pancreas to exclude a tumour.

Sites Duodenal ulcer recurs at its original site following proximal gastric vagotomy without drainage and on or near the suture line

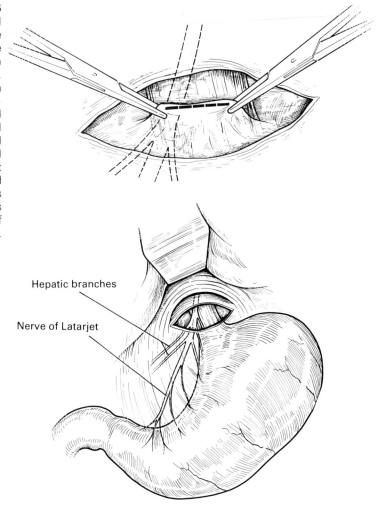

Hepatic branches

Nerve of Latarjet

following vagotomy and pyloroplasty. After Polya gastrectomy, or vagotomy and gastroenterostomy, ulcers recur on or just beyond the gastroenterostomy suture line.

Features The pain of recurrent ulcer resembles that of the original ulcer, but it may not be periodic, nor situated as expected. Stomal ulcer is sometimes felt in the central abdomen or even the left iliac fossa. Local tenderness may be detected.

Investigations Endoscopy is the most valuable investigation because the ulcer can be confidently seen. Barium radiography is less certain. In addition to basal and pentagastrin-stimulated acid-secretion studies, the Hollander insulin test should be carried out if vagotomy was performed. If as a result of hypoglycaemia the acid

Figure 9.37
Posterior truncal
vagotomy: definition
of the anatomy.

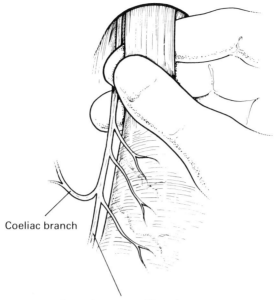

Coeliac branch

Posterior nerve of Latarjet

secretion increases, this suggests that there are intact vagal fibres. Zollinger–Ellison syndrome is typified by high basal and maximum acid secretion: whenever there is doubt estimate the serum gastrin, and also the serum calcium level to exclude hyperparathyroidism.

Management Before the advent of H2-receptor blocking drugs, further surgery was usually mandatory following recurrent ulceration. Recurrence is not, however, necessarily persistent and a course of cimetidine or ranitidine may induce healing which is permanent. However, if the drug fails to heal the ulcer, if the ulcer recurs rapidly following adequate treatment, or if bleeding or perforation occur, surgery is indicated.

Recurrence following surgery for a duodenal ulcer demands the combination of truncal vagotomy and gastric resection. Thus a patient who has already been subjected to a Polya gastrectomy should have a truncal vagotomy carried out. If the ulcer has not caused severe stenosis, do not carry out a further resection. Sometimes only a portion of the anastomosis is distorted, narrowing the efferent loop. In this case place occluding, non-crushing clamps above and below the anastomosis. Excise the ulcer and resuture the stomach and jejunum (Fig. 9.38). If the gastroenterostomy is stenosed, perform a higher gastrectomy. Do not attempt to use the existing defect in the jejunum, but trim the edges and close it in two layers as a transverse suture line (Fig. 9.39). Employ a segment of jejunum just distal to the previous stoma, or if the afferent loop was long, use a proximal segment.

Figure 9.38
Ulcer excision and
resuture with truncal
vagotomy.

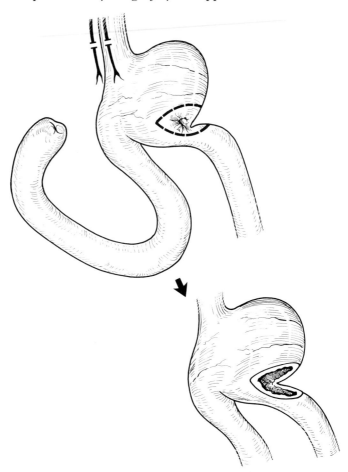

Figure 9.38
Ulcer excision and resuture with truncal vagotomy.

Very rarely a fistula forms between the ulcer and the transverse colon—a gastrojejunocolic fistula. Disconnect the colon without contaminating the wound and close it in two layers (Fig. 9.40). Then perform truncal vagotomy and hemigastrectomy.

Recurrence following proximal gastric vagotomy is appropriately treated by truncal vagotomy and Polya gastrectomy. First of all, carefully perform the vagotomy. If the highly selective vagotomy was correctly carried out, the trunks should be in their correct sites, but be prepared for some distortion. Preferably make a fresh transverse incision through the peritoneum and phreno-oesophageal ligament in an unscarred area higher than the transverse part of the previous vagotomy (Fig. 9.41).

Partial gastrectomy by the Polya method is usually appropriate, but first carefully ensure that the spleen was not removed at the previous operation or damaged during the truncal vagotomy. Provided the spleen is intact—and with it the short gastric

Figure 9.39
To perform a higher gastrectomy, resect the stomach more proximally, close the trimmed margins of the jejunal defect as a transverse suture line and create a fresh gastroenterostomy. Carry out truncal vagotomy.

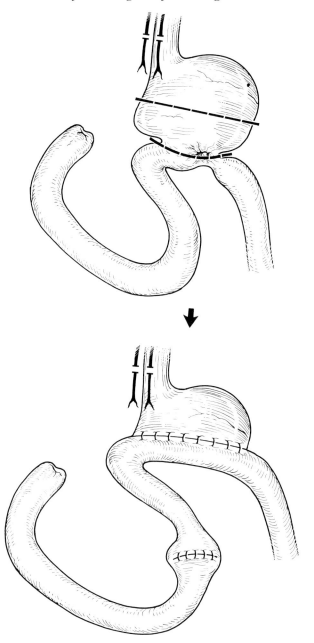

and left gastroepiploic vessels—carry out hemigastrectomy and gastrojejunostomy.

If the spleen has been removed, do not perform partial gastrectomy, since the proximal stomach will have no local blood supply, the left gastric vessels having been previously disconnected from it. In these circumstances I (RMK) perform a

Figure 9.40
Gastrojejunocolic
fistula. The colon is
disconnected and
repaired. Polya partial
gastrectomy and
truncal vagotomy are
carried out.

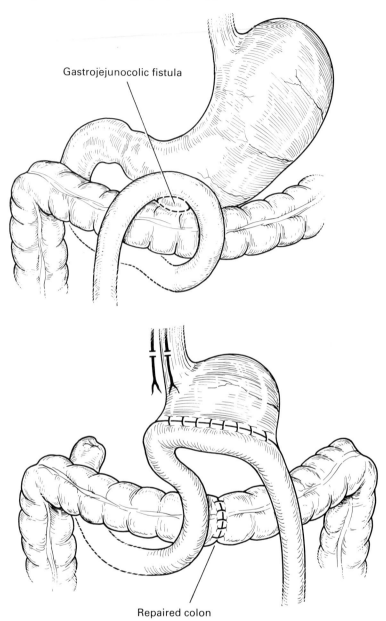

Figure 9.40
Gastrojejunocolic
fistula. The colon is
disconnected and
repaired. Polya partial
gastrectomy and
truncal vagotomy are
carried out.

Gastrojejunocolic fistula

Repaired colon

mucosal gastric resection, since this avoids further vascular
ligation. First carry out a full mobilization of the duodenum by
Kocher's manoeuvre. Make an anterior gastroduodenotomy
similar to the incision for pyloroplasty but extending 7–8 cm
proximal to the pylorus (Fig. 9.42). Infiltrate 250–300 ml, 1 in
300 000 adrenaline in saline into the gastric submucosa from the

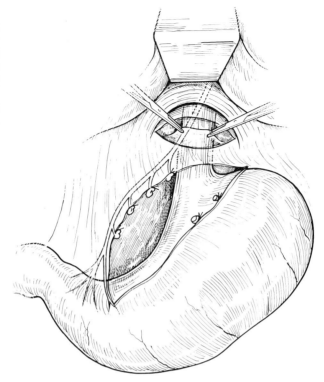

pylorus to a line 7–8 cm proximal to it (Fig. 9.43). This lifts the mucosa and constricts the blood vessels. Incise the mucosa along the pyloric ring and strip it up as an intact sheet, cutting through the distended submucosa. When the sheet has been fully lifted, cut it off along a line parallel to the pylorus (Fig. 9.44). The denuded submucosa bleeds surprisingly little, but carefully pick up each vessel with fine diathermy forceps and seal it using the lowest setting for the minimum time. Now draw the posterior cut edge of gastric mucosa and submucosa down to the cut pyloric mucosa and submucosa using 2/0 chromic catgut sutures, folding posteriorly the intact seromuscularis (Fig. 9.45). When this is completed (Fig. 9.46), start at the ends and work towards the middle, drawing the anterior gastric cut edge down to the edges of the duodenotomy with all-coats stitches (Fig. 9.47). Insert a second layer of seromuscular sutures. The intact folds of sero-muscularis produce 'dog ears' above and below. Insert sutures to draw the 'dog ears' over the front as an extra loose cover for the anterior suture line (Fig. 9.48).

This operation achieves a gastrectomy without dividing a single major vessel and I use it routinely in place of gastrectomy when operating for the cure of recurrent duodenal ulcer. It is only the mucosa that one wishes to remove, and because the posterior wall remains intact, and the anterior suture line is reinforced by the excess stomach wall, leakage is virtually

Figure 9.42
Recurrent ulcer
following proximal
gastric vagotomy with
splenectomy. Truncal
vagotomy has been
carried out. The
incision for gastric
mucosal resection is
indicated by the
broken line.

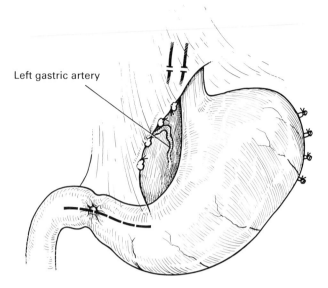

Left gastric artery

Figure 9.42
Recurrent ulcer following proximal gastric vagotomy with splenectomy. Truncal vagotomy has been carried out. The incision for gastric mucosal resection is indicated by the broken line.

prevented. The technique has the additional advantage that the sometimes dense adhesions between the stomach and the liver need not be dissected. I have never experienced leakage or postoperative bleeding in approximately 150 operations, nor has there been a single duodenal ulcer recurrence.

If the patient has previously been treated for duodenal ulcer by truncal vagotomy and a drainage operation, first explore the cardiac area to determine if the vagotomy was complete (see p. 232). Explore the anterior surface of the oesophagus from the angle of His down to the upper part of the gastrohepatic omentum. Encircle the oesophagus to determine whether the dorsal 'mesentery', in which there could lie an intact posterior vagal trunk, is still present. Display the whole of the hiatus in case an undivided nerve is displaced.

Now perform Polya gastrectomy, removing at least half the stomach. If gastroenterostomy was previously carried out, the recurrence will be at the stoma. Disconnect the anastomosis, excise the ulcer and close the defect in the jejunum as a transverse suture line in two layers, then temporarily close the gastric stoma with sutures to prevent leakage. If a pyloroplasty was previously performed, the recurrence lies on or near the suture line. It will be necessary to mobilize and transect the duodenum, ensuring that no gastric mucosa remains.

I employ gastric mucosal resection in such patients (see p. 236). An anterior juxtapyloric gastroenterostomy stoma can be extended distally through the pylorus. A pyloroplasty can be opened along the suture line, restored to its original longitudinal alignment and continued proximally.

Recurrent gastric ulcer may follow an emergency procedure such as excision or biopsy, a drainage operation and vagotomy

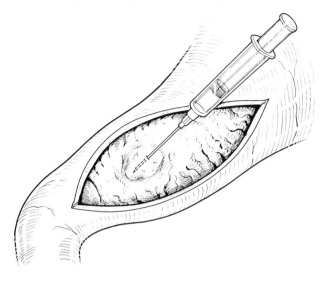

Figure 9.43
Submucosal injection
of adrenaline in saline
solution.

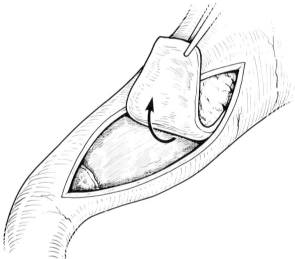

Figure 9.44
Raise the flap of
mucosa proximally for
7–8 cm and excise it.

for the control of bleeding or perforation. Carry out Billroth I gastrectomy. If the previous operation was a Billroth I gastrectomy, perform a higher resection. If this is technically difficult because the ulcer is high or because of adhesions, a Polya gastrectomy may be performed distal to the ulcer, provided that adequate preoperative endoscopic biopsies excluded neoplasia. This is the Kelling–Madlener procedure.

Zollinger–Ellison syndrome
Recurrent ulcer warns of the possibility of gastric hypersecretion because the original operation was inadequate, because there is hyperparathyroidism, antral G-cell hyperplasia or Zollinger–

Figure 9.45
The stitches draw the mucosal edges together as the seromuscularis is folded posteriorly.

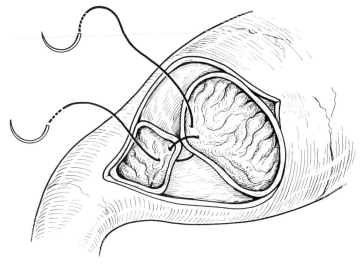

Figure 9.46
The posterior wall is completed.

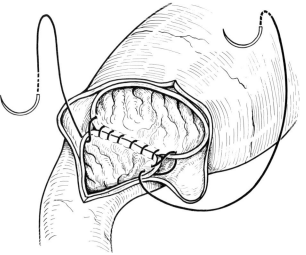

Ellison syndrome. In Zollinger–Ellison syndrome the original or recurrent ulceration may be in an unusual site, especially postbulbar or jejunal, and may be multiple. Estimate basal, insulin-stimulated and pentagastrin-stimulated acid secretion. In Zollinger–Ellison syndrome and G-cell hyperplasia, the basal acid secretion is very high, with little or no rise on maximal pentagastrin stimulation. Serum gastrin tests reveal high levels. The fasting gastrin level is elevated by at least 200 ng/ml within 30 seconds of infusing 2 units/kg body weight of secretin. Antral biopsies distinguish G-cell hyperplasia. The insulin test will determine whether vagotomy is complete. Serum calcium, phosphate, and if indicated parathormone levels, should exclude hyperparathyroidism. Always check the serum prolactin levels to evaluate pituitary function in such patients.

Figure 9.47
The anterior all-coats stitch is completed.

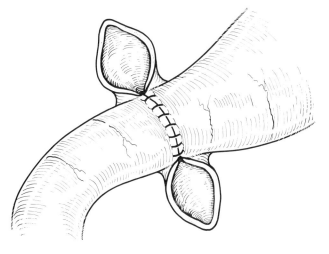

Figure 9.48
The 'dog ears' are folded over the anterior suture line.

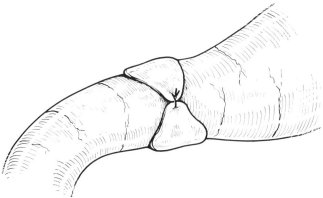

The management of Zollinger–Ellison syndrome is unsettled, but it is best determined by those who have considerable experience and facilities to investigate it satisfactorily.

Computed tomography and selective angiography help to identify the tumour and any metastases. Selective venous sampling of pancreatic veins can be carried out by percutaneous, transhepatic, portal vein catheterization to determine the site of release of gastrin.

It was formerly advised that every patient should be submitted to total gastrectomy. If investigation reveals multiple metastases, then cimetidine or ranitidine in high continuous dosage may control the symptoms of what is often a slowly growing tumour. Total gastrectomy is reserved in such patients for those who cannot be controlled with H2-receptor blocking drugs.

If there is no evidence of metastases, exploration is indicated. The pancreas is carefully mobilized and palpated. The whole abdomen is completely explored. A solitary tumour of the body or tail is excised by distal pancreatectomy, but in the head, enucleation is preferable.

If a solid tumour has been removed, the syndrome will be cured, but if not, and if cimetidine or ranitidine has failed to control the symptoms, carry out abdominal total gastrectomy.

Nutritional and haematological complications

Causes Vagotomy alone has few nutritional effects, although gastric retention may adversely affect digestion. An accompanying drainage operation does increase the intestinal transit rate, so digestion is impaired. The loss of part or all of the stomach reduces or abolishes contact of the food with gastric acid, the mixing and storage function of the stomach, the addition of intrinsic factor, and the important selective metering of fluid and chyme from the stomach into the duodenum through the pylorus, either because it is destroyed, bypassed or denervated. For reasons not entirely clear, fat digestion and absorption are prejudiced so that absorption of fat-soluble vitamins may be impaired. Calcium metabolism is also disturbed. The effects are somewhat proportional to the amount of stomach resected.

Sometimes previously undetected coeliac disease, and inflammatory bowel disease, produce malnutrition. When the afferent loop is long in Polya gastrectomy it may act as a 'blind loop', producing malabsorption. Many of the bizarre 'remedial' operations intended to improve postgastrectomy and postvagotomy syndromes introduce blind-loop features. Inadvertent, iatrogenic gastroileostomy causes devastating diarrhoea and malabsorption.

Features The most obvious feature is weight loss or failure to regain preoperative weight. The effects of anaemia produce lethargy. Osteoporosis occasionally results in fractures.

Investigations After many years about half the patients who have had a partial gastrectomy, and almost all patients who have had a total gastrectomy, become anaemic. This is initially microcytic, and later often macrocytic. Check the blood haemoglobin and red cells every year and include serum iron and vitamin B_{12} estimations if necessary. Three-day faecal fat content should not exceed 6 g, but most partial gastrectomy patients have a degree of steatorrhoea.

Some surgeons check the serum calcium, phosphate and protein levels at intervals after 5 to 10 years following gastrectomy. Osteoporosis is best assessed on plain X-rays of long bones. If nutritional deficiency is associated with marked steatorrhoea, exclude inflammatory bowel disease by sigmoidoscopy, barium meal and follow-through X-ray and barium enema. In the presence of demonstrable small bowel changes, arrange a small bowel biopsy. Barium meal and follow-through X-ray demonstrates the anatomical features following previous surgery, the rate of gastric emptying and small bowel transit time; it also demonstrates the mucosal pattern. It must be remembered that the efferent loop undergoes adaptive changes following Polya partial gastrectomy. If steatorrhoea is severe, assess it with the radioactive vitamin B_{12} absorption test before and after a course of antibiotics.

Preoperative weight is rarely a good benchmark in our modern, overfed Western society. The patient's assessment of his energy is of greater concern, but this is determined in part by his psychological make-up.

Treatment   If the anaemia is hypochromic, give oral iron supplements, and if macrocytic anaemia develops, give in addition intramuscular injections of 250 μg of vitamin B_{12} every two months, together with 5 mg of folic acid each day. For many years I (RMK) have given all patients who have had a total gastrectomy a single intramuscular injection of vitamin B_{12} annually and have not encountered macrocytic anaemia among them.

It it doubtful whether added vitamins and calcium are necessary in a patient who takes a good mixed diet. Some surgeons give vitamin D supplements in the hope of protecting patients against osteomalacia. If gluten sensitivity or inflammatory bowel disease are discovered, treat them on their own merits.

Severe malabsorption responds to antibiotics and their good effect can be monitored by the use of the radioactive vitamin B_{12} absorption test before and after giving antibiotics. If there is a mechanical blind loop, then it should be treated surgically.

Primary carcinoma

Recurrent carcinoma following gastrectomy for carcinoma is considered in Chapter 10. In the past carcinoma was occasionally treated as benign ulcer and proved to be malignant only after excision. Endoscopic biopsy and cytology should prevent this error.

Following partial gastrectomy, and possibly also vagotomy, there appears to be an increased risk of developing gastric carcinoma, often after a considerable interval. It would be expected that patients who have had gastrectomy for gastric ulcer, with associated dysplasia, would be at the highest risk, but this is not proven.

Radical surgical treatment is often possible and long-term survival is recorded, so a hopeless attitude is not justified.

Gastritis

Following gastric operations mucosal changes occur. The gastric mucosa atrophies following vagotomy. Following gastroenterostomy or pyloroplasty, bile reflux into the stomach appears to cause hypertrophic gastritis. This may be associated with epigastric burning pain and vomiting. However, the symptoms, endoscopic appearances and histology do not correlate.

As a rule symptomatic treatment is appropriate. Metoclopramide is usually prescribed, but I (RMK) have seen little benefit from this. Mucosal protecting substances such as sucralfate may also help. Illogically, in my experience antacid preparations often give the most relief. Operations to prevent bile reflux are inappropriate because its connection with the symptoms is uncertain.

Persisting Controversies

- Place of surgery in elective treatment of uncomplicated duodenal ulcer.
- Best technique for control of ulcer bleeding.
- Indications for surgery in recurrent peptic ulcer after surgery, including Zollinger–Ellison syndrome.
- Indications for reoperation for dumping and diarrhoea following surgery for peptic ulcer, and choice of operation.

Further reading

Cuschieri, A. (1977) Isoperistaltic and antiperistaltic jejunal interposition for the dumping syndrome. *Journal of the Royal College of Surgeons of Edinburgh, 22,* 319–324.

Ebied, F.H., Ralphs, D.N.L., Hobsley, M. & Le Quesne, L.P. (1982) Dumping symptoms after vagotomy treated by reversal of pyloroplasty. *British Journal of Surgery, 69,* 527–528.

Herrington, J.L. & Sawyers, J.L. (1972) A new operation for the dumping syndrome and post-vagotomy diarrhoea. *Annals of Surgery, 175,* 790–801.

Johnson, A.G. & Baxter, H.K. (1977) Where is your vagotomy incomplete? Observations on operative technique. *British Journal of Surgery, 64,* 583–586.

Kirk, R.M. (1976) Exploration of the abdomen. *Annals of the Royal College of Surgeons of England, 58,* 452–456.

Kirk, R.M. (1979) Antrectomy with vagotomy for duodenal ulcer. *World Journal of Surgery, 3,* 249.

Kirk, R.M. (1984) Drainage operations to accompany vagotomy. In Schwartz, S. & Ellis, H. (Eds) *Maingot's Abdominal Surgery,* 8th Edn. New York: Appleton Century Crofts.

Lancet (1980) Dumping syndrome and gut peptides. *Lancet* (Editorial), *ii,* 1173.

Leeds, A.R., Ebied, F.H., Ralphs, D.N.L., Metz, G. & Dilawari J.B. (1981) Pectin in the dumping syndrome: reduction of symptoms and plasma volume changes. *Lancet, ii,* 1075–1078.

Logan, R.F.A. & Langman, M.J.S. (1983) Screening for gastric cancer after gastric surgery. *Lancet, ii:* 667–670.

Long, R.G., Adrian, T.E. & Bloom, S.R. (1985) Somatostatin and the dumping syndrome. *British Medical Journal 290,* 886–888.

Thompson, J.C., Lewis, B.G., Weiner, I. & Townsend, C.M., Jr. (1983) The role of surgery in the Zollinger–Ellison syndrome. *Annals of Surgery, 197,* 594–607.

Totten, J., Burns, H.J.G. & Kay, A.W. (1983) Time of onset of carcinoma of the stomach following surgical treatment of duodenal ulcer. *Surgery, Gynecology and Obstetrics, 157,* 431–433.

Wyllie, J.H., Clark, C.G., Alexander-Williams, J., Bell, P.R.F., Kennedy, T.L., Kirk, R.M. & Mackay, C. (1981) Effect of cimetidine on surgery for duodenal ulcer. *Lancet, i,* 1307–1308.

10 Complications Specific to Gastrectomy

Early Complications

Biliary leak

Causes   A biliary leak following gastrectomy is most likely to develop from a burst duodenal stump or gastroduodenal anastomosis (p. 196). Rarely the retroduodenal or supraduodenal common bile duct is injured or transected while dissecting the duodenum. Both are more likely to occur during duodenal ulcer operations than cancer surgery.

Prevention   Since duodenal stump leaks and common bile duct injury most frequently follow dissection around a duodenal ulcer rather than mobilization in cancer surgery, the likely explanation is that the ulcer scar probably distorts the anatomy and this is not appreciated by the surgeon. The best way to prevent an injury therefore is to choose an alternative operation for duodenal ulcer whenever this is possible.

During dissection the surgeon must take great care to keep strictly on the duodenal wall, not damaging it, nor wandering away from it. Unless he does so, he runs the risk of damaging the wall so that it leaks, of injuring the common bile duct, or of injuring the pancreas.

If the injury of the common bile duct is noted at the time, it should be repaired immediately and a T-tube drain inserted (see *Complications of Biliary and Pancreatic Surgery*).

Features   Biliary peritonitis often, though not inevitably, causes profound collapse, with peripheral vascular shutdown, weak thready pulse, low blood pressure and adynamic ileus of the bowel, within a few hours of operation if the bile duct is directly injured or after a few days if the duodenal stump leaks. If a drain is in place, the bile may track to the surface, though not reliably so.

Management   The collapsed patient in whom the true diagnosis may not yet be made, apart from the recognition of an acute abdominal catastrophe, should be resuscitated and returned to the operating theatre (see p. 204). The abdomen is re-explored, all the bile is aspirated and a careful assessment is made of the cause. If the duodenal stump has leaked, it should be drained (see p. 205). If the bile duct is injured, it may be possible to repair it, but as a rule the best that can be done is to insert a T-tube into the supraduodenal part to drain it, and explore the patient at a later date to carry out a definitive repair or create a choledochojejunostomy.

Jaundice

The onset of jaundice in a patient recovering from gastrectomy is very disconcerting to the surgeon, who is often obsessed by the possibility of a technical failure.

Causes The anxious surgeon fears obstruction of the common bile duct and possibly also the pancreatic duct following a difficult duodenal closure. Maximal mobilization of the duodenum to facilitate a high anastomosis may temporarily obstruct the bile duct. Deeply placed sutures intended to stop bleeding of an ulcer may obstruct the duct. However, haemolysis from incompatible transfusion and sepsis or hepatotoxicity and liver failure may result in jaundice, as may absorption of leaked bile. Remember that drugs may produce cholestatic, hepatotoxic or haemolytic jaundice. Remember also that the patient may have had unsuspected biliary tract disease and that a displaced stone could have obstructed the bile duct: an operator's ability to exclude gallstones is poor.

Prevention Since damage is most likely to occur in the presence of severe duodenal ulcer, is there an alternative operation that would avoid the risk?

The rule when dissecting around the duodenal bulb is to stick scrupulously to the duodenal wall without damaging it. If it is damaged, it will leak. If the surgeon allows the dissection to wander away from the duodenal wall, he risks damaging the bile duct and the pancreas, causing leakage, obstruction or inflammation. If the bile duct is at risk, display the supraduodenal portion and insert a Bakes' dilator that can be felt below as a guide to the bile duct (Fig. 10.1). At the end of the operation insert a 'T-tube' drain.

At an operation to control duodenal ulcer bleeding, the stitches of non-absorbable material must be accurately inserted to encompass the gastroduodenal artery, while avoiding the bile duct and pancreatic ducts.

If damage to the bile duct is noted, repair it carefully and insert a T-tube.

Features In the early stage the appearance of the jaundice may be difficult to categorize. The patient is usually not yet passing stools to allow their colour to be noted, and if there is any dehydration, the rather dark urine may be misinterpreted. An external leak of bile

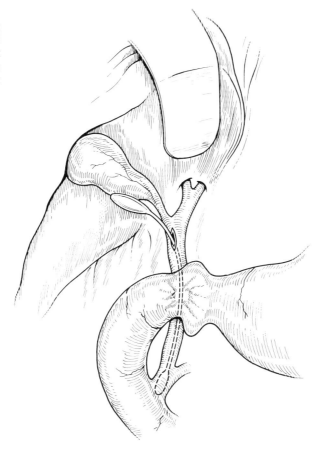

suggests that some is being absorbed. Following Polya type gastrectomy, the absence of bile in the nasogastric aspirate suggests biliary obstruction.

Investigations Liver function tests and urine biochemistry usually distinguish the type of jaundice. If a bile leak is suspected but not demonstrable, ultrasound or CT scanning usually displays a collection. Percutaneous cholangiography clarifies suspected mechanical obstruction. Check the drug list carefully. If haemolysis is suspected, obtain help from the haematologists. In the presence of pyrexia, send blood cultures to exclude sepsis.

Management Depending on the cause, stop blood transfusions and any drug likely to be producing jaundice, drain any bile collection and treat the cause. If liver failure is evident, obtain advice from a hepatologist.

Transient obstructive jaundice following maximum duodenal mobilization to allow oesophagoantral anastomosis after upper partial gastrectomy or gastroduodenal anastomosis following extensive Billroth I gastrectomy is presumed to be from kinking of the bile duct, but could be caused by oedema, collections or mild pancreatitis.

Persisting obstructive jaundice following the underrunning of a bleeding duodenal ulcer, duodenal closure in the presence of an extensive duodenal ulcer or extensive duodenal resection in the presence of a distal gastric carcinoma may also result from pancreatitis or the pressure from a collection, but if it is not resolved within 10–14 days, it is almost certainly from mechanical bile duct obstruction. If gastroduodenal or oesophagoduodenal anastomosis was performed, carry out a HIDA scan (hippo-iminodiacetic acid labelled with technetium-99m scintigraphy) or ERCP (endoscopic retrograde cholangiopancreatography) to elucidate the site of obstruction. Exclude hyperamylasaemia, check the clotting factors and order a percutaneous cholangiogram if necessary. If obstruction is not complete, the radiologist may be able to introduce a guide-wire through the stenotic segment and gently dilate it. If the obstruction is complete, reoperate on the patient and bypass it after an interval of two weeks, with a choledochoduodenostomy or choledochojejunostomy. In a cancer patient following extensive duodenal mobilization, I (RMK) should perform cholecystojejunotomy if the obstruction is distal to the cystic duct entry into the common bile duct, but in other cases choledochojejunostomy may be more appropriate (see *Complications of Biliary and Pancreatic Surgery*).

Pancreatitis

Acute, haemorrhagic pancreatitis is an infrequent but disastrous complication of gastrectomy. Lesser degrees are probably missed.

Causes   It is reported that pancreatitis develops following gastrectomy, with injury to the pancreas, to the duct of Santorini, or from back pressure in the pancreatic ductal system caused by afferent loop obstruction.

It is very often impossible to know what caused acute pancreatitis, since it is relatively rare. In my experience it has occurred only following Polya gastrectomy for duodenal ulcer, yet transection and closure of the duodenum may be accomplished well distal to the pylorus in the presence of distal gastric cancer without provoking pancreatitis. I (RMK) have not seen it following Billroth I gastrectomy. Pancreatitis does not necessarily occur following difficult gastrectomies, but can unexpectedly develop after a straightforward procedure.

Prevention   On the assumption that pancreatic parenchymal or ductal damage may trigger the attack, take great care when mobilizing the pancreas and when mobilizing and closing the duodenal stump. Look in or near the base of the ulcer for the opening of the duct of Santorini and avoid it. Do not insert stitches into the head of the pancreas. The pancreas is liable to damage when elevating the head together with the duodenal loop in Kocher's manoeuvre, when mobilizing the first part of the duodenum, and while inserting stitches to close it or unite the duodenum to the stomach.

Features The patient deteriorates or collapses, but epigastric pain passing through to the back, tenderness and guarding may be absent or modified. If gut function has not yet returned, the ensuing paralytic ileus is not recognized.

Investigations The diagnosis is usually made in a patient who suddenly deteriorates, by discovering a serum amylase level of well over 1000 IU. Ultrasound or CT scanning may demonstrate pancreatic enlargement. In case of doubt, the diagnosis may be made at an exploratory operation, when free fluid, fat necrosis and a swollen, possibly haemorrhagic pancreas is found, and no other lesion is discovered.

Management Provided that the diagnosis is confidently made, postgastrectomy pancreatitis is managed conservatively by restoring the circulatory volume with intravenous fluid, electrolytes, plasma and if necessary blood. Defunction the gut by continuing nasogastric suction. Although prophylactic antibiotics probably have no effect, most surgeons give them to these patients, who are very vulnerable if they develop any infection. Administer pethidine in small repeated intramuscular doses as an analgesic. It is wise to insert a central venous catheter so that the venous pressure can be monitored. Check and if necessary correct diabetes and hypoglycaemia. Cystic cavities and abscesses may develop. They can be localized using CT or ultrasound scans and drained percutaneously or if necessary by operation.

If the diagnosis is in doubt, explore the patient in the early phase, especially if he does not respond to vigorous conservative treatment. Explore the whole abdomen, and carefully examine the pancreas, gallbladder, bile duct, duodenal stump and afferent jejunal loop. Note any fat necrosis and pancreatic swelling. Perform operative cholangiography after aspirating bile for culture from the common duct. If there is biliary obstruction, remove the gallbladder, explore the common duct for stones and insert a T-tube drain. If there is afferent loop obstruction, correct it. Peritoneal lavage is currently under trial for the management of acute pancreatitis, but its value is not yet settled.

Late Complications

Recurrent carcinoma

Cause and prevention   However radical is the resection for gastric carcinoma, recurrence may occur. It is not even possible to predict who will develop recurrence, since only tissue that has been removed can be examined and the remaining tissue may look and feel normal and appear normal when tests or scans are applied, yet have microscopic disease. On the whole, however, recurrence is more likely if the resection was inadequate. Radical resection must be intelligently performed; many surgeons consider that splenectomy converts a palliative into a radical gastrectomy, but this is not so. A distal carcinoma is but a few centimetres from the liver along the hepatoduodenal ligament and is almost in direct contact with the hepatic and right gastroepiploic arteries; in addition, the propensity for gastric carcinoma to spread into the duodenum is greater than was previously realized. Polya gastrectomy is preferable to Billroth I gastrectomy to exclude the possibility of stomal recurrence from residual tumour in the duodenum (Fig. 10.2). The hepatic artery should be stripped clean of all lymphatic tissue from the porta hepatis to the coeliac axis. The right gastroepiploic artery and right greater omentum must be radically cleared, bearing in mind that the middle colic artery lies but 1 cm from the right gastroepiploic artery, which will be tied at its origin from the gastroduodenal artery. The left gastric vessels are tied at their origins.

More proximal gastric carcinoma demands radical total gastrectomy, and since the tumour readily invades the oesophagus the operation is most successfully accomplished by a thoracoabdominal approach, although in elderly or poor risk patients a compromise may be necessary. Radical clearance of the left gastric and splenic vessels, the spleen, distal pancreas and omentum should be carried out. Reconstruction by oesophagojejunostomy is appropriate.

The place of postgastrectomy radiotherapy of known residual tumour, or cytotoxic chemotherapy in preventing or delaying recurrence has not yet been determined.

Features   Recurrent tumour may present in one of two ways—gastrointestinal symptoms, usually of obstruction, or gradual and general deterioration from metastases in the liver and elsewhere.

Investigations   It is not possible to screen every patient who has had a gastrectomy for carcinoma of the stomach to detect presymptomatic recurrence. Once suspicious symptoms occur, then clinical examination, endoscopy and radiological examination are appropriate. If ascites is suspected, insert a fine needle percutaneously in each abdominal quadrant to seek fluid, which is then sent for cytological examination. Ultrasound or CT scans are valuable if

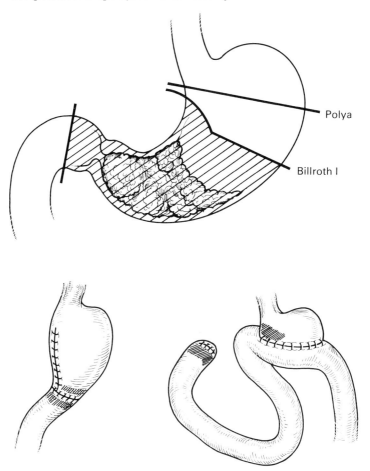

Figure 10.2
The advantages of Polya reconstruction with full-width stoma, over Billroth I gastrectomy for distal gastric carcinoma. The shaded portions show possible sites for local recurrence.

liver metastases are suspected, and should be carried out if further palliative surgery is contemplated.

Management　　Cure is unlikely, but useful palliation is often possible. Avoid surgery in patients with extensive metastatic disease and no mechanical gastrointestinal symptoms. Re-explore patients with mechnaical obstruction or other features. There is no evidence about the prognosis following local recurrence early or late after initial resection. Early recurrence may represent inadequate resection, lymphatic spread, microscopic satellite tumour, or highly malignant tumour. The surgeon tends to feel justified in an aggressive approach to local recurrence developing late, and most of us would treat this as though it were a local primary tumour. Be prepared to radically resect a local recurrence, since long-term palliation is possible. I (RMK) have on occasion resected part of an invaded liver lobe, a segment of transverse colon, and the distal pancreas, in continuity with a local recurrence, when this was the only detectable tumour.

Local recurrence of a distal gastric carcinoma with obstruction is suitable for resection if possible, or high gastroenterostomy if it is extensive (Fig. 10.3). Remember that the high gastroenterostomy leaves a sump below, often lined with malignant ulcerating tumour, so the patient will often not be entirely relieved, because the gastroenterostomy will drain only when the distal stomach has filled and overflows. Devine, a famous Australian surgeon, transected the stomach below the gastroenterostomy to exclude the distal stomach in such cases, but I have rarely performed this extra procedure, since the patients usually have such extensive local or distant disease that short-term palliation of the obstruction has seemed all that was justified.

Patients who have had total gastrectomy or upper partial gastrectomy and develop recurrence with dysphagia can rarely be helped by further resection, though bypass is occasionally useful. An isolated colonic or jejunal segment can be taken up beyond the blockage and joined to the oesophagus, and to the duodenum or jejunum below.

The insertion of an oesophageal tube is often worth while, since no surgeon would wish to close the abdomen while leaving the patient with severe dysphagia. Make an incision in the stomach or bowel below the recurrence and pass a gum-elastic bougie from below upwards to the pharynx. It is usually necessary to insert a finger through the gastrotomy or enterotomy to identify the passage, and then to insert the bougie alongside, to be guided in the correct direction. Often it is

Figure 10.3
Efferent loop stomal obstruction from recurrent carcinoma following Polya partial gastrectomy. A second, high, gastroenterostomy is fashioned.

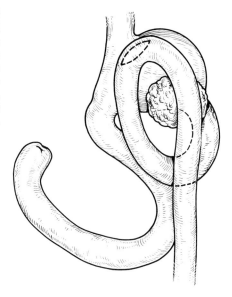

necessary to use the finger as a dilator—occasionally the tumour splits as it is pushed upwards. Do not despair, but pass up the bougie, ask the anaesthetist to attach the leader of a Mousseau–Barbin or Celestin tube and draw it down. Carefully impact the tube in the split and cut off the excess. The tube forms an obturator to prevent free leakage through the split. Close the incision into the stomach or bowel.

The place for radiotherapy is not certain but sometimes produces excellent palliation of adenocarcinoma. Unless there are extensive metastases in the liver or peritoneum, I always mark the limits of recurrent localized tumour with metal clips. Postoperative radiotherapy may give striking improvement and is nearly always worth trying. Patients who have extensive inoperable tumour with impending dysphagia may be spared a surgical procedure by local radiotherapy to the obstructing tumour. As a rule the dysphagia gets initially worse as the tumour swells, and it may be necessary to give a fluid diet, pass a fine-bore tube or carry out endoscopic dilatation. Gradually, swallowing improves. Of course the resulting fibrosis impairs peristaltic action but the relief is nevertheless often dramatic.

The difficulty comes with patients who have a proved recurrence but are relatively asymptomatic. If the recurrence appears to be localized, it is certainly worth re-exploring the patient after discussing the problems with him. In the past, a few surgeons re-explored their cancer patients deliberately after an interval, for a 'second look.' Indeed, Owen Wangensteen, the great American surgeon who popularized the technique, took further looks for as long as the patients survived. The advent of radiological improvements, more versatile endoscopes and scanning techniques have made this type of exploration unnecessary.

Adjunctive methods of treatment are under trial. Palliative chemotherapy is improving but is not yet fully accepted for the management of advanced recurrent gastric adenocarcinoma. Much depends on the skill and good sense of the physician who administers the treatment. If the patient is improving, and is not suffering side-effects, then treatment should be continued. The effect on his morale of feeling that something is being done about his disease is profound. However, if he suffers side-effects, is deteriorating and has lost confidence in the treatment, it should be stopped. The preferred combinations of drugs change rapidly and it is wise to have the advice of an expert. If one combination fails, another may bring benefit.

Persisting Controversies

- Management of postgastrectomy obstructive jaundice.
- Cause of postgastrectomy pancreatitis.
- Place of chemotherapy as adjuvant treatment for gastric carcinoma.

Further reading

Akiyama, H. (1979) Thoracoabdominal approach for carcinoma of the cardia of the stomach. *American Journal of Surgery, 137,* 345–349.

Kirk, R.M. & Williamson, R.C.N. (1986) *General Surgical Operations*, 2nd Edn. Edinburgh: Churchill Livingstone.

Kodama, Y., Sugimachi, K., Soejima, K., Matsusak, T. & Inokuch, K. (1981) Evaluation of extensive lymph node dissection for carcinoma of the stomach. *World Journal of Surgery, 5,* 241–248.

Papachristou, D.N. & Shiu, M.H. (1981) Management by en bloc multiple organ resection of carcinoma of the stomach invading adjacent organs. *Surgery, Gynecology and Obstetrics, 152,* 483–487.

11 Complications Specific to Vagotomy

Most of the undesirable long-term sequelae of vagotomy and drainage are a consequence of the drainage procedure and not the vagotomy. Loss of pyloric control of gastric emptying following either pyloroplasty or gastroenterostomy may result in symptoms of dumping or diarrhoea due to rapid postprandial gastric emptying. The enterogastric bile reflux, which occurs frequently after pyloroplasty and inevitably after gastroenterostomy, may cause bilious vomiting or epigastric pain due to gastritis and has been implicated as an aetiological factor in the development of operated stomach cancer. The incidence of these postoperative problems is significantly lower after highly selective vagotomy because preservation of antral vagal innervation makes a drainage procedure unnecessary. The majority of complications specific to the vagotomy present in the immediate postoperative period and are due either to damage to an adjacent structure or to ischaemia of the stomach. There are conflicting reports on the long-term effects of truncal vagotomy on gallstone formation and gastro-oesophageal reflux.

Ideally an operation for a benign gastric or duodenal ulcer should have no mortality. The reported mortality rate for elective vagotomy and drainage varies between 0.5 and 2% (Cox, Spencer and Tinker, 1969) and for highly selective vagotomy is less than 0.5% (Johnston, 1975). This rate is higher after emergency vagotomy for complications of ulcer disease such as perforation or bleeding. The mortality rate for vagotomy and oversewing of a bleeding duodenal ulcer in patients over the age of 60 years exceeds 10%.

Oesophageal Complications

Perforation

During mobilization the lower oesophagus may be damaged at the level of the oesophageal hiatus. This is usually the result of blunt finger dissection in obese patients or in those with perioesophageal inflammation secondary to reflux oesophagitis. It is more likely to occur during truncal or selective vagotomy. Highly selective vagotomy demands a more careful and precise dissection in this region. Digital injury usually involves the posterior wall of the oesophagus, but the anterior wall can also be damaged during over enthusiastic attempts to divide the fine anterior vagal fibres. Minor oesophageal damage can lead to complete circumferential disruption if excessive force is applied to a sling around the gastro-oesophageal junction. The most frequent type of injury is a posterior perforation affecting 20–30% of the oesophageal circumference.

Prevention   The risk of oesophageal damage can be virtually eliminated by careful sharp dissection in the oesophageal hiatus. Using scissors divide the peritoneal reflection over the anterior wall of the oesophagus, 2–3 cm above the gastro-oesophageal junction. This incision is continued laterally in both directions: to the left, into the angle of His and continuing 1–2 cm onto the anterior border of the gastric fundus; and to the right, over the ascending branch of the left gastric artery and into the lesser omentum (Fig. 11.1). With downward traction on the stomach continue the dissection in the angle of His round onto the posterior aspect of the oesophagus. Now pass the right index finger behind the oesophagus; only a single layer of peritoneum on the right lateral margin remains to be divided by blunt dissection. Sharp dissection with

Figure 11.1
The peritoneal reflection must be divided with scissors from the lesser omentum, over the oesophagus and into the angle of His.

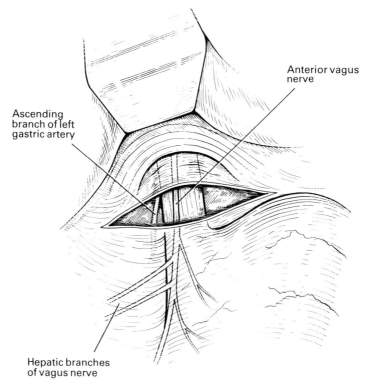

Anterior vagus nerve

Ascending branch of left gastric artery

Hepatic branches of vagus nerve

scissors is the key to success. Blunt digital dissection of all tissues laterally and posterior to the oesophagus puts the oesophageal wall in jeopardy.

Presentation   The mode of presentation is dependent on the time at which the oesophageal damage is recognized. This may:

1 Be recognized intraoperatively.
2 Present as a postoperative pyrexia due to mediastinitis or a subphrenic abscess.
3 Present weeks or months after operation, with rigors, pyrexia and a subphrenic abscess (uncommon).

Oesophageal damage recognized during operation should be repaired immediately. Postoperatively oesophageal damage may be more difficult to detect. Perform a penetrated chest X-ray, looking for mediastinal widening or surgical emphysema. Screen the oesophagus whilst the patient drinks a water-soluble contrast medium, looking for evidence of a perforation. A mediastinal or subphrenic abscess may be detected by ultrasound, CT scan or radionuclide scanning using gallium or labelled leucocytes.

Treatment   *Intraoperatively* oesophageal damage can be repaired by a variety of manoeuvres (see Chapter 5). A small tear can be repaired transabdominally, but major damage, including total disruption, requires extension of the abdominal incision into a left thoracoabdominal exposure. Ask the anaesthetist to replace the normal endotracheal tube with a double-lumen tube which will permit collapse of the left lung. Expose, prepare and drape the left chest and extend the incision across the costal margin between the seventh and eighth ribs. The oesophageal defect can be repaired in one or two layers using inner absorbable and outer non-absorbable sutures. The repair can be reinforced by suturing the phreno-oesophageal ligament to the oesophagus or alternatively by fundoplication or a Thal patch.

Postoperatively a mediastinal or subphrenic abscess should be drained transabdominally and a wide-bore drain inserted. Do not attempt to close the perforation, for the sutures will simply cut through the oesophageal wall. Put the patient on broad-spectrum antibiotics and begin total parenteral nutrition. Radiological screening at weekly intervals will determine when the perforation has closed and when oral feeding can be reintroduced.

Dysphagia
Mild dysphagia is a common problem following vagotomy, occurring in 15–20% of patients. It is usually transient in nature, beginning on the fourth or fifth postoperative day, when solid food is first taken, and resolving by the fourteenth day in all but 1% of patients. It is due to oedema or haematoma formation at the

oesophageal hiatus. Barium swallow and endoscopy are unnecessary in patients with mild dysphagia in the early postoperative period. However, if the dysphagia is severe, limiting the patient to a liquid diet, or persists for more than two weeks, then a barium swallow *should* be performed. If an intrinsic oesophageal stricture is present so soon after vagotomy, it may be the result of intraoperative oesophageal damage and a careful look for radiological evidence of a perforation is required. Extrinsic compression from a perioesophageal haematoma produces a smooth tapered narrowing with a normal mucosal pattern. If the dysphagia is due to extrinsic compression, perform oesophageal dilatation using Maloney's, Celestin's or Hurst's dilators. Investigate the patient with an oesophageal stricture endoscopically, using the minimum of air insufflation, looking for evidence of oesophagitis or oesophageal trauma. If no perforation is observed, gently dilate the stricture using Celestin's dilators passed over a guide-wire and with radiological screening. The dysphagia will resolve completely after one or two dilatations in over 90% of patients. In a small minority of patients the dysphagia does not improve after dilatation and may progress relentlessly to complete oesophageal obstruction within a few weeks of operation. Endoscopically there is no evidence of oesophagitis and on manometry the lower oesophageal sphincter can be seen to relax on swallowing. Repeated dilatation is contraindicated and early laporotomy should be performed. These patients usually have a tough fibrotic collar encircling the lower oesophagus and this should be excised. This intense fibrous reaction is due either to organization and fibrosis of a haematoma or to an excessive foreign body reaction, most frequently owing to the presence of suture material in the vicinity.

Very rarely the barium swallow shows the characteristic appearance of achalasia. On manometry the lower oesophageal sphincter pressure may be high, but this relaxes with swallowing, and peristaltic waves are present in the body of the oesophagus. This problem has been associated more frequently with transthoracic than with transabdominal vagotomy. Such patients generally respond to a standard oesophageal dilatation. Forceful dilatation or oesophagomyotomy are unnecessary.

Gastro-oesophageal reflux

Gastro-oesophageal reflux is not a complication of vagotomy. The lower oesophageal sphincter is not dependent on the vagus for its intrinsic tone and there is no fall in sphincter pressure following vagotomy. Reflux symptoms are present in 50% of preoperative duodenal ulcer patients and over 30% have macroscopic and/or microscopic oesophagitis on endoscopy (Flook and Stoddard, 1985). If a careful history is taken from patients with postoperative reflux symptoms, the majority will have had similar symptoms before operation, which were either overlooked or incorrectly attributed to their ulcer. Although gastro-oesophageal reflux symptoms improve in many patients after vagotomy, 30% still have abnormal 24-hour intraoesophageal pH recordings. Careful preoperative assessment of duodenal ulcer patients is necessary, for vagotomy does not abolish gastro-oesophageal reflux and those with significant reflux symptoms and oesophagitis need an antireflux procedure in addition to their vagotomy.

Patients with postoperative reflux symptoms should have endoscopy to determine whether there is oesophagitis and to ensure that the reflux is not secondary to gastric outlet obstruction. Medical treatment should be initiated and antireflux surgery reserved for the small group of patients whose symptoms cannot be controlled by a long, intensive course of such treatment. If surgery is necessary, the surgeon should perform his usual antireflux procedure. Although patience will be necessary to separate the stomach from the undersurface of the liver and diaphragm if a transabdominal approach is used, a previous vagotomy is not a specific indication for a transthoracic operation.

Splenic Injury

Splenic injury is either due to traction on an adhesion between the spleen and omentum which results in a tear in the splenic capsule or to traction on the hilum which damages a branch of the splenic vein. Splenic preservation is preferable to splenectomy. The different methods of splenic repair are described in detail in Chapter 12. Damage to the spleen can be avoided by dividing adhesions between the spleen and omentum early in the operation or by inserting a pack behind the spleen to displace it anteromedially, thus avoiding traction on the splenic vein in the hilum. Capsular tears should be repaired by a simple manoeuvre such as the application of diathermy or local haemostatic substances. Hilar bleeding may require partial or total splenectomy.

Lesser Curve Necrosis

Aetiology This rare complication occurs exclusively after highly selective vagotomy. It is due to an ischaemic necrosis of the lesser curve of the stomach following division of the branches of the left gastric artery along with the vagal branches to the body and fundus. Although there is an extensive intramural anastomosis between the left and right gastric and gastro-epiploic arteries, division of the branches of the left gastric artery leaves a relatively ischaemic area 1 cm in width in the long axis of the stomach, along the lesser curvature. This area is at risk of ischaemic necrosis. Splenectomy and highly selective vagotomy are a potentially dangerous combination, for the former also involves division of the short gastric vessels. Suturing the lesser omentum onto the lesser curve of the stomach after highly selective vagotomy does not appear to reduce the prevalence or risks of lesser curve necrosis.

Presentation and treatment

Patients initially make an uneventful recovery following operation, but then suddenly develop severe abdominal pain and peritonitis on, or about, the third or fourth postoperative day. Hypovolaemia is absent and the diagnosis of intra-abdominal bleeding is thus unlikely. An erect chest X-ray may show a substantial amount of air under the diaphragm. A small amount of free air may merely represent unabsorbed air following the initial laparotomy. Radiological screening using a water-soluble contrast material is valuable in any patient in whom there is doubt about the diagnosis or the need for a second laparotomy.

All patients with a suspected lesser curve necrosis following highly selective vagotomy should have a laparotomy after prior resuscitation with intravenous fluids. Re-explore the abdomen through the original incision. An area of necrotic gastric wall with a perforation surrounded by area of ischaemia will be found on the lesser curvature (Fig. 11.2). The leaked gastric contents should be aspirated and peritoneal lavage performed with warm

Figure 11.2
Lesser curve necrosis following highly selective vagotomy.

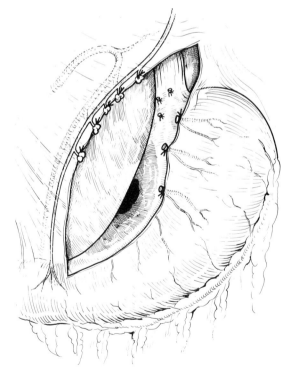

saline containing 1 g of tetracycline per litre. Do not simply suture the perforation, for the leak was due to ischaemia and healing is unlikely. Excise the wall until healthy bleeding stomach is reached and then close the defect in two layers. If the ischaemic area is extensive, a Polya gastrectomy may be the safest procedure.

Abnormalities of Gastric Emptying

Aetiology Gastric motility, as well as acid and pepsin output, is reduced after all forms of vagotomy. The extent of the motility disturbance is related to the type of operation, being less after highly selective vagotomy, in which antral innervation is preserved, than after truncal or selective vagotomy. The need for a drainage procedure after truncal or selective vagotomy is attributable to this reduction in motor activity.

 The motility change affects the rate of emptying of both liquid and solid meals. Gastric emptying rates can be measured by giving a radioisotope-labelled meal and scanning the upper abdomen with a gamma camera for the following 90 minutes. The rate of emptying of liquids is controlled by the proximal stomach, which has the capacity to relax to accommodate large volumes of ingested fluid, with only a small rise in intragastric pressure. This accommodation reflex is vagally mediated. The forceful contractions of the distal stomach control the rate of emptying of solids. Vagal denervation reduces the strength of the antral contractions. Thus after vagotomy the rate of emptying of solids is delayed, because of the weaker antral contractions, but liquid emptying is enhanced, because of the loss of receptive relaxation. The delay in the emptying of solids is greatest immediately after operation and in the majority of patients returns towards normal over the next six months.

Symptoms Although all patients have disordered gastric motility after vagotomy, only a few have any symptoms of gastric stasis. The majority of these patients will have had a truncal or selective vagotomy and pyloroplasty. Symptomatic gastric stasis after highly selective vagotomy is suggestive of inadvertent antral denervation. The onset, duration and severity of these symptoms is variable. Some patients present in the early postoperative period with persistent large volumes of gastric aspirate. Spontaneous motility returns within a few days in most patients, but in some the gastric stasis can persist for two to three weeks. Other patients present weeks after operation with symptoms of epigastric fullness, flatulence, early satiety, or vomiting. On examination, a succussion splash may be elicited and there may be evidence of weight loss. Gastric stasis occurs most frequently after truncal vagotomy and drainage. Patients with pyloric stenosis are more prone to postoperative gastric stasis because of the chronic gastric dilatation and overstretching of the gastric musculature.

<table>
<tr><td>*Investigation and treatment*</td><td>A mechanical obstruction of the gastric outlet must be excluded by endoscopy or barium meal. The latter also permits a diagnosis of gastric atony to be made by demonstrating absent gastric peristalsis. Immediate postoperative gastric stasis should be treated expectantly with nasogastric aspiration and intravenous fluid replacement. Intravenous H2-receptor blocking drugs will reduce gastric acid production and hence electrolyte loss. Daily electrolyte estimations are essential. If gastric atony lasts more than seven days, intravenous parenteral nutrition should be commenced. Restoration of motility can be stimulated pharmacologically. The best drug is bethanechol chloride, a parasympathomimetic agent, given subcutaneously in a dose of 2.5 mg six-hourly. Once motility returns, as evidenced by reduced volume of nasogastric aspirate or relief of symptoms, oral bethanechol 5 mg q.d.s. before meals can be substituted. In the absence of gastric contractions metoclopramide is ineffective in initiating peristalsis.</td></tr>
</table>

Patients presenting with gastric stasis weeks after operation have some gastric motor activity rather than complete atony. These patients generally *do* respond to metoclopramide, 10 mg t.d.s., or domperidone before meals.

If the gastric stasis persists after three days of pharmacological manipulation, consider a second laparotomy. Persevere with medical treatment as long as possible for the symptoms will generally resolve. The exact timing of a second operation is dependent on an absence of reduction of the volume of gastric aspirate, failure of response to pharmacological manipulation, and the patient's general heath and fitness for another procedure. After a previous truncal or selective vagotomy and pyloroplasty the stasis can be relieved by performing a retrocolic posterior gastroenterostomy. If the stasis follows a highly selective vagotomy, add a pyloroplasty.

Bleeding

Significant intra-abdominal bleeding after vagotomy occurs in 0.2–1% of patients and is one of the principal causes of postoperative death. The bleeding may be *intraluminal* from a pyloroplasty, gastroenterostomy or the ulcer itself, or *intraperitoneal* from the edge of a mobilized left lobe of the liver, the spleen or a slipped ligature or clip on the lesser curve of the stomach after highly selective vagotomy.

Serious intraluminal bleeding presents with haematemesis and/or melaena, but intraperitoneal bleeding may be more difficult to detect. Patients develop signs of hypovolaemia—tachycardia, peripheral vasoconstriction, poor urine output and eventually hypotension. Measurement of abdominal girth as a means of detecting intra-abdominal bleeding is useless, but peritoneal lavage using 1 litre of saline run into the abdominal cavity through a peritoneal dialysis catheter (inserted away from the incision), allowed to equilibrate, and then run out again, may be valuable.

Treatment of anastomotic bleeding has been described on p. 192. Patients with a major intraperitoneal bleed require an emergency second laparotomy after prior resuscitation with a combination of colloidal and crystalloid solutions whilst blood is being crossmatched. Open the abdomen through the original incision, evacuate the blood clot and identify and ligate the bleeding point(s). Patients who require massive transfusions should have a clotting screen performed and may require platelets and fresh frozen plasma in addition to the blood.

Gallstones

There is considerable clinical evidence that truncal vagotomy predisposes to the formation of cholesterol gallstones and that this can be prevented by preservation of the hepatic branches of the vagus nerve. Truncal vagotomy results in the division of not only the vagal efferent fibres to the stomach but also those to the liver and gallbladder. Stimulation of the hepatic vagal branches results in contraction of the gallbladder. Dilatation of the gallbladder following truncal vagotomy was observed over 30 years ago and it was suggested that this dilatation was due to hypotonia and might lead to biliary stasis and hence gallstone formation. The hepatic vagal branches are not divided during selective or highly selective vagotomy and these patients are not at increased risk. There have been conflicting reports relating to the incidence of gallstones after truncal vagotomy. These have ranged from a negligible increase to six times the incidence in an age and sex matched group of non-vagotomized control patients.

It was suggested that the increased gallstone formation after truncal vagotomy was due to an alteration in the composition of bile, leading to an increased lithogenicity, but this hypothesis has now been disproven. Changes in gallbladder motility or in the flow of bile into the duodenum are believed to be responsible for the increase in gallstones. Increased resistance to flow through the sphincter of Oddi has been demonstrated after truncal vagotomy in the prairie dog, but not in man. Ihasz and Griffith observed that 50% of patients had a radiologically dilated gallbladder with impaired or absent contractility four to seven years after truncal vagotomy and that 19.5% of these patients had gallstones, compared with only 2.2% of the other patients who had a normal, non-distended gallbladder.

Hitherto gallbladder contraction has been assumed to occur in response to the emptying of food into the duodenum. Using a double-isotope technique to measure gastric and biliary empty-ing simultaneously, it has been shown that some normal patients empty their gallbladders spontaneously, probably in relation to the passage of an interdigestive myoelectrical complex. How-ever, in the majority, biliary emptying commences within a few minutes of eating a meal, some patients having a rapid, large-volume ejection and others a small, low-volume ejection. Abnor-mal gallbladder emptying patterns are observed in approxima-tely half the patients after truncal vagotomy, the gallbladder emptying either incompletely or in an irregular manner. Thus, when studied radiologically or using a radioisotope technique, approximately 50% of patients have abnormal gallbladder emp-tying after truncal vagotomy and this group probably represents those at greatest risk of gallstone formation.

Highly selective vagotomy is associated with a lower incidence of dumping, diarrhoea, bile vomiting and gallstone formation than truncal vagotomy. The lower risk of gallstone formation is another reason for believing that highly selective vagotomy is the best operation for patients with duodenal ulceration.

The presentation, investigation and management of patients with gallstones follows the same pattern, irrespective of whether a vagotomy has or has not been performed previously. If cholecystectomy is advised, a right subcostal incision is to be preferred, for it avoids the intra-abdominal adhesions related to the previous surgery.

Conclusions

Intraoperative oesophageal and splenic injury during vagotomy can be avoided by careful operative technique. Partial oeso-phageal tears can be repaired from the abdomen, but total oesophageal disruption will require extension of the incision into a thoracoabdominal exposure to permit surgical correction. Dysphagia is a common, but usually transient, complication of vagotomy. Many patients with duodenal ulceration also have gastro-oesophageal reflux symptoms, but reflux per se is not a complication of the vagotomy. Lesser curve necrosis, delayed gastric emptying and gallstone formation are potential, but technically unavoidable, complications of certain types of vago-tomy.

Persisting Controversies

- Is there a need for reperitonealization of the stomach follow-ing highly selective vagotomy?
- What is the best method of oesophageal repair following iatrogenic injury?
- What is the most appropriate drug treatment of gastric stasis?

● What is the aetiology and prevalence of gallstones after truncal vagotomy?

Further reading

Baxter, J.N., Grime, J.S., Critchley, M. & Shields, R. (1985) Relationship between gastric emptying of solids and gallbladder emptying in normal subjects. *Gut*, *26*, 342–351.

Cox, A.G., Spencer, J. & Tinker, J. (1969) In Williams, J.A. & Cox, A.G. (Eds) *After Vagotomy*. London: Butterworth.

Flook, D. & Stoddard, C.J. (1985) Gastro-oesophageal reflux and oesophagitis before and after vagotomy for duodenal ulcer. *British Journal of Surgery*, *72*, 804–807.

Ihasz, M. & Griffith, C.A. (1981) Gallstones and vagotomy. *American Journal of Surgery*, *141*, 48–50.

Johnston, D. (1975) Operative mortality and post-operative morbidity of highly selective vagotomy. *British Medical Journal*, *ii*, 545–547.

Jordan, P.H., Jr & Condon, R.E. (1970) A prospective evaluation of vagotomy-pyloroplasty and vagotomy-antrectomy for treatment of duodenal ulcer. *Annals of Surgery*, *172*, 547–560.

Postlethwaite, R.W., Kim, S.K. & Dillon, M.L. (1969) Oesophageal complications of vagotomy. *Surgery, Gynecology and Obstetrics*, *128*, 481–488.

Sheiner, M.J. & Catchpole, B.N. (1976) Drug therapy for post-vagotomy gastric stasis. *British Journal of Surgery*, *63*, 608–611.

Skellenger, M.E. & Jordan, P.H., Jr (1983) Complications of vagotomy and pyloroplasty. *Surgical Clinics of North America*, *63*, 1167–1180.

Spencer, J.D. (1975) Post vagotomy dysphagia. *British Journal of Surgery*, *62*, 354–355.

Wirthlin, L.S. & Malt, R.A. (1972) Accidents of vagotomy. *Surgery, Gynecology and Obstetrics*, *135*, 913–916.

12 Complications of Splenectomy

Splenectomy has a significant morbidity and mortality rate. The spleen should never be removed unnecessarily either in a child or in an adult. In patients with splenic trauma, iatrogenic or otherwise, the spleen should be repaired and preserved whenever possible. The occurrence of some postoperative complications is related to the indication for splenectomy. The complication rate is highest in patients undergoing splenectomy for trauma, secondary hypersplenism or as an incidental part of another operation. The risk of thromboembolic phenomena and overwhelming postsplenectomy sepsis may persist for many years after the operation.

Splenic Structure and Function

The normal adult spleen weighs 150 g and lies in the left upper abdomen, protected by the ninth, tenth and eleventh ribs. Its blood supply is from the splenic artery, which divides into segmental branches in the hilum, before entering the substance of the spleen. This segmental arrangement is responsible for the transverse fractures along the intersegmental planes, which occur with major blunt splenic injuries. Transection of the segmental vessels is uncommon with blunt injuries, although they may be seriously disrupted by a penetrating injury. The anatomical arrangement also enables the surgeon to control bleeding to individual segments of the spleen and to perform partial, as opposed to total, splenectomy following ligation of the appropriate segmental vessels.

The spleen normally plays a minor role in haemopoiesis, this being confined to the mid trimester of intrauterine life. It can resume this function during childhood if the capacity of the bone marrow is exceeded and in adult life in patients with myelofibrosis. The spleen plays a major role in red cell maturation. Here the cells are converted to biconcave discs; damaged and mis-shapen cells are removed and cellular inclusions are extracted. The spleen is important in both cell mediated and humoral immunity. It stimulates the production of immunoglobulin M (IgM) antibodies in the germinal centres, which are active against circulating bacterial antigens, and is also important in the regulation of T and B lymphocytes. It is the source of the opsonins, tuftsin and properdin, which are essential for maximal stimulation of neutrophil phagocytic activity.

Effects of Splenectomy

Haematological
The number of circulating abnormal red blood cells increases. Howell–Jolly bodies (nuclear remnants) and target cells are seen in the peripheral blood. There is a leucocytosis, which is maximal between the fifth and fourteenth postoperative days. This is due to a transient rise in neutrophils and a more prolonged rise in lymphocytes and eosinophils. At the same time the platelet count rises owing to increased platelet production, rather than to the decreased rate of removal, and may rise to over 1000×10^9 per litre. A thrombocytosis is defined as a platelet count exceeding 400×10^9 per litre, and when present can persist for anything from a few weeks to a few years.

Immunological
The effect of splenectomy on immunological status is age dependent, being most marked in the infant. IgM levels fall postoperatively and rise again slowly over the next four or five years. There is a marked reduction in the ability to opsonize and phagocytose encapsulated organisms. This is due to the immediate and prolonged fall in the plasma tuftsin levels and also to defective complement activation via the alternative pathway because of the fall in properdin levels.

Splenic Preservation

The extent of splenic injuries ranges from minor capsular tears to complete avulsion from the splenic pedicle. Whenever possible the spleen should be repaired and not removed because of the risk of late postsplenectomy sepsis. The feasibility of splenic preservation is dependent on the magnitude of the damage, the skill and experience of the surgeon, and associated injuries to adjacent structures. The alternatives to splenectomy for a damaged spleen are shown in Table 12.1.

Table 12.1
Alternatives to splenectomy in patients with a splenic injury

Non-operative treatment
Topical agents
Splenorrhaphy
Arterial ligation
Partial splenectomy
Autotransplantation

Non-operative treatment
Splenic injuries can be managed non-operatively in children. The child must be haemodynamically stable on admission and facilities must be available for regular, careful, inpatient observation and assessment. Non-operative treatment is not applicable to adults because of the risk of damage to other organs or structures and because arrest of haemorrhage is less likely to occur. Adult patients with suspected splenic trauma should undergo laparotomy.

Topical agents
Bleeding from minor capsular tears can be controlled by direct pressure, coagulation diathermy or the application of haemostatic substances such as gelatin sponge, thrombin or microfibrillar collagen (Avitene).

Splenorrhaphy
A deeper splenic laceration may be repaired by splenorrhaphy. This can be a direct suture of the splenic tissue using chromic catgut sutures on a large atraumatic round-bodied needle either with (Fig. 12.1a) or without (Fig. 12.1b) ox fibrin buttresses. Alternatively omentum may be used to pack a splenic laceration or be sutured directly onto the spleen (Fig. 12.1c).

Arterial ligation
Segmental bleeding can be controlled by ligation of a segmental

Figure 12.1
Methods of splenorrhaphy. (a) Simple suture of spleen. (b) Suture over ox fibrin buttresses. (c) Omentum sutured onto the spleen.

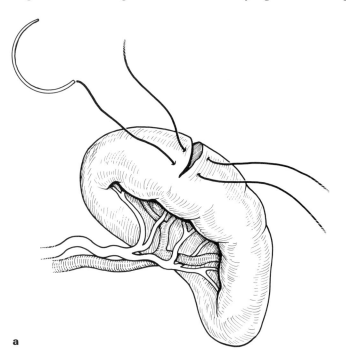

a

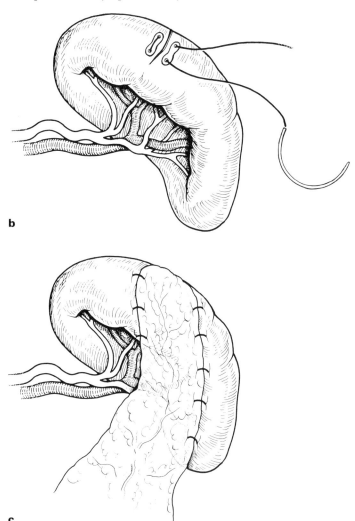

b

c

artery in the hilum. The main splenic artery can also be ligated to control haemorrhage. This does not necessarily produce splenic infarction because of arterial inflow via the short gastric arteries. Although the spleen can be preserved by this manoeuvre, it has been suggested that its immunological function may be depressed and the patient is at increased risk of postsplenectomy sepsis. Thus ligation of the main splenic artery as a means of controlling haemorrhage is not to be recommended.

Partial splenectomy
The nature of the arterial supply allows partial splenectomy, most frequently a hemisplenectomy, to be performed. The segmental artery to the damaged half of the spleen is ligated and the splenic pulp divided by the 'finger-fracture' technique. The

bleeding from the cut end of the spleen is controlled by suture using ox fibrin buttresses and omentum or microfibrillar collagen.

Autotransplantation
If splenectomy is necessary because of major disruption, the spleen can be diced and reimplanted into an omental pocket. These splenic cells remain viable, but their functional capacity is difficult to determine. They may have some protective value against septic complications, but at the present time the evidence for this is inconclusive and passive immunization is probably safer.

Operative technique for splenic preservation
Selection of the surgical technique to be used for the control of bleeding depends primarily on the extent of the splenic damage. Repair of a damaged spleen is a delicate procedure and adequate access to the left upper quadrant and good exposure of the spleen is essential. The abdomen will have been opened with a vertical incision in the vast majority of patients and access to the spleen may initially be poor. This difficulty is worst in obese patients or when the anteroposterior diameter of the chest is particularly large. Do not open the left chest solely to suture and repair a damaged spleen. The morbidity and mortality associated with thoracoabdominal incisions are greater than the potential benefits of splenic preservation as opposed to splenectomy. If improved exposure is necessary, enlarge the abdominal incision vertically. Alternatively a horizontal muscle-cutting incision extending from the vertical incision to the left upper quadrant may be used. If splenorrhaphy or partial splenectomy are to be performed, the spleen must be mobilized prior to insertion of the sutures. Bleeding should be controlled by direct pressure with an abdominal pack during the mobilization. The lienorenal ligament should be divided first and the spleen and tail of the pancreas reflected medially.

   If the splenic damage is just a capsular tear or involves only the superficial layer of the red pulp, topical agents can be applied and splenic mobilization is unnecessary. A deep laceration should be treated by splenorrhaphy or partial splenectomy. If there is a major splenic laceration (usually a stellate fracture), serious damage to other structures or circulatory problems due to hypovolaemia, do not waste time trying to repair the spleen. In these situations splenectomy should be performed.

Complications following splenic preservation procedures
The main complications are rebleeding and a subphrenic abscess.

Rebleeding
It is important that complete haemostasis be achieved in a normotensive patient before the abdomen is closed after sple-

norrhaphy or partial splenectomy. Thereafter careful monitoring of pulse, blood pressure and, if necessary, central venous pressure should be performed for the next 24 hours, looking particularly for evidence of hypovolaemia due to rebleeding. If this occurs, the patient should initially be given a blood transfusion and be placed under careful observation. Further hypovolaemia within the next six hours suggests a major splenic bleed, and an emergency laparotomy is necessary. If rebleeding has occurred, do not risk a second failure of conservative surgery but rather proceed to splenectomy.

Subphrenic abscess

A haematoma in the vicinity of the spleen is far more likely after splenic preservation than after splenectomy. This haematoma may become the nidus for a subphrenic abscess, the diagnosis and treatment of which are discussed later in this chapter

Prevalence and Aetiology of Complications of Splenectomy

Splenectomy is performed for a variety of reasons (Table 12.2) and some of the complications are related to the indication for operation. Complications are highest in patients undergoing splenectomy for trauma, incidental splenectomy during another operation, or because of secondary hypersplenism. This reflects the effects of injuries to other organs and structures (chest wall, liver, kidney, gastrointestinal tract) and of complications related to the other procedures. The morbidity and mortality are lowest in patients having splenectomy for diagnostic purposes, Hodgkin's disease, or for primary hypersplenism.

Factors that influence the occurrence of postoperative complications are:

- Indication for splenectomy
- Associated surgical procedures
- Other injuries (in cases of trauma)
- Haematological changes following splenectomy (thrombosis)
- Impaired immunity

Table 12.2
Indications for splenectomy

Trauma	
Incidental	—during other operations, e.g. gastrectomy, distal pancreatectomy
Primary hypersplenism	
Secondary hypersplenism	
Haematological disorders	e.g. anaemias, thrombocytopenia
Neoplasia	e.g. Hodgkin's, non-Hodgkin's lymphoma, leukaemia
Miscellaneous conditions	e.g. splenic cyst or abscess

In a number of large published series the overall mortality rate following splenectomy ranged from 6 to 13% and the morbidity rate was between 15 and 61% (Table 12.3). The mortality rate has been falling over the past 20 years, not solely because of improved anaesthesia, surgery and postoperative care, but because of the changing indications for surgery. Splenectomy is now performed more frequently for diagnostic purposes or as a staging procedure for Hodgkin's disease, which are associated with a lower morbidity and mortality. It may be followed by serious postoperative complications and the spleen should be removed only if:

- It is specifically advantageous for the patient, e.g. in spherocytosis, ITP (idiopathic thrombocytopenic purpura) or during radical gastrectomy for carcinoma
- It may affect subsequent treatment, e.g. for Hodgkin's disease
- It is irreparably damaged

Respiratory Complications

Postoperative respiratory problems are the commonest complication of splenectomy. Atelectasis, pleural effusion and pneumonia may occur. These develop most frequently in patients having splenectomy for secondary hypersplenism, because of the associated disease, and after splenectomy for trauma, because of chest wall injuries and rib fractures.

Take all possible precautions to reduce the chance of chest problems in patients who are at increased risk. Intercostal nerve blocks with a long-acting local anaesthetic, such as 0.5% Marcain, are valuable in patients with rib fractures or after thoracotomy. Chest physiotherapy with incentive spirometry will reduce the occurrence of atelectasis. If the patient develops a pleural effusion, consider the possibility of a subphrenic abscess. A pyrexia is suggestive of an abscess, but a leucocytosis is less helpful in making the diagnosis because of the increased white cell count that invariably follows splenectomy. An erect X-ray of the subphrenic area, diaphragmatic screening or ultrasound scan may confirm the presence of an abscess, treatment of which is considered later in this chapter.

Table 12.3
Morbidity and
mortality of
splenectomy

Author	Years	No. of patients	Morbidity (%)	Mortality (%)
Fabri	1949–1973	1944	39	9.5
Traetow	1973–1980	473	15	6
Eïsenberg	1972–1976	50	20	6
Coltheart	1968–1973	150	61	13

Haemorrhage

Bleeding may occur from a slipped ligature on the splenic pedicle, from the raw surface of the diaphragm or from a short gastric vessel. Adhesions between the surface of the spleen and under-surface of the diaphragm are often found in patients with massive splenomegaly. These adhesions provide an alternative blood supply for the enlarged spleen or develop because of recurrent splenic infarcts due to the spleen outgrowing its blood supply. A large bleeding surface may be left following splenectomy and blood accumulates in the subphrenic area. Bleeding from the splenic pedicle may occur immediately after operation, as the patient's blood pressure rises or as a secondary haemorrhage seven to ten days after operation, usually in association with a subphrenic abscess.

The haemorrhage may be visible externally if a peritoneal drain is in situ or the patient may develop hypovolaemic shock. It can be prevented by separate double ligation or transfixion of the splenic artery and vein at the time of surgery and by careful attention to haemostasis, particularly when the spleen is adherent to the diaphragm. A subphrenic drain may be inserted at the end of the operation if there has been any particular problem with bleeding intraoperatively. Only closed drainage systems should be used. The drain should be removed 24 hours postoperatively for fear of contamination of the subphrenic space and later abscess formation.

If the patient becomes shocked following splenectomy, perform an ECG to exclude myocardial infarction and look for signs of pulmonary embolism secondary to deep vein thrombosis. If the ECG is normal and the patient is hypovolaemic, blood should be cross matched and arrangements made for a repeat laparotomy. When the haemorrhage is due to a slipped ligature, the splenic artery and vein should be transfixed separately. If the haemorrhage occurs from the splenic pedicle in association with a subphrenic abscess, resuture of the pedicle will be difficult, because sutures tend to cut out. Drain the abscess. Extend the opening into the lesser sac and locate the splenic artery and vein above the upper border of the mid-point of the pancreas (Fig. 12.2). The vessels can be separately ligated at this point, and the sutures are unlikely to cut out.

Subphrenic Abscess

Factors associated with the development of a subphrenic abscess after splenectomy are:

- Subphrenic haematoma
- Opening the gastrointestinal tract
- Use of intraperitoneal drains
- Damage to other structures—stomach; colon; pancreas

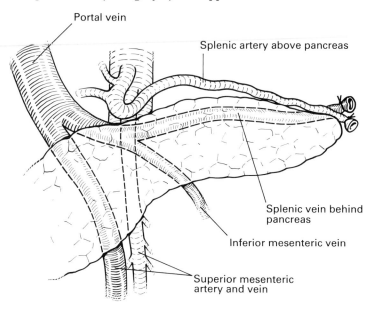

Figure 12.2
Site for ligation of the splenic artery in the lesser sac above the upper border of the pancreas.

The prevalence of subphrenic abscesses can be reduced. Ensure that there is no bleeding in the splenic area before the abdomen is closed. When the gastrointestinal tract has been opened during the course of an operation such as oesophagogastrectomy, the bacterial contamination in the area can be reduced by peritoneal lavage with a litre of normal saline containing 1 g of tetracycline. Intraperitoneal drains should be used as infrequently as possible, for they increase the risk of a subphrenic abscess by up to ten times. Only closed drainage systems are permissible and the drain should be removed 24 hours postoperatively if there is no excessive drainage. A subphrenic drain is only necessary when there is a large raw area on the undersurface of the diaphragm or when splenectomy has been combined with pancreatectomy.

The stomach, pancreas and splenic flexure of the colon are all in close proximity to the spleen and may be damaged, leading to a subphrenic abscess and subsequent fistula. A gastric fistula can arise because a ligature is tied around the gastric wall rather than around the short gastric vessels, because of an intramural haematoma, or because of ischaemia of the greater curve, which is extremely rare. Postoperative gastric dilatation increases the risk of fistula formation and should be avoided by the insertion of a nasogastric tube for 24 hours. A pancreatic fistula is usually the result of inadvertent transection of the tail of the pancreas during ligation of the splenic vessels. It can be avoided by careful identification of the margins of the pancreas before the splenic vessels are clamped and tied. A colonic fistula results either from a direct cut or by a splitting, with tearing of the bowel wall, which usually occurs along one of the taenia coli.

Presentation and investigation

The patient with a subphrenic abscess develops a swinging pyrexia five to ten days postoperatively. There may be tenderness over the left costal margin and a left pleural effusion. Perform an erect chest X-ray, looking for the pleural effusion and bubbles of gas in the left subphrenic space. The gastric air bubble may be displaced downwards by the abscess, between the diaphragm and fundus. Screening the diaphragm may show decreased diaphragmatic movement. If there is still doubt, a subphrenic abscess may be demonstrated by ultrasound or CT scan. Blood cultures should be performed.

Treatment

The timing of an operation to drain a subphrenic abscess is determined by the patient's clinical condition. A balance must be reached between premature drainage of a well-localized immature subphrenic abscess and unnecessary delay in operation in a toxic patient with increasing sepsis. If the abscess is confined to the subphrenic space and the patient has little evidence of generalized sepsis other than a mild pyrexia and/or tachycardia, then abscess drainage can be delayed until the ninth or tenth postoperative day. By this stage the abscess cavity will be well walled off and it is possible to drain it through a small left subcostal incision, without entering the general peritoneal cavity. This reduces the risk of spreading infection within the abdomen. Broad-spectrum antibiotics, chosen either empirically or on the result of a positive blood culture, should be given whilst the abscess is reaching maturity. We (CJS and RMK) have not been impressed by percutaneous abscess drainage using an ultrasound or CT-guided needle. The abscess is usually multilocular, the locules needing to be broken down by digital exploration to give adequate drainage, and the pus is often too thick to be aspirated easily. Similarly a posterior approach to the subphrenic abscess is not always successful. The surgeon will be less familiar with the incision and inadvertent opening of the pleura may lead to an empyema of the chest. Once the pus has been drained, irrigate the abscess cavity and insert a large drain. An F28 chest drain is ideal. This should be connected to a closed drainage system.

Earlier drainage of the abdomen may be required if the patient becomes 'toxic', with a high fever, rapid tachycardia, confusion, hypoxia and signs of spreading intra-abdominal infection. This situation is usually associated with contamination from the gastrointestinal tract, either the greater curvature of the stomach or the splenic flexure of the colon. In these circumstances the abscess has not been localized in the subphrenic space and urgent peritoneal toilet and effective drainage of the subphrenic area is required. Delay in laparotomy may be fatal. The patient should be resuscitated with intravenous fluids, the requirements being based on regular measurement (at least hourly at first) of central venous pressure and urine output. Antibiotics active against aerobic and anaerobic bacteria should be given intravenously prior to operation. The abscess should be drained through the original (usually midline) incision when feasible, and thorough peritoneal lavage performed with saline containing 1 g of tetracycline per litre. Colonic damage is obvious from the smell as the abscess is drained. A gastric fistula is less distinctive, but food particles may be seen in the fluid in the abscess cavity intraoperatively, or gastric contents appear in the drainage fluid postoperatively.

Colonic fistula. The presence of faecal material in the abscess cavity indicates a communication with the colon, usually the splenic flexure. Resection of the colonic perforation will be extremely difficult because of faecal contamination and local oedema. *Do resect* the splenic flexure if this is possible, but *do not* attempt a primary colonic anastomosis, because of the high risk of a further anastomotic leak. The proximal transverse colon should be exteriorized as an end colostomy and the descending colon as a mucous fistula. When all signs of sepsis have resolved, alimentary continuity can be re-established three months later by laparotomy and colo-colo anastomosis.

If resection of the splenic flexure is impossible, drain the abscess cavity and perform a defunctioning loop transverse colostomy or alternatively a caecostomy. The colonic perforation should close if the transverse colon is completely defunctioned and the abscess cavity adequately drained. Drainage from the abscess will decrease and the patient become afebrile. Six weeks later perform a distal loop barium enema to ensure that:

● The perforation has sealed
● There is no residual communication with the abscess cavity
● There is no colonic stricture at the site of perforation

If the perforation *has* closed and there is no stricture, the colostomy should be closed. However, if there is a persistent colonic leak or a stricture, a left hemicolectomy should be performed after thorough preoperative bowel preparation. The entire left colon should be mobilized to ensure that the anastomosis is not under tension when the splenic flexure has been resected. If possible, the transverse colostomy should not be closed at this stage, as it will serve to decompress the anastomosis. Should the colostomy be too close to the splenic flexure for the latter to be resected with a safe colonic anastomosis without tension, then the two options are:

1 Close the colostomy at the same time as the left hemicolectomy.
2 Perform a subtotal colectomy, with formation of an ileosigmoid anastomosis.

We (CJS and RMK) would favour option 2, for this results in one, rather than two, colonic anastomoses and ensures that the anastomosis is well away from the abscess cavity in the left upper quadrant.

Gastric fistula. The opening between the stomach and abscess cavity may be recognizable at operation and if so should be closed with a single layer of interrupted, non-absorbable sutures. The stomach should be decompressed with a nasogastric tube and total parenteral nutrition given for a minimum of one week. If a gastric fistula is suspected postoperatively following drainage of an abscess, the diagnosis should be confirmed by a Gastrografin meal or by giving the patient oral methylene blue. If a fistula is present, the dye will appear in the drainage fluid within a few minutes. Insert a nasogastric tube, begin intravenous nutrition, and if the fistula output exceeds 0.5 litre per day, give intravenous H2 receptor blocking drugs. In the absence of distal obstruction the fistula will eventually close.

Pancreatic fistula. The fluid from a pancreatic fistula is slightly opalescent and has a high amylase content, often greater than 40 000 units per litre. If there is no pancreatic duct obstruction, an external fistula from the tail of the pancreas will generally close. If a pancreatic fistula develops after splenectomy, stop all oral intake and begin total parenteral nutrition. The skin around the external opening should be protected and the effluent collected and measured. Skin excoriation is less of a problem than with an intestinal fistula because the pancreatic enzymes are inactive. Monitor the serum electrolytes daily and correct any abnormality due to external loss with intravenous fluids. A fistulogram should be performed to exclude the presence of an enterocutaneous fistula.

Atropine, acetazolamide and glucagon have an inhibitory effect on pancreatic secretion and can be used if the fistula output remains high. Unfortunately each has only a short duration of action and has undesirable side-effects. Atropine affects the parasympathetic nervous system, causing pupillary dilatation, difficulty with micturition and disturbed gastrointestinal motility. Acetazolamide, a carbonic anhydrase inhibitor, increases urinary bicarbonate loss, resulting in metabolic acidosis. Glucagon decreases gastrointestinal motility and promotes renal loss of sodium, potassium and chloride. Intravenous cimetidine or ranitidine indirectly decreases pancreatic secretion by reducing acid-induced release of pancreatic stimulating hormones in the duodenum. Somatostatin 250 μg hourly by intravenous infusion has been recently shown to reduce the output of pancreatic fistulae dramatically. However, this hormone is expensive and not readily available in many centres. Beta-adrenergic agonists will also inhibit pancreatic exocrine secretion. Isoproterenol has undesirable chronotropic and inotropic effects on the heart.

Terbutaline has fewer myocardial side-effects and when given orally in a dose of 5 mg eight-hourly combined with 0.25 mg subcutaneously eight-hourly will reduce pancreatic secretion and fistula output.

If the fistula output shows no evidence of diminishing, then pancreatic duct obstruction should be considered and endoscopic retrograde pancreatography performed. If there is duct obstruction or the fistula output fails to decrease after three to four weeks, surgical treatment will be required. The tail of the pancreas should be mobilized and a pancreaticojejunostomy constructed using a Roux-en-Y anastomosis (Fig. 12.3). Referral of the patient to a unit specializing in pancreatic surgery should be considered.

Damage to the Diaphragm

Intraoperative damage to the left diaphragm is uncommon and usually occurs in patients with massive splenomegaly, as the spleen is being mobilized. The enlarged spleen becomes attached to the diaphragm and there is no clear plane of cleavage between them. Beware of this possible complication when the spleen is adherent and ensure that during blunt mobilization a major tear does not occur in the dome. Keep the diaphragm constantly in view, and if a small tear develops, use sharp dissection to separate it from the spleen, thus preventing removal of a

Figure 12.3
Pancreaticojejunostomy using Roux-en-Y anastamosis for persistent pancreatic fistula.

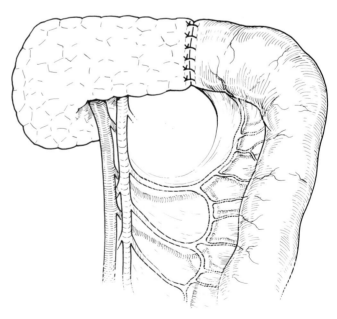

substantial part of the diaphragm itself. Intermittent positive pressure ventilation will stop the left lung collapsing.

Treatment   Tell the anaesthetist what has happened. Remove the spleen, which will allow complete exposure of the diaphragm and accurate assessment of the extent of the damage. Insert a chest drain and repair the laceration. The diaphragm should be closed with a layer of continuous 0-chromic catgut sutures reinforced at 2–2.5 cm intervals with interrupted sutures of the same material. Even if some of the diaphragm has been excised, there will be enough remaining to perform an effective repair. The chest drain should remain in position for two to three days postoperatively.

Thrombocytosis and Thrombotic Phenomena

The platelet count rises following splenectomy, reaching a maximum five to 14 days after operation, and thereafter gradually returns to normal within a few months. In a minority of patients the thrombocytosis may persist for many years. Ten per cent of patients have a persistent platelet count of over 1000×10^9 per litre. Although the rise in the platelet count is widely believed to be associated with an increased risk of thrombotic complications, particularly deep vein thrombosis and pulmonary embolism, there is little evidence to support this assumption. Platelet function and kinetics are normal in the majority of patients and there is no increase in platelet aggregation or adhesion. Only patients with myeloproliferative disorders (chronic myeloid leukaemia, myeloid metaplasia and polycythaemia rubra vera) have abnormal platelet function following splenectomy and this group has the highest prevalence of thrombosis. Thromboembolic phenomena occur in 3–6% of patients following splenectomy, which is greater than would normally be expected after laparotomy. However, if the patients with myeloproliferative disorders are excluded, then there is no substantial increase in risk of thromboembolism (Boxer et al, 1978).

Thromboembolic phenomena are commoner in patients with a preoperative thrombocytosis than in those with a normal platelet count, although in some series the difference is not statistically significant (Traetow, Fabri and Carey, 1980). There is no evidence that the risk of thromboembolism increases further if the platelet count exceeds 1000×10^9 per litre.

Prevention of Thromboembolic Complications

The prevalence of postoperative thromboembolic phenomena in patients over the age of 40 years undergoing laparotomy can be reduced by the use of prophylactic subcutaneous heparin. Patients in this age group undergoing splenectomy should receive heparin preoperatively and for seven days postoperatively. It is more difficult to be dogmatic about the role of antiplatelet drugs such as aspirin and dipyridamole. Much of the evidence is anecdotal: there have been some retrospective reviews but no prospective studies. Certainly patients with myeloproliferative disorders have a greater risk of thromboembolic complications and the use of aspirin 300 mg daily and dipyridamole 100 mg t.d.s. would seem justified, especially if there is a postoperative thrombocytosis. The use of platelet inhibitors in other patients with thrombocytosis is controversial. The three options, all of which have their proponents are:

1 No treatment.
2 Aspirin 300 mg daily.
3 Aspirin 300 mg daily + dipyridamole 100 mg t.d.s.

Treatment with aspirin alone is neither expensive nor an onerous burden for the patient, and since it may confer some advantage it is probably the most logical option. There is no firm evidence that antiplatelet therapy is definitely indicated if the platelet count exceeds 1000×10^9 per litre.

Mesenteric Vascular Thrombosis

This is a rare complication of splenectomy, with a mortality rate in excess of 70%. Most cases have occurred in patients undergoing splenectomy for haematological disorders, particularly myeloproliferative diseases. The presenting symptoms and signs are central abdominal pain, bloody diarrhoea, oliguria and subsequently peritonitis. The white blood cell count is elevated over $20\,000 \times 10^9$ per litre and abdominal X-rays may show distended fluid-filled loops of small bowel. After resuscitation, laparotomy should be performed and gangrenous bowel resected. The thrombosis is usually venous rather than arterial and the prognosis is unlikely to be improved by thrombectomy. Thrombosis affecting the entire small bowel is invariably fatal. Heparin and streptokinase infusions have been used but with little success.

It has been suggested that patients with myeloproliferative disorders and preoperative thrombocytosis who are at greatest risk of this complication should be treated preoperatively with busulphan or other alkylating agents to reduce the platelet count below 200×10^9 per litre prior to operation. Evidence that this treatment is effective in reducing the incidence of postoperative thrombosis is unproven at the present time.

Postsplenectomy Sepsis

Splenectomy is followed by an increased susceptibility to late overwhelming infection. This was first observed in 1919 by

Morris and Bullock, whose rat experiments demonstrated that after splenectomy there was a fourfold greater mortality rate from infection with the rat plague bacillus. More than 30 years elapsed before this risk of late postsplenectomy sepsis in humans was recognized. In 1952, in a retrospective review, King and Shumaker reported that children were at increased risk of fulminant infections. Despite some conflicting views and reports, it is now widely recognized that this same risk of sepsis also applies to adults. The infective problems are the result of impaired immunity. Splenectomy results in decreased production of the IgM antibody opsonin tuftsin and loss of helper T cells which are involved in antibody production, particularly to encapsulated organisms. The filtration function of the spleen in removing particulate antigens and bacteria is also lost.

In the early postoperative period pneumonia and subphrenic abscesses occur more frequently in patients with an underlying malignancy or receiving immunosuppressive therapy. These infections are usually caused by common organisms such as *Escherichia coli*, *Staphylococcus aureus* or *Klebsiella*, but occasionally rare organisms may be isolated.

Although the occurrence of late postsplenectomy sepsis is well recognized in children, the disagreement about the risk in adults is due to the fact that fulminant infections may occur up to 40 years after operation, the true risk having been underestimated in some studies because the follow-up period has been too short. Nevertheless, 50% of infections occur within the first year of operation and less than 15% over three years. The mortality rate is high, between 50 and 80%. The shorter the interval between splenectomy and infection, the higher the chance of a fatal outcome. Although the overall risk of developing a serious postsplenectomy infection is only 4.0% the mortality rate is 2.4%. The risk is age related, being greatest in children under the age of one year. It is also related to the indication for operation, being lowest after splenectomy for trauma, ITP or spherocytosis, and highest for thalassaemia, hypersplenism or acquired haemolytic anaemias.

Postsplenectomy sepsis is usually due to infection by encapsulated organisms such as pneumococci, *Haemophilus influenzae* or *Neisseria meningitides*, but other organisms, staphylococci, *E. coli*, pseudomonas or viruses may be responsible. Pneumococcal infections are the commonest (50%) and have the highest mortality rate (80%). Different pneumococcal capsular antigens occur and types 4, 6, 13, 18, 22 and 23 are responsible for a higher rate of sepsis in splenectomized patients than in the general population.

Clinical features   The term overwhelming postsplenectomy infection syndrome (OPSI) has been applied to this condition. It often begins as a nonspecific illness with nausea and confusion, but rapidly progresses and may be fatal within 24 hours, unless treated vigorously. After the initial symptoms patients develop signs of severe infection, with pyrexia, rigors, tachycardia, hypotension and oliguria. Disseminated intravascular coagulation may occur. If the condition is suspected, perform a blood culture and look at a peripheral blood smear. There may be more than 10^6 organisms per ml of blood and these can be seen under the microscope. Intravenous antibiotics such as the newer penicillins should be given immediately in large doses and hypotension corrected with intravenous fluids.

Prophylaxis   Prevention of postsplenectomy sepsis may be achieved by prophylaxis. Preserve the spleen in patients with splenic trauma, if possible. When splenectomy cannot be avoided, vaccination and long-term antibiotics are the alternatives. Polyvalent vaccines active against 23 different pneumococcal capsular types are currently available. Children under the age of two years do not respond to the vaccine and there is some evidence that the response is suboptimal below the age of five. The response to the antigens in the vaccine is poorer after splenectomy or when the patient is receiving chemotherapy or radiotherapy. Ideally, if splenectomy is being performed as an elective procedure, the patient should be vaccinated at least one month preoperatively; 0.5 ml of the vaccine is given either intramuscularly or subcutaneously. The vaccine does not provide universal protection against pneumococcal infection, for not all the capsular types are included. However, 90% of pneumococcal infections are due to the capsular types contained within the currently available vaccine.

Long-term prophylactic antibiotics may be used following splenectomy. Either penicillin or amoxycillin, which has greater activity against haemophilus, are the first-choice antibiotics. Erythromycin or co-trimoxazole are alternatives for penicillin-sensitive patients. The duration of antibiotic therapy is controversial. The risk of and mortality rate for sepsis is highest in the first three years after operation and antibiotic prophylaxis is thus probably most important at this stage. The difficulties of long-term patient compliance have led some authors to the conclusion that early intermittent antibiotic treatment for all minor infective events is preferable to continuous prophylaxis.

Splenic preservation, vaccination and prophylactic antibiotics will all reduce the incidence of severe postsplenectomy sepsis. Do not remove all the spleen unless absolutely necessary, particularly in a child. All splenectomized patients should be vaccinated and this should be given preoperatively in patients undergoing elective splenectomy. Prophylactic penicillin should be given to all children under the age of five years, to patients who develop a chest infection and to those patients receiving chemotherapy or radiotherapy. Patients should be warned of the risks of postoperative sepsis and the need for urgent medical treatment.

Conclusions

Splenectomy should be avoided in patients with splenic injuries, particularly children, because of the risks of postoperative complications. The incidence of haemorrhage and subphrenic abscess formation can be reduced by careful operative technique. Late postsplenectomy sepsis can occur in adults and children and has been observed more than 30 years after operation. Encapsulated bacteria, especially pneumococci, are normally responsible for the infection, which can become life threatening within 24 hours, unless immediate antibiotic treatment is given. Polyvalent pneumococcal vaccines reduce the risk of pneumococcal septicaemia. Alternatively patients may be given long-term prophylactic antibiotics. The rise in platelet count that follows splenectomy is not usually associated with an increased risk of thromboembolic phenomena unless the patient has a preoperative thrombocytosis or a myeloproliferative disorder.

Persisting Controversies

- Is there a need for splenic preservation?
- What is the risk of thromboembolic complications?
- Is there a need for antiplatelet treatment in patients with thrombocytosis?
- Is there a risk of postsplenectomy sepsis in adult patients?
- What is the role of pneumococcal vaccine and prophylactic antibiotics?

Further reading

Boxer, M.A., Brown, J. & Ellman, L. (1978) Thromboembolic risk of post-splenectomy thrombocytosis. *Archives of Surgery, 113,* 808–809.

Coltheart, C. & Little, J.M. (1976) Splenectomy: a review of morbidity. *Australia and New Zealand Journal of Surgery, 46,* 32–36.

Cooper, M.J. & Williamson, R.C.N. (1984) Splenectomy: indications, hazards and alternatives. *British Journal of Surgery, 71,* 173–180.

Eisenberg, B.L., Andreassy, R.J., Haff, R.C. et al (1976) Splenectomy in childhood. A correlative review of the indications and complications in fifty patients. *American Journal of Surgery, 132,* 720–722.

Ellison, E.C. & Fabri, P.J. (1983) Complications of splenectomy. Aetiology, prevention and management. *Surgical Clinics of North America, 63,* 1313–1329.

Fabri, P.J., Metz, S.N. & Nick, W.V. (1974) A quarter century with splenectomy. *Archives of Surgery, 108,* 569–574.

Francke, E.L. & Neu, H.C. (1981) Postsplenectomy infection. *Surgical Clinics of North America, 61,* 135–155.

King, H. & Shumaker, H.B., Jr (1952) Splenic Studies 1. Susceptibility to infection after splenectomy performed in infancy. *Annals of Surgery, 136,* 239–242.

Morris, D.H. & Bullock, F.D. (1919) The importance of the spleen in resistance to infection. *Annals of Surgery, 70,* 513–521.

Schwartz, S.I. (1981) Splenectomy for hematologic disease. *Surgical Clinics of North America, 61,* 117–125.

Sherman, R. (1981) Rationale for and methods of splenic preservation following trauma. *Surgical Clinics of North America, 61,* 127–134.

Traetow, W.D., Fabri, P.J. & Carey, L.C. (1980) Changing indications for splenectomy. *Archives of Surgery, 115,* 447–451.

13 Complications of Laparotomy

The postoperative complications of laparotomy are usually related to the intra-abdominal procedure, such as gastrectomy or colectomy, and not to the laparotomy per se. With current methods of investigation, particularly CT scanning, exploratory laparotomy in the investigation of abdominal pain or weight loss, which has eluded diagnosis, is becoming increasingly uncommon. The complications of operations on specific intra-abdominal structures are described in the relevant chapters of this, and three other books in this series, namely, *Complications of Surgery in General*, *Complications of Surgery of the Lower Gastrointestinal Tract* and *Complications of Biliary and Pancreatic Surgery*. This chapter summarizes some of the topics covered elsewhere, such as wound infection and wound healing, but also discusses the investigation and treatment of other complications of laparotomy, such as postoperative intraperitoneal sepsis and acute pancreatitis.

Wound Infection

Bacterial contamination of an abdominal incision can occur from a number of different sources (Table 13.1). Certain operations carry a higher risk of wound infection than others. Abdominal operations can be divided broadly into three categories:

1 *Clean* abdominal operations, which are those that do not involve opening the gastrointestinal tract and which are not performed in the presence of intraperitoneal infection. The wound infection rate for these operations should be less than 3%.

2 Those in which *potential contamination* of an incision can occur, e.g. during elective operations such as gastrectomy, vagotomy and pyloroplasty and colonic resection, when the gastrointestinal tract is opened. The risk of a wound infection in this group can be reduced by the use of prophylactic antibiotics and, in patients undergoing colectomy, by preoperative bowel preparation.

3 Those in which *contamination* of a wound is inevitable, e.g. when surgery is performed in the presence of intra-abdominal infection such as a perforated gangrenous appendix or faecal peritonitis. The majority of operations that fall into this category are emergency rather than elective procedures.

Table 13.1		
Potential sources of abdominal wound infection.	Patient him/herself	-skin -gastrointestinal tract -septic intra-abdominal focus
	Other patients	
	Attendants	-doctors, nurses
	Unsterile instruments	
	Poor operative technique	

Prevention Efforts should be made to reduce the risk of wound contamination, and thus wound infection, in all patients undergoing abdominal surgery.

The patient. Obese patients are at greater risk of wound infection, and pre-operative weight reduction is advantageous if this is feasible. Drug treatment, particularly with steroids and immuno-suppressive drugs, should be reviewed. Steroids impair macrophage motility and phagocytic function and thus predispose to wound infection. Diabetes mellitus should be controlled. H_2 receptor blockers should not be given for 48 hours preoperatively, for they result in an increase in the intragastric pH. Bacterial contamination of the gastric contents occurs when the pH rises above pH4, and if the stomach is opened intraoperatively (pyloroplasty or gastroenterostomy), the incision may also become contaminated. Hot baths and shaving the skin in the vicinity of the incision within 12 hours of operation increase the wound infection rate and should be avoided. Patients awaiting elective colonic resection should have thorough bowel preparation.

Operating theatre. Modern theatre design, with air circulation to the outside, and central sterilization of instruments have contributed to a reduction in the risk of wound contamination. Masks, gloves and gowns reduce the spread of organisms from surgeons and nursing staff to the patient. Chlorhexidine or iodine should be used for skin preparation. Adhesive transparent drapes and wound protectors inserted over the edges of the skin incision and into the peritoneal cavity have not been shown to reduce the incidence of wound infection. Peritoneal lavage with saline containing 1 g of tetracycline per litre and local application of povidone-iodine after peritoneal closure have both been shown to be beneficial.

Prophylactic antibiotics
Prophylactic antibiotics should be given perioperatively to all patients with contaminated or potentially contaminated wounds. Ideally, the antibiotic chosen should be given intravenously 15 minutes before skin incision, so that the maximum tissue levels of

antibiotic are achieved intraoperatively at the time of inoculation of the bacteria into the wound. A single dose of antibiotic is usually sufficient unless the patient has gross peritoneal soiling due to gastrointestinal perforation. In this case the antibiotics should be continued for five days post operatively. The choice of antibiotic depends on a number of factors including the type of surgery being performed, the infecting organism, the history of antibiotic allergy, and individual preference.

Presentation and treatment

A wound infection is defined as the discharge of pus or serum from a wound and if Gram staining or bacteriological culture confirms the presence of pathogenic bacteria. A developing wound infection usually causes increasing discomfort in the vicinity of the incision, combined wih a pyrexia, mild tachycardia and neutrophil leucocytosis. There is erythema, induration, swelling and tenderness around the wound.

Inspect the abdominal wound daily following laparotomy, looking for signs of infection. If a wound infection occurs, ensure adequate drainage of pus by removal of some skin sutures and separation of the wound edges over a distance of a few centimetres with sinus forceps. Irrigate the wound once or twice daily, depending on the degree of contamination, with either hydrogen peroxide alone or a mixture of hydrogen peroxide and povidone-iodine. The wound edges should be kept open by gentle packing with gauze soaked in eusol and paraffin or by a silastic foam stent to allow an exit route for any further discharge and to prevent premature skin healing. A bacteriological swab should be taken from all infected wounds to identify the infecting organism(s) and determine its antibiotic sensitivity. It also permits identification of the emergence of multiple infections with the same organism on a single ward or surgical unit.

Antibiotics are unnecessary in the majority of patients once the wound has been drained. However, there are certain infections where antibiotics *should* be used. Rapidly spreading cellulitis is usually due to a streptococcal infection and should be treated with penicillin or erythromycin. Crepitus in subcutaneous tissue or muscle is characteristic of a clostridial infection. The wound should be explored immediately under general anaesthetic and any necrotic subcutaneous tissue excised. High-dose intravenous antibiotics, penicillin 3 g four-hourly, tobramycin (or gentamicin) and metronidazole, should be given. Bacterial synergistic (Meleney's) gangrene is due to a combined infection with aerobic and anaerobic bacteria. It begins as a small patch of purplish erythema on the abdominal wall and spreads rapidly to give an area of frank gangrene within the space of a few hours. This is a surgical emergency. Intravenous antibiotics should be given immediately and the wound explored in theatre. All gangrenous skin and the extensive necrotic tissue beneath *must* be excised if the patient is to survive. At a later date, when the infection has resolved and the wound is clean and granulating, split skin grafting may be used to speed convalescence.

Failure of Wound Healing

Impairment or failure of abdominal wound healing may result in either dehiscence of all layers of the abdominal wall (a 'burst abdomen') or an incisional hernia. The frequency with which these complications occur has decreased during the past 10–15 years. This is because of an increasing awareness of the mechanics of wound healing and wound suture techniques and also because of an improvement in suture materials used for abdominal closure. They occur less frequently in transverse, as opposed to vertical, laparotomy incisions and are very uncommon in paediatric surgical practice.

Predisposing factors The factors that increase the risk of wound failure are shown in Table 13.2.

General factors
Nutritional status. Weight loss, hypoalbuminaemia, and vitamin and trace element deficiencies may contribute to poor wound healing. Weight loss of greater than 20% of the ideal body weight, as may occur in patients with gastrointestinal tract carcinoma, is associated with an increased morbidity, owing to failure of wound and anastamotic healing. Albumin has a long half-life of 10–21 days and is a poor indicator of the rapid changes in nutritional status that occur in the postoperative response to major surgery. However, hypoalbuminaemia may be the result of chronic protein malnutrition (protein catabolism) and is associated with an increased incidence of major postoperative complications, including failure of wound healing. In patients undergoing resection for gastrointestinal cancer, 85% of the major complications occur in patients with an initial serum albumin level of under 35 g/litre. Ascorbic acid (vitamin C) is necessary for collagen maturation and in vitamin C depleted

Table 13.2 Factors that predispose to failure of abdominal wound healing.

General	Local
Nutritional status	Infection
Age	Haematoma
Malignant disease	Obesity
Drugs	Raised intra-abdominal pressure
Diabetes mellitus	Irradiation
Jaundice	Poor surgical technique
Uraemia	Suture material

animals wound tensile strength has been shown to be diminished. Similarly, deficiency of trace elements such as zinc, copper and iron also results in impaired wound healing. There is no evidence that dietary supplementation of these trace elements results in improved wound healing.

Age. The contribution of age alone to wound healing is difficult to determine, for many other factors, such as malignancy and malnutrition, may also be present in this group. Compared with young adults, collagen production is slower and the prevalence of wound dehiscence is four of five times greater in the elderly.

Malignant disease. Patients with an intra-abdominal malignancy are at increased risk of wound failure. The reasons for this are incompletely understood at the present time. Age, anorexia, weight loss, and hypoproteinaemia may all contribute, as do uptake of dietary protein and carbohydrate by the tumour. The concept that tumour cells produce substances that interfere with wound healing is unproven.

Drugs. Steroids adversely affect wound healing by a number of different mechanisms. The risk of infection is increased because of decreased phagocytic activity. Capillary fragility increases, probably because of lack of supportive connective tissue, and this reduces capillary ingrowth during the early stages of repair and increases the risk of haematoma formation. The mineralocorticoid effect increases extracellular fluid and glucocorticoid effect stimulates gluconeogenesis from amino acids, which reduces their availability for wound repair. Chemotherapeutic drugs, if given too soon after surgery, also affect the multiplying cells in the wound, as well as the tumour cells, and thus adversely affect the process of wound healing.

Diabetes mellitus. Diabetics are more prone to wound infection. They are also prone to obliterative disease of small arteries, which may impair nutrition and oxygenation of the wound.

Jaundice. Hyperbilirubinaemia per se does not affect wound healing. However, extrahepatic biliary obstruction results in:

(a) decreased absorption of vitamin K and hence clotting abnormalities, which increase the risk of a wound haematoma;
(b) eventual impairment of protein synthesis in the liver;
(c) a possible association with ascites and postoperative protein loss through the wound,
(d) stagnation and thus infection of the bile, which increases the risk of wound infection.

In many patients biliary obstruction is due to malignancy. This, and all the factor listed above, increases the risk of wound failure.

Uraemia. In vitro, fibroblast activity is inhibited by high concentration of urea.

Local factors

Infection. This is the commonest cause of wound failure. The mere presence of infection delays the healing process. The wound becomes oedematous, thus increasing the tension on the sutures and the risk that they will cut through the tissues.

Haematoma. A wound haematoma provides a perfect nidus for development of a wound infection.

Obesity. Obliteration of dead space in the subcutaneous tissues is more difficult and increases the risk of haematoma formation or collection of serous fluid. Intertrigo is common in the obese patient and the risk of wound contamination from the surrounding skin is greater. Fat has a relatively poor blood supply and thus the body's natural defence against infection here is poorer.

Raised intra-abdominal pressure increases the force at the suture/tissue interface and thus increases the chance of the suture material cutting through the musculoaponeurotic tissues. A postoperative chest infection, paralytic 'ileus', ascites and vomiting all increase intra-abdominal pressure.

Irradiation. Previous irradiation results in endarteritis obliterans and this has an adverse effect on wound healing if the incision passes through the irradiated tissue.

Surgical technique and suture material. Non-absorbable sutures should be used for closure of all abdominal wounds, with the possible exceptions of appendicectomy and Pfannensteil incisions. Either a mass closure technique using interrupted sutures or a continuous suture technique (usually of two separate layers) are acceptable methods of abdominal closure (Figures 13.1 and

Figure 13.1
Far-and-near method of mass closure using interrupted sutures.

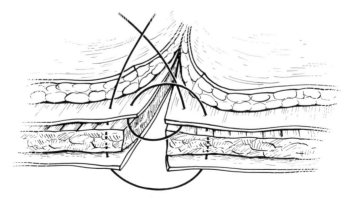

Figure 13.2
Abdominal wall
closure using two
layers of continuous
non-absorbable
sutures and also deep
tension sutures. The
peritoneal layer also
incorporates the deep
tension sutures, thus
preventing loops of
bowel being caught
between the tension
suture and abdominal
wall.

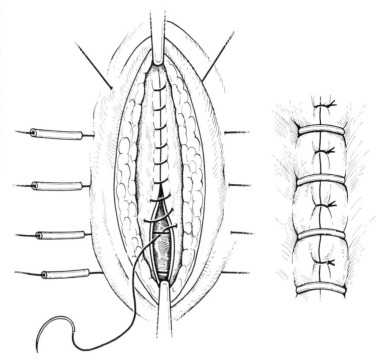

Figure 13.2 Abdominal wall closure using two layers of continuous non-absorbable sutures and also deep tension sutures. The peritoneal layer also incorporates the deep tension sutures, thus preventing loops of bowel being caught between the tension suture and abdominal wall.

13.2). Through-and-through deep tension sutures may also be used to give increased support to the abdominal wall. Jenkins has shown that when a continuous suture technique is used, the tissue 'bites' should be 1 cm deep and 1 cm apart and that the ratio between suture and wound length must be 4:1 or greater. The suture should approximate, but not strangulate, the two edges of the abdominal wall. The incision will become oedematous following surgery, and if the suture is pulled tight at the time of operation, it may cut through the tissues a few days later.

Complete wound dehiscence ('burst abdomen')

The incidence of complete wound dehiscence in vertical laparotomy incisions should be less than 1%. Any surgeon whose own figure is higher than this should re-examine his surgical technique for abdominal wound closure. Wound disruption is a serious complication, requiring a second operation, and carries a mortality rate of between 25 and 45%. Moreover, more than 50% of patients who survive will develop an incisional hernia.

Wound dehiscence is preventable. The author's (CJS's) preference for closure of vertical incisions is a continuous suture technique using two layers of 2/0 Prolene. Deep tension sutures are also inserted as an extra precaution in patients:

- with intra-abdominal malignancy
- over the age of 70 years

- taking steroids
- having a second laparotomy through an old incision
- in the presence of intra abdominal sepsis

This method of closure has resulted in only one dehiscence over a period of ten years.

Presentation   The characteristic sign of impending disruption is a serosanguineous discharge from the wound which begins six or seven days after laparotomy. There are usually no signs of a wound infection (erythema, induration, swelling) and the discharge is invariably sterile on bacteriological culture. Removal of some skin sutures and gentle opening of the superficial layers over a distance of a few centimetres may reveal omentum or loops of small intestine in the base of the wound. Less frequently wound disruption occurs suddenly after an episode of coughing or abrupt movement. The patient may experience sudden pain in the incision, or if the skin sutures/clips have been removed, small intestine may protrude through the skin. Understandably this is accompanied by severe anxiety, particularly if the event occurs after the patient has been discharged from hospital. Deep tension sutures will reduce the risk of dehiscence but do not completely prevent the problem. Too few tension sutures may have been used or they may have been removed too early after operation.

Treatment   It is too late to correct any of the factors that predispose to abdominal dehiscence. The patient should be calmed, with intravenous sedatives if necessary. First explain what has happened and the proposed plan of treatment, and obtain signed consent. Cover the wound with a moist pack to minimize trauma and fluid loss from the exposed abdominal contents and the risk of exogenous contamination. Pass a nasogastric tube and recommence intravenous fluid therapy, having first taken blood for serum electrolytes and urea estimation.

Once the stomach is empty and the electrolytes deemed satisfactory, a second laparotomy is performed under general anaesthesia. Reopen the wound completely and remove all suture material. Gently re-explore the abdomen, separating the filmy adhesions by blunt dissection with the hand, and look for possible intra-abdominal abscess formation. Complete exteriorization of the small bowel is unnecessary, but peritoneal lavage with warm saline containing 1 g of tetracycline per litre is beneficial. The abdominal wall should then be resutured. A conventional layered closure is rarely possible because of difficulty in identifying the separate layers, oedema and failure of the wound to support the sutures. The preferred resuture technique is with multiple through-and-through deep tension sutures inserted at 1 cm intervals. Insert all the sutures and then lift them vertically en masse (Figure 13.3). The abdominal wall is thus elevated off

Figure 13.3
En masse elevation of
deep tension sutures
prior to their separate
ligation to avoid
trapping a loop of
small intestine
between the
abdominal wall and
the sutures.

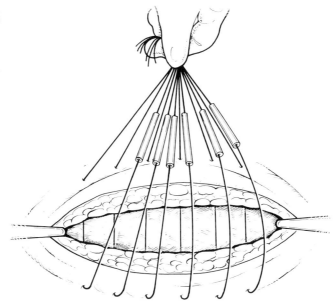

the underlying bowel and this reduces the risk of trapping a loop of small intestine as the individual sutures are tied. It may be possible to insert a single layer of a continuous non-absorbable suture into the linea alba or anterior rectus sheath before the tension sutures are tied, if the small intestine is not distended. Once the tension sutures are tied, the skin edges lie opposed. The risk of wound contamination and subcutaneous infection is high and thus there is little advantage to be gained by primary suture of the skin. However, a delayed primary suture of the skin will usually result in satisfactory healing without wound infection. Interrupted mattress sutures are inserted into the skin edges, their ends being left long and not tied. The subcutaneous fat is exposed, and the wound loosely packed with gauze pads. The swabs should be kept moist by pouring saline onto their exposed surface every six to eight hours. The skin sutures are tied four or five days postoperatively.

Post-operative abdominal distension should be minimized by use of a nasogastric tube and avoiding oral feeding until good bowel motility has returned. There is no evidence that an abdominal binder helps to reduce the risk of a subsequent incisional hernia. The tension sutures must not be removed for at least three weeks after insertion.

Incisional hernia
The incidence of an incisional hernia in vertical laparotomy incisions is between 2 and 6%. Fifty per cent occur within a year and the other 50% between one and five years after operation,

indicating the length of follow-up that is required in assessment of wound healing.

The three options for treatment are:

1 No treatment.
2 Provision of a surgical corset.
3 Surgical repair.

The treatment selected depends on a number of factors:

- the prognosis of the initial operation
- symptoms of pain or intestinal obstruction
- size of the neck of the hernial defect
- patient's general health
- patient's desire for further surgery
- cosmetic appearance

Surgery should be advised for a fit patient with a small defect and episodes of recurrent abdominal pain. Overweight patients who continue to smoke and have large defects may be treated satisfactorily with a corset. The principles of surgical repair of an incisional hernia are to dissect out and mobilize the margins of the aponeurotic defect and the skin edges for the whole length of the incision. The defect can then be repaired using the overlapping Mayo technique or a Keel repair. Induction of a preoperative pneumoperitoneum for 10–14 days may be beneficial in patients with large defects. Avoid the use of synthetic materials inserted into the wound, e.g. Marlex mesh, because of the risk of infection.

Intra-abdominal Abscesses

The common sites for postoperative intra-abdominal abscesses are in the subphrenic, subhepatic and pelvic regions and between loops of small intestine. The three major factors that contribute to an intrabdominal abscess are:

1 Anastamotic leakage.
2 Peritoneal contamination, e.g. perforated duodenal ulcer.
3 Intraperitoneal haematoma.

Presentation   The commonest presentation is with a swinging pyrexia that begins on the fourth or fifth postoperative day and gradually increases in magnitude. There may be an associated tachycardia, confusion and tachypnoea. An intra-abdominal abscess should be suspected in the absence of signs of infection in more common sites (chest, wound, urinary tract). The neutrophil count will be elevated.

Subphrenic abscess. This usually follows gastroduodenal or splenic operations and is commoner on the left than the right.

Figure 13.4
Gastrograffin swallow
showing an
anastamotic leak (✐)
following
oesophagogastrectomy
and multiple air fluid
levels in a subphrenic
abscess (↟↟).

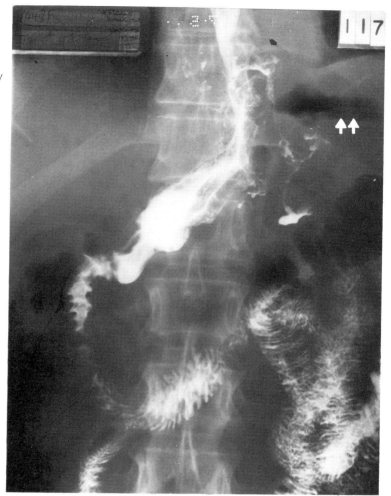

Figure 13.4 Gastrograffin swallow showing an anastamotic leak (✐) following oesophagogastrectomy and multiple air fluid levels in a subphrenic abscess (↟↟).

The patient may develop chest pain on deep inspiration, hiccups owing to diaphragmatic irritation, shoulder tip pain, a pleural effusion or tenderness over the left costal margin. Chest X-ray may show diaphragmatic elevation, a pleural effusion or subphrenic air-fluid levels. If the patient has had an oesophagogastric or gastrojejunal anastomosis, radiological studies using a water-soluble contrast medium may reveal an anastomotic leak (Figure 13.4). Ultrasound, CT and radionuclide scans may also help to localize an abscess in difficult cases.

Subhepatic abscess. Laparotomy for a perforated duodenal ulcer, leakage from the duodenal stump following Polya gastrectomy, and operations on the biliary tract, particularly in the presence of infection, are the commonest causes of a subhepatic abscess.

The pus forms in Morrison's pouch between the undersurface of the liver and anterolateral surface of the duodenum and hepatic flexure of the colon. Chest signs are absent, but there may be tenderness in the right upper quadrant on deep inspiration.

Pelvic abscess. A pelvic abscess usually occurs after rectal excision, appendicectomy or in the female after pelvic operations. Rectal examination reveals a tender boggy swelling in the rectovesical pouch in the male or rectovaginal pouch in the female. Associated diarrhoea is due to irritation of a loop of adjacent bowel, usually the sigmoid colon, or to perforation and discharge of the abscess into the rectal lumen. If the abscess develops after anterior resection of the rectum, a water soluble contrast enema may reveal an anastamotic leak. Whether a pelvic abscess is the cause, or end result, of an anastamotic leakage is controversial.

Treatment *Subhepatic or subphrenic abscess*
Antibiotics. Broad-spectrum antibiotics should be given and may result in resolution of an infection in its early stages. Once the subphrenic abscess is well established, antibiotics alone are insufficient to effect a cure but will control the systemic effects and reduce the risk of septicaemia. Either a third-generation cephalosporin or a combination of penicillin, tobramycin and metronidazole should be used.

Surgery. Drainage of a mature subphrenic abscess is usually required. The indications for surgery are failure of resolution, increase in size of the abscess, or septicaemia. Ultrasound or CT guided percutaneous drainage has been used, with mixed success. I (CJS) have not been impressed with this technique, for the abscesses are invariably multilocular and the pus thick, which makes complete drainage difficult. I prefer an anterior extraperitoneal approach through a small subcostal incision. Loculi are broken down digitally and a large drain inserted. If a gastrointestinal communication is present (e.g. following oesophagogastrectomy or gastrectomy), oral feeding should be withheld and intravenous nutrition given. Do not attempt to close the perforation, for the sutures will cut out. A posterior or anterior transperitoneal approach is an acceptable alternative method of drainage, but less desirable on account of the potential risk of pleural or more extensive peritoneal contamination.

Pelvic abscess
An untreated pelvic abscess will usually drain spontaneously into the rectum or the vault of the vagina as it increases in size. Daily digital examination will allow the development of the abscess to be monitored. Digital pressure on the anterior rectal wall may encourage drainage into the rectum. If the patient becomes septic, formal incision and drainage under general

anaesthetic may be necessary. The patient is placed in the lithotomy position and the abscess drained through its softest point into either the rectum or vagina.

Acute Pancreatitis

Acute pancreatitis in the early postoperative period may complicate any laparotomy. It is seen most frequently after biliary tract operations, particularly exploration of the common bile duct or transduodenal sphincteroplasty. It can also complicate gastrectomy, especially when there is afferent loop distension following Polya gastrectomy. Acute postoperative pancreatitis probably occurs more frequently than is recognized, the pain due to the pancreatitis being attributed to normal postoperative pain and treated with narcotic analgesics without a serum amylase estimation being performed.

The patient may experience particularly severe postoperative pain, usually in the epigastrium, which may radiate through to the back. On examination there may be marked upper abdominal tenderness. Alternatively, the patient may become shocked with hypotension and tachycardia for which there is no obvious cause. On examination look for signs of intraluminal or intra-abdominal bleeding and perform an ECG, looking for signs of an acute myocardial infarction. If all of these are normal, consider acute pancreatitis and check the serum amylase. A level of greater than 1000 IU should be considered diagnostic. A value in excess of 6000 IU may be recorded in patients with pancreatitis secondary to afferent loop obstruction after gastrectomy. The mortality rate of postoperative pancreatitis is high. Blood gas estimation should be performed whilst the patient is receiving oxygen by face mask and assisted ventilation considered if the Pao_2 is less than 7·5 kPa. The pancreatitis should be treated along conventional lines. Aprotinin and glucagon are probably of no benefit, but there is some recent evidence that somatostatin may be of value.

Postoperative Paralytic Ileus

A period of temporary quiescence of intestinal peristalsis is common following abdominal surgery. Generally this is no more than a few hours, or at most a few days, in duration. However, the loss of normal gastrointestinal motility may persist, sometimes for as long as 7–14 days, this condition being termed a 'paralytic ileus'. This term is a misnomer for two reasons. Firstly, the bowel is not paralysed but the contractions merely inhibited, and secondly, following laparotomy peristalsis returns first in the small bowel, gastric and colonic peristalsis being delayed.

Paralytic ileus is a serious complication, which significantly increases the morbidity and mortality rate of surgery. It may follow any abdominal procedure, but is commonest after gastric or colonic operations or in the presence of peritonitis. It can also occur in patients with septicaemia, retroperitoneal bleeding or injury, electrolyte imbalance, particularly hypokalaemia; metabolic disorders; or in patients in the intensive care unit receiving assisted ventilation.

The loss of peristaltic activity and muscular tone in the intestinal wall leads to distension of the bowel with gas and fluid. The gaseous component is derived initially from swallowed air, but later gas-forming organisms contribute, as bacterial overgrowth occurs in the stagnant intraluminal contents. The distension of the bowel increases as water and electrolytes, mainly sodium and chloride ions, accumulate in the lumen. A vicious circle is established, for increasing distension results in decreased intestinal absorption and the bowel becomes more distended and even more adynamic. This increasing distension is a major factor in the development of a paralytic ileus, for exclusion of swallowed air or intestinal decompression often results in resolution of the condition.

Aetiology   The aetiology of paralytic ileus is somewhat obscure, but it is probably a sympathetically mediated nervous reflex. Stimulation of sympathetic nerves to the gut decreases intestinal motility. Using experimental animal models it has been shown that postoperative paralytic ileus can be abolished by prior division of the splanchnic (sympathetic) nerves. Spinal cord destruction or high spinal anaesthesia, which blocks the sympathetic outflow from the spinal cord, results in increased small bowel motility and inhibits the development of postoperative ileus. The mere presence of peritonitis does not in itself result in paralytic ileus, but the latter does develop if the intestine becomes distended with fluid and gas. It can be prevented in animals with peritonitis by previous splanchnicectomy, again suggesting that the condition is due to a sympathetically mediated mechanism. The intestinal smooth muscle is not actually 'paralysed', but rather inhibited by sympathetic overactivity.

Clinical features   Some abdominal distension and absence of bowel sounds for 24–48 hours are common after laparotomy and require no specific treatment, for they are self-limiting in the majority of patients. However, if this situation persists for more than four or five days, it may perpetuate itself as fluid and gas accumulate in the bowel. The patient becomes distended, passes no flatus per rectum and may vomit. The presence of intestinal colic suggests a mechanical rather than an adynamic obstruction. Abdominal X-rays show distended loops of small bowel and also a distended stomach. In some patients the distension is predominantly due to intestinal fluid rather than gas and the X-rays may be misinterpreted.

Prevention   It has been suggested that the risk of paralytic ileus can be reduced by avoiding intra-abdominal infection and unnecessary intestinal handling at the time of operation, and by postoperative gastrointestinal decompression using a nasogastric tube. Routine insertion of a nasogastric tube after all laparotomies is not to be recommended because of the problems that are associated with their use. The tube may be difficult to insert, cause pharyngeal discomfort and make the gastro-oesophageal junction incompetent, leading to reflux oesophagitis. Nasogastric tubes are unnecessary where the risk of postopertive ileus is low, such as after cholecystectomy or highly selective vagotomy. However, it would be prudent to keep the stomach decompressed for a few days after gastrectomy, small bowel resection or colectomy or following laparotomy for a gastrointestinal perforation. The tube can be safely removed when active bowel sounds return or when the aspirate falls below 300 ml in 24 hours.

Treatment   If the abdominal distension persists and bowel sounds are absent for more than five days, further investigation and treatment are needed. Ensure that there is no mechanical obstruction of the bowel, which is much more common than a paralytic ileus and is more likely if the patient has intestinal colic. Check the hernial orifices for the presence of a previously unsuspected hernia. Check the parastoma region after operations involving ileostomy or colostomy formation, looking for a paraostomy hernia, and review the X-rays in these patients, looking carefully for evidence of an internal hernia adjacent to the stoma.

The gastrointestinal tract should be decompressed using a nasogastric tube of reasonable size, such as F16. Fluids should be given intravenously to correct dehydration and electrolyte depletion, particularly in hypokalaemia. As a simple rule of thumb the patient's nasogastric aspirate in the preceeding 24 hours should be replaced with an equal volume of normal saline, in addition to the standard daily requirements for an average 70 kg patient of approximately 3 litres of fluid, of which one litre should be normal saline. The Miller Abbott tube, which was designed for per oral decompression of the small intestine, is of little value in an established paralytic ileus, for there is no intestinal peristalsis to carry the tube along the bowel.

The possibility of a mechanical obstruction must be constantly borne in mind. Mechanical obstruction often requires further laparotomy for its relief, whereas in adynamic obstruction, laparotomy may worsen the situation. If there is doubt about the diagnosis or if the ileus has not resolved after 48 hours' gastrointestinal decompression, a barium meal and follow-through or small bowel enema should be performed. There are conflicting views on whether a water-soluble contrast medium or a dilute barium solution should be used. The former may stimulate intestinal motility, but, by virtue of its high osmolarity, draws fluid into the bowel lumen, thus exacerbating intestinal distension. There is no doubt that the quality of the X-rays is far better with barium. Consider the possibility of intra-abdominal sepsis, particularly a subhepatic, subphrenic or a pelvic abscess.

If the ileus is still present more than a week after surgery, has not responded to gastric decompression and there are no symptoms or signs of mechanical obstruction, pharmacological stimulation of intestinal peristalsis should be considered, although the necessity for this to be used will be extremely rare. Cathartics, enemata, rectal washouts and even electrical stimulating devices in the duodenum have been tried, but without success. As the condition is due to a relative sympathetic overactivity, a reasonable pharmacological approach would be:

1 Augmentation of the parasympathetic drive to the gut
     (a) by blocking the removal of acetylcholine with an anticholinesterase;
     (b) by stimulating with a cholinergic drug.
2 Blockade of the sympathetic nervous system.

Neostigmine has a longer half-life and fewer side-effects than physostigmine and is the most effective of the anticholinesterases. Of the cholinergic drugs, bethanechol is the most useful. Its action is predominantly muscarinic and it lacks the nicotinic side-effects of carbachol, from which it is derived. Dopamine antagonists, such as domperidone or metoclopramide, are less useful in the treatment of paralytic ileus, for although they increase gastrointestinal motility, they are relatively ineffective in initiating peristalsis in the paralysed bowel. Both alpha and beta sympathetic receptors are present in the gut and both inhibit motility. Small bowel inhibition is mediated predominantly by alpha adrenergic receptors, the colon by beta receptors and the stomach equally by alpha and beta receptors. Guanethidine blocks both alpha and beta adrenergic receptors.

Before any attempt is made to stimulate the bowel pharmacologically, ensure that the patient is not hypokalaemic or in negative fluid balance. Sympathetic blockade results in a fall of blood pressure, and severe hypotension could occur in a hypovolaemic patient. The most effective drugs for stimulation of gut motility are bethanechol and guanethidine. Bethanechol 2·5 mg is given subcutaneously and the dose repeated 30 minutes later if the patient has not passed flatus. This can be continued at a maximum dose of 5 mg subcutaneously 6-hourly for the next 24 hours or until adequate gut motility is obtained. If there has been no response after 24 hours, this regimen should be repeated after prior infusion of guanethidine 20 mg in an intravenous solution over a period of 40 minutes, beginning 1 hour before the bethanechol. Regular monitoring of pulse and blood pressure is necessary. The patient may experience mild abdominal colic, a desire to pass urine and a slight fall in blood pressure. Once the intestinal inhibition has been overcome, contractions return and usually persist even though the pharmacological stimulus is withheld.

Intra-abdominal adhesions

Intra-abdominal adhesions may be responsible for a number of postoperative sequelae, including acute small bowel obstruction, chronic recurrent abdominal pain due to an incomplete obstruction, and pain due to traction on an adhesion between the parietal peritoneum and/or an intra-abdominal structure. Intra-abdominal adhesions are now the commonest cause of intestinal obstruction in the adult population (Ellis, 1971). In the UK and USA at the turn of the century strangulated groin hernias accounted for a large proportion of cases of intestinal obstruction, obstruction due to adhesions being relatively uncommon. Improvements in anaesthetic and surgical techniques have resulted in a dramatic increase in the number of patients undergoing laparotomy and elective herniorrhaphy, and as a direct consequence the prevalance of intestinal obstruction due to adhesions has risen, while that due to incarcerated hernias has fallen. In primitive communities, where abdominal operations are rare, strangulated hernias are still the commonest cause of small bowel obstruction.

Over 75% of patients with intra-abdominal adhesions have undergone prior abdominal surgery. Adhesions can also occur under other circumstances (Table 13.3). Although adhesions are an inevitable consequence of every laparotomy, the number of patients who develop postoperative problems from adhesions is very small compared with the total number undergoing laparotomy. Not all abdominal operations carry the same risk of postoperative small bowel obstruction. Adhesions to the under-surface of the liver are common following gastroduodenal or biliary surgery. Although they may make re-operation in the upper abdomen more difficult, they are rarely the cause of intestinal obstruction. Lower abdominal procedures such as appendicectomy, gynaecological operations and colorectal resections are responsible for the majority of cases of adhesive obstruction.

Table 13.3. Aetiology of intra-abdominal adhesions.	1. Previous laparotomy 2. Congenital adhesions 3. Intra-abdominal inflammatory conditions, e.g. appendicitis, diverticulitis, salpingitis, Crohn's disease, tuberculosis 4. Side-effect of specific drugs, e.g. practolol (Eraldin) 5. Chronic ambulatory peritoneal dialysis

Pathogenesis of postoperative adhesions

Ischaemia. Adhesions are the end result of healing by fibrosis. Immediately after laparotomy fibrinous adhesions form between adjacent loops of bowel, the omentum and parietal peritoneum. These may be completely reabsorbed or become organized into fibrous adhesions by ingrowth of capillaries and fibroblasts. Initially it was believed that the stimulus for adhesion formation (rather than reabsorption) was peritoneal injury. Great emphasis was placed on minimizing damage to the visceral peritoneum, suturing parietal peritoneal defects and covering intestinal anastomoses with omental flaps. It has since been shown that peritoneal defects heal rapidly without necessarily causing intra-abdominal adhesions. Creation of a peritoneal defect in an experimental model causes an inflammatory response, followed by intense fibroblastic activity. This results in the generation of a new mesothelium within a few days of the original injury, but without adhesion formation. It is the presence of ischaemic tissue within the abdominal cavity that causes the development of adhesions. Such ischaemic tissue can be produced by excessive diathermy, mass ligation of large amounts of tissue, or, experimentally, by ligation of mesenteric vessels. Adhesions form between the ischaemic tissue and adjacent structures and provide the means by which revascularization can occur. In animal models short segments of devascularized bowel do not become ischaemic if adhesions are allowed to develop, but if the devascularized segment is wrapped in polythene sheeting, it becomes gangrenous. The stimulus to adhesion formation is not damage to the perotineum, but the presence of ischaemic tissue.

Foreign body granulomas and adhesions. Foreign bodies introduced into the abdomen at the time of laparotomy can also stimulate adhesion formation. Primarily these originate from the surgeon's gloves or abdominal gauze packs. Talc, magnesium silicate, was the first substance used as a glove dusting powder and the first to be implicated, following identification of talc particles within the adhesions, using polarized light. Talc was replaced by starch powder on the basis that the latter would be absorbed from the peritoneal cavity. However, starch granules have also been identified within intra-abdominal adhesions. Washing the gloves in water or saline prior to operation will remove some of the surface powder, but may cause clumping of the starch. This effect can be reduced by incorporation of a small amount of magnesium oxide into the dusting powder, but this in itself may be a factor in adhesion development. Starch-free gloves are available, but some varieties have a different 'texture' to powdered gloves and may be less acceptable to the surgeon.

Clinical features

Small bowel obstruction is the commonest complication of intra-abdominal adhesions. The patient presents with a history of colicky, central abdominal pain, abdominal distension and vomiting. The vomitus initially contains food, but then becomes faeculent. On examination the patient is dehydrated, the abdomen distended and bowel sounds increased. Palpate the abdomen carefully, looking for an area of localized peritonitis, which suggests that a loop of small bowel has become gangrenous. Examine the hernial orifices.

Chronic abdominal pain due to incomplete small bowel obstruction secondary to adhesions is a less common problem. The pain is usually episodic, exacerbated by food and associated with abdominal distension but less frequently with vomiting. Diarrhoea occurs because of bacterial overgrowth. The patient may lose weight because of the fear that eating will exacerbate the pain. These symptoms and signs also occur in patients with Crohn's disease or colonic carcinoma, from which it must be differentiated.

Patients admitted as an emergency with small bowel obstruction should have a sigmoidoscopy, a full blood count, urea and electrolyte estimation and erect and supine abdominal X-rays performed. A relative polycythaemia is common because of haemoconcentration. A white cell count of over 25×10^9 per litre should alert the surgeon to the possibility of intestinal ischaemia. Sigmoidoscopy is very important. In some patients with a carcinoma of the sigmoid colon or rectosigmoid junction colonic distension may occur late and in these patients plain abdominal X-rays suggest small bowel obstruction. Chronic abdominal pain demands upper and lower gastrointestinal radiology to determine the level and degree of obstruction and to exclude other pathology

Treatment   *Initial treatment.* The patient with small bowel obstruction should be resuscitated with intravenous fluids and a nasogastric tube inserted. With this treatment the symptoms and signs will resolve within 48 hours in the majority of patients and a second, and often unnecessary, laparotomy can thus be avoided. However, re-operation after resuscitation is necessary in those patients who have an area of localized peritonitis, a white cell count in excess of 25×10^9 per litre, or if a solitary loop of distended small bowel is present on abdominal X-rays. In these three situations there may be a loop of ischaemic small bowel and operation should not be delayed. If dehydration is extreme, resuscitation should be prompt and a compromise reached between the risk of delaying surgery and that of operating too early in a patient with hypovolaemia.

Operative treatment. If a patient has a lower midline or paramedian incision, this should be reopened. If a Pfannenstiel or appendicectomy incision was performed previously, use a right paramedian incision. Start at the caecum and follow the small bowel cranially until the point of obstruction is found. If this is due to a solitary band, it should be divided. Obstruction due to multiple adhesions between adjacent loops of bowel is a more difficult problem. All the adhesions should be divided by a combination of sharp and blunt dissection. However, when the abdomen is closed further adhesions may form and the obstruction can recur. If the patient has not undergone previous laparotomies for small bowel obstruction, then probably nothing needs to be done other than to divide these adhesions. However, if the intestinal obstruction is a recurrent problem, then steps should be taken to prevent a further recurrence. The aim of treatment should be to prevent the adhesions causing acute angulation of the bowel. This can be done in two ways. Adjacent loops of small bowel can be plicated together in zigzag fashion, beginning at the duodenojejunal junction and continuing along the whole length of the small intestine (Noble's plication). This is a slow and tedious process. An alternative method is to thread a long Jones tube through the small bowel from the jejunum to the caecum. This is a long intestinal tube with an inflatable balloon at the distal end. The tube is inserted into the proximal jejunum in an identical manner to the insertion of a feeding jejunostomy tube, and when the balloon is inflated it is milked along the small intestine and into the caecum. The bowel is held in smooth coils by the tube, and when adhesions form between adjacent loops in the postoperative period, acute angulation does not occur. The jejunostomy is sutured to the undersurface of the anterior abdominal wall and the tube is anchored to the skin. It is kept in situ for two weeks and then removed, the enterocutaneous fistula thus created usually closing within 48 hours.

Insertion of a Jones tube is less time consuming than Noble's plication and in my (CJS's) opinion is the preferred method of treatment. Its use is recommended when the patient has had more than two previous operations for intestinal obstruction due to adhesions.

The occurrence of sub-acute intestinal obstruction due to adhesions is a less common problem. If the proximal small bowel is dilated on barium studies, then the obstruction must be considered significant and a further laparotomy performed. This type of obstruction is usually due to multiple adhesions rather than a single band. These adhesions should be divided and a Jones tube inserted to prevent a recurrence of the problem.

Granulomatous starch peritonitis

Granulomatous starch peritonitis is a very uncommon complication of laparotomy, which occurs two to six weeks after operation. The patient presents with generalized malaise, abdominal pain and a pyrexia. On investigation, the erythrocyte sedimentation rate and plasma viscosity are usually raised, but there are no specific diagnostic haematological tests that can substantiate the diagnosis.

This granulomatous reaction is probably an immunological response to the starch powder on the surface of surgical gloves (Grant et al, 1982). Skin testing with an intradermal injection of 1 mg of starch glove powder in 0.1 ml of sterile pyrogen-free water usually results in an intense erythematous reaction 5 mm or more in diameter at the inoculation site, which appears between three and eight days after the injection. A similar injection into control subjects who have not undergone either surgery or laparotomy may result in a mild reaction in a few patients, but the area of erythema is less than 5 mm in diameter, and the reaction which occurs within 24 hours of inoculation is less intense and fades within three to four days. Skin biopsies from patients with starch peritonitis show a dense perivascular exudate in the dermis at the site of inoculation of the starch. Giant cell or epithelioid granulomata may be present, accompanied by a large number of monocytes and polymorpholeucocytes.

In the past the only means of confirming this suspected diagnosis was a second laparotomy. The intradermal skin test described may be useful in confirming the diagnosis, although its major drawback is the lag between the inoculation and the appearance of the skin reaction. If the diagnosis can be established without laparotomy, then steroids should be given in the form of hydrocortisone 100 mg three times daily; dramatic responses have been observed. It is important that other infective causes of peritonitis are excluded before treatment with steroids is commenced.

Starch glove powder thus has three distinct pathological effects. It has a direct irritant effect when in high concentration in the peritoneum and may be the aetiological factor behind the development of some intra-abdominal adhesions. Granulomatous peritonitis is probably an immunological delayed hypersensitivity response. Thirdly, some patients may have an accelerated reaction to injection of intradermal starch, and this probably represents an antibody-mediated hypersensitivity reaction.

Reoperation through existing incisions

Three potential hazards are associated with a reoperation through a previous laparotomy incision:

1. Damage to intra-abdominal contents

Intra-abdominal structures beneath an incision may adhere to the posterior aspect of the anterior abdominal wall and are at risk of inadvertent damage if the incision is reopened. Those structures at risk vary with different abdominal incisions (Table 13.4). The damage may be caused either by a scalpel, as the linea alba, rectus sheath or peritoneum are incised, or by scissors, as the initial incision is enlarged. This complication is totally avoidable with careful surgical technique. Do not rush the reopening of an old abdominal incision. If possible open the

Incision	Structures at risk
Upper midline	1. Liver
	2. Stomach
	3. Omentum
	4. Small intestine
	5. Transverse colon
Subcostal/upper right paramedian	1. Liver
	2. Heptic flexure of colon
	3. Omentum
	4. Small intestine
Lower midline/paramedian/Pfannenstiel	1. Small intestine
	2. Omentum

Table 13.4 Intra-abdominal contents at risk of inadvertent damage during reopening of an abdominal incision.

peritoneum in 'virgin' territory just above or below the previous incision. Use a scalpel to open the linea alba or rectus sheath and then carefully and slowly incise the peritoneum beneath. There is always a plane between peritoneum and intra-abdominal contents that can be located and opened without damaging the latter.

A hepatic laceration is immediately obvious by the colour of the incised liver tissue. Coagulate any bleeding points with diathermy. If the laceration is large, it should be sutured using a chromic catgut suture on an atraumatic, round-bodied hand needle, supported by ox-fibrin buttresses. Brisk arterial bleeding just beneath the peritoneum is typical of an omental tear or laceration. The bleeding vessel should be identified and ligated rather than diathermized. Damage to the small intestine or colon, although usually recognized by the visible appearance or odour of gastrointestinal contents in the wound, may be missed, the patient developing unexplained postoperative peritonitis. A small laceration of the small intestine or colon should be repaired immediately in two layers, by careful approximation of the edges of the bowel using either chromic catgut and silk or two layers of catgut. If the laceration is large, the bowel should be closed transversely to prevent luminal narrowing. Irrigate the wound with warm saline to minimize bacterial contamination and give a prophylactic broad-spectrum antibiotic intravenously to reduce the risk of postoperative wound infection. If the transverse colon is completely, or almost completely, transected and there is significant faecal loading in the proximal bowel, it may be necessary to bring out a double-barrelled colostomy rather than risk an anastamotic leak following a primary closure. This situation is extremely rare, a colonic laceration generally being small and amenable to immediate resuture.

2. Wound failure   The risk of wound failure, either a burst abdomen or incisional hernia, is greater after reoperation through a previous incision more than a few weeks old. This risk can be reduced by appreciation of the danger and careful closure of the abdominal wall after the second laparotomy. Any non-absorbable suture material can be used for abdominal closure, according to the surgeon's preference. My (CJS's) preference in this situation is for two layers of continuous polypropylene (Prolene) reinforced with deep tension sutures.

3. Ischaemia of the abdominal wall The other complication that may occur in relation to reoperation through an adjacent parallel incision is ischaemic necrosis of the abdominal wall and skin between the two incisions. The abdominal wall receives its arterial input from penetrating branches of the intercostal arteries, with little cross boundary flow across the midline. If a vertical laparotomy incision is followed within a few weeks by a second parallel incision, the skin in between the incisions is liable to undergo necrosis because of ischaemia. Thus it would be unwise to perform two vertical parallel incisions within three months of each other. After this time new vessels grow across the primary incision and the risk of ischaemia in relation to a second incision diminishes.

Intraperitoneal Bleeding

Postoperative intra-abdominal bleeding can occur from any gastrointestinal anastomosis, a slipped ligature on a vessel, or from any part of the abdominal wall denuded of peritoneum. The bleeding is either primary, reactionary or secondary in type and can occur at any time, from a few hours to two weeks after operation. Clinically significant bleeding usually occurs within the first 24 hours of operation. Anastomotic bleeding, which is almost without exception intraluminal, and postsplenectomy bleeding have been discussed in other parts of this book.

Bleeding into the peritoneal cavity may be overt, if an abdominal drain is in situ, or concealed. The presence of an abdominal drain is not an absolute safeguard in the detection of intraperitoneal bleeding, for the internal opening of the drain may become blocked by blood clot. Postoperative hypotension and tachycardia are the cardinal signs of intra-abdominal bleeding. Shoulder tip pain due to subdiaphragmatic irritation by blood may be present. Hypotension may also occur because of hypovolaemia secondary to inadequate intraoperative fluid replacement, recent administration of narcotic analgesics or a myocardial infarction. Review the drug and intravenous fluid charts and perform an ECG. Give 500 ml of warm saline intravenously over a period of 20–30 minutes. An initial improvement in tachycardia and hypotension, followed by a deterioration, is suggestive of intra-abdominal bleeding. If there is still doubt about the diagnosis, insert a CVP line for measurement of central venous pressure and/or perform peritoneal lavage using a peritoneal dialysis catheter. A moderately or heavily blood-stained effluent on peritoneal lavage indicates the need for a repeat laparotomy after emergency blood cross-matching. Perform a clotting screen to detect a coagulation disorder. Measurement of abdominal girth as a means of detecting intra-abdominal bleeding is a complete waste of time. Pints of blood can collect in the abdomen without any significant change in the girth measurement. Similarly, gaseous distension of the bowel owing to the presence of a 'paralytic ileus' may result in an increase in abdominal girth without there being any intra-abdominal bleeding. If the patient has persistent hypotension and tachycardia, with no evidence of narcotic overdosage or myocardial infarction, it is safer to re-explore the abdomen than risk missing a major intraperitoneal bleed.

Abdominal Trauma

Abdominal trauma may be due to a penetrating injury, usually a knife wound, or a blunt non-penetrating injury. The latter may be the result of a blow from a moving object or due to sudden deceleration of the patient, usually during a road traffic accident. With penetrating injuries any intra-abdominal structure may be traversed and injured. With blunt abdominal injuries the intra-abdominal damage occurs at the junction of a fixed and a relatively mobile structure, for example at the duodenojejunal flexure or the junction of the hepatic veins and the liver. Compression of intra-abdominal structures, such as the pancreas or colon, between the abdominal wall and vertebral column may occur in patients wearing seat belts at the time of a road accident.

The usual indications for laparotomy following abdominal trauma include, signs of peritonitis, hypotension or heavily bloodstained peritoneal lavage fluid. The most serious, and also the most common, complication of laparotomy for trauma is the failure to recognize that more than one structure has been damaged. This is particularly true of penetrating wounds. A long knife thrust into a victim's left upper quadrant may damage the omentum, multiple loops of small bowel, the splenic flexure of the colon, the spleen, the diaphragm and even the lung. Before any patient with an upper abdominal stab wound is anaesthetized, examine the chest carefully and perform an erect chest X-ray, looking for evidence of a haemopneumothorax. When the abdomen is opened a thorough laparotomy should be performed, inspecting all the intraperitoneal and retroperitoneal structures. If the knife is found to have penetrated one loop of small bowel, do not assume that this is the only injury and look for other damage.

A minor splenic laceration can be repaired by the techniques described in Chapter 12. Small bowel lacerations should be repaired with two rows of sutures, preferably a layer of inner continuous absorbable sutures followed by a layer of outer interrupted sutures. Major abdominal trauma due to penetration with a large blunt object, as may occur in a road traffic accident, may require resection of either small or large intestine. If resection of the left side of the colon is required, a primary anastomosis is unwise and a right transverse colostomy should be performed. The peritoneal cavity should be lavaged with saline containing 1 g tetracycline per litre prior to abdominal closure.

Failure to recognize a second bowel injury will result in the development of peritonitis in the postoperative period. There may be no abnormal signs in the first six to eight hours after operation because the hole in the bowel is sealed by a mucosal plug, thus preventing major leakage of intestinal contents. However, within a few hours of laparotomy a localized peritonitis develops within the vicinity of the second injury. The small bowel then distends and the mucosa retracts, thus allowing spillage of gastrointestinal contents into the peritoneal cavity. Over the next 24 hours the patient will develop a tachycardia, pyrexia and signs of spreading peritonitis. Abdominal X-rays will be unhelpful, for air will be present in the peritoneal cavity following the laparotomy. After resuscitation with intravenous fluids and administration of broad-spectrum antibiotics the abdomen should be reopened.

Following abdominal trauma, damage to any part of the gastrointestinal tract that requires surgery may be followed by the development of a subphrenic, subhepatic or pelvic abscess. This risk can be minimized by thorough peritoneal lavage prior to abdominal closure. The recognition and treatment of intra-abdominal abscess is dealt with in an earlier part of this chapter.

Abdominal Drains

Abdominal drains are inserted for a variety of reasons:

- Drainage of blood, bile, pancreatic juice or serous fluid from the abdominal cavity following a variety of surgical operations, including biliary procedures, gastrectomy, pancreatectomy or rectal excision.
- As a precaution against anastomotic leakage following intestinal, particularly colonic, resection.

There are basically two types of abdominal drain.

- *A passive drain*, such as a latex tube drain or Penrose drain. The intra-abdominal fluid tracks along the drain to the exterior.
- *An active suction drain*. This may be a sump drain or a suction drain connected to either a glass 'Redivac' bottle or a disposable bottle. The fluid is actively sucked from the peritoneal cavity.

Complications associated with the use of abdominal drains

Injury to intra-abdominal contents

The instrument used to bring the drain through the abdominal wall (either a heavy-duty artery clip or a sharp pointed introducer) may be inadvertently thrust into the bowel or, very rarely, a vascular structure in the abdomen. The injury should be recognized immediately. Close an intestinal perforation with two layers of sutures. Repair a vascular injury by ligation or suture of the vessel, depending on its size and importance. Major vessels should be repaired using a vascular suture such as 4/0 or 5/0 Prolene. Smaller vessels, so long as they are not end arteries to an important structure, should be ligated. Be sure to ligate the vessel as shown in Figure 2.1, on page 12. The superior or inferior epigastric vessels may be damaged as the introducer is brought through the abdominal wall. Bleeding from this source can always be controlled by direct pressure.

Suction injuries

Negative pressures exceeding 600 mmHg can be reached in glass suction bottles. The pressures in disposable plastic bottles are much lower. High-pressure suction can result in a loop of small intestine or colon being sucked onto the tube and this may result in a series of ischaemic perforations at the points where the suction holes in the intraperitoneal tubing are in contact with the bowel. In my (CJS's) opinion high-pressure suction drains should not be used within the peritoneal cavity, where they may come into contact with loops of small bowel. However, they can be used safely in the post-rectal space after an extraperitoneal colorectal anastamosis has been performed following anterior resection of the rectum. Indeed, suction drains are preferable to passive drains in this situation. Use a disposable suction bottle rather than a 'Redivac' system, because of the lower pressures that the former generates.

Intestinal perforation due to a suction injury presents three or four days after operation, with signs of increasing peritonitis. Laparotomy should be performed. If a series of longitudinal perforations are found in a loop of bowel, it is safer to resect that short segment of bowel with an end-to-end anastamosis rather than individually to close a series of perforations that are the end result of ischaemic injury.

Infection

Only closed drainage systems should be employed. Open drainage systems can result in bacteria being drawn into the peritoneal cavity, in which case any haematoma within the vicinity of the drain would be an ideal site for an infection to develop.

Persistent drainage of peritoneal fluid

Intra-abdominal drains should be kept in position for as short a period as possible. Once any discharge of blood or bile has decreased to less than 100 ml in 24 hours the drain should be removed. If the drain is left in situ for more than four days, a track will develop, and following drain removal intraperitoneal fluid may continue to leak to the exterior for a number of days. If the drainage fluid is simply serous intraperitoneal fluid, then the skin at the site of insertion of the drainage tube should be sutured using interrupted mattress sutures, following injection of a local anaesthetic.

Anastomotic leakage The use of intra-abdominal drains adjacent to a colonic anastomosis in an attempt to minimize the risks of an anastomotic dehiscence is controversial. There is good evidence to suggest that latex tube drains may actually *increase* the chance of a leak. There is no need to insert a drain adjacent to any small bowel anastomosis. However, some surgeons prefer to drain the duodenal stump following Polya gastrectomy and also the left colon following a left hemicolectomy or sigmoid colectomy. There is no evidence that these drains will diminish the risks of an anastomotic leakage.

If a drain is used and peritoneal fluid continues to drain following removal of the tube, the skin at the site of the drainage hole should be sutured using interrupted mattress sutures, following injection of a local anaesthetic. Treatment of an intestinal fistula following small or large bowel resection is covered in the book *Complications of Surgery of the Lower Gastrointestinal Tract.*

Tumour implantation in the abdominal wall Tumour cells may be deposited in the abdominal wall along the track of an intraperitoneal drain in patients undergoing laparotomy for intra-abdominal malignancy. These patients present some months after operation with a hard nodule, usually 2–4 cm in diameter, just beneath the skin at the site of insertion of the drain. Often they have other signs of recurrent carcinoma within the abdomen. If the patient has no other evidence of recurrence, it is wise to resect the abdominal wall deposit under general anaesthetic, to prevent fungation of the tumour through the skin.

General Precautions Following Laparotomy

Some postoperative complications of laparotomy can be avoided by performing a number of simple checks immediately prior to abdominal closure.

Bleeding Intra-abdominal bleeding following laparotomy may arise from an anastomosis, a raw surface or cut edge of the peritoneum, the omentum or a slipped ligature. The presentation, diagnosis and management of patients with postoperative bleeding from the upper gastrointestinal tract has been discussed fully in Chapter 2. The principles of management, including the indications for re-laparotomy, are identical for bleeding that arises from other sites. At laparotomy ligate all vessels carefully and do not gather large bunches of tissue into the ligature. Re-examine the abdominal contents in the vicinity of the operation before the abdomen is closed, looking for bleeding points. The bleeding may be primary, reactionary or secondary in type. Check with the anaesthetist that the patient is not hypotensive at the time of abdominal closure. Reactionary bleeding may occur as the blood pressure rises with postoperative intravenous fluid replacement. Perform a clotting screen and give fresh frozen plasma if there is any suggestion that continued postoperative bleeding is the result of a coagulation problem.

Internal herniation   Loops of small bowel may herniate through any mesenteric defects or around an ostomy stoma postoperatively, leading to small bowel obstruction. In my (CJS's) view all mesenteric defects should be closed and not left open. Be careful not to damage the vessels in the cut edges of the mesentery as the mesenteric defect is closed. Wherever possible an anterior resection anastomosis should be reperitonealized. This limits the spread of any infection if an anastomotic leakage occurs and also prevents loops of small bowel being trapped deep in the pelvis. The risk of internal herniation in the neighbourhood of an ostomy can be reduced by bringing out an extraperitoneal, rather than a transperitoneal, ileostomy or colostomy, whichever is appropriate.

Omentum   If present, omentum should be drawn downwards into the pelvis, thus covering the abdominal viscera, before the abdomen is closed. This reduces the risk of inadvertent damage to the bowel and also prevents the small intestine becoming attached to the posterior aspect of the abdominal wall. The risk of damaging the small bowel if the abdomen has to be reopened in future years is also reduced. The omentum may also be valuable in walling off postoperative intra-abdominal infection.

Persisting Controversies

- Indications for antibiotics in postoperative wound and intra-abdominal abscesses.
- Method of abdominal closure following wound dehiscence.
- Indications for preoperative pneumoperitoneum in patients with an incisional hernia.
- Percutaneous or open drainage of a subphrenic abscess.
- Indications for pharmacological stimulation of the bowel in patients with a paralytic ileus.
- Techniques for prevention of recurrence of intestinal obstruction secondary to adhesions.

Further reading
Ellis, H. (1971) The cause and prevention of post-operative intraperitoneal adhesions. *Surg. Gynecol. Obstet.*, *133*, 497–511.

intraperitoneal adhesions. *Surg. Gynecol. Obstet., 133*, 497–511.

Grant, J.B.F., Davies, J.D., Espiner, H.J. & Eltringham, W.K. (1982) Diagnosis of granulomatous starch peritonitis by delayed hypersensitivity skin reactions. *Br. J. Surg., 69*, 197–199.

Irvin, T.T. (1981) *Wound healing. Principles and Practice.* London and New York: Chapman and Hall.

Jenkins, T.P.N. (1976) The burst abdominal wound—a mechanical approach. *Br. J. Surg., 63*, 873–876.

Jones, P.F. & Munro, A. (1985) Recurrent adhesive small bowel obstruction. *World J. Surg., 9*, 868–875.

Neely, J. & Catchpole, B. (1971) Ileus: the restoration of alimentary-tract motility by pharmacological means. *Br. J. Surg., 58*, 21–28.

Smith, J.A.R. (1984) *Complications of Surgery in General.* London: Baillière Tindall.

Stoddard, C.J. & Smith, J.A.R. (1985) *Complications of Minor Surgery*. London: Baillière Tindall.

Smith, J.A.R. & Taylor, I. (1985) *Complications of Surgery of the Lower Gastrointestinal Tract*. London: Baillière Tindall.

Index